# Medical Application of Functional Biomaterials (2nd Edition)

*Guest Editors*

Cristian Scheau
Department of Physiology
The "Carol Davila"
University of Medicine and
Pharmacy
Bucharest
Romania

Andreea Cristiana Didilescu
Department of Embryology
and Microbiology
Faculty of Dentistry
The "Carol Davila"
University of Medicine and
Pharmacy
Bucharest
Romania

Constantin Caruntu
Department of Physiology
The "Carol Davila"
University of Medicine and
Pharmacy
Bucharest
Romania

*Editorial Office*
MDPI AG
Grosspeteranlage 5
4052 Basel, Switzerland

This is a reprint of the Special Issue, published open access by the journal *Journal of Functional Biomaterials* (ISSN 2079-4983), freely accessible at: https://www.mdpi.com/journal/jfb/special_issues/23B4A70YLZ.

For citation purposes, cite each article independently as indicated on the article page online and as indicated below:

| Lastname, A.A.; Lastname, B.B. Article Title. *Journal Name* **Year**, *Volume Number*, Page Range. |
|---|

**ISBN 978-3-7258-4207-0 (Hbk)**
**ISBN 978-3-7258-4208-7 (PDF)**
**https://doi.org/10.3390/books978-3-7258-4208-7**

Cover image courtesy of Cristian Scheau

# Medical Application of Functional Biomaterials (2nd Edition)

Guest Editors

**Cristian Scheau**
**Andreea Cristiana Didilescu**
**Constantin Caruntu**

MDPI

Basel • Beijing • Wuhan • Barcelona • Belgrade • Novi Sad • Cluj • Manchester

# Contents

Journal of
*Functional Biomaterials*

*Editorial*

# Functional Biomaterials: Scaffolds for Innovative Treatments

**Cristian Scheau [1,2], Andreea Cristiana Didilescu [3,*] and Constantin Caruntu [1,4]**

1 Department of Physiology, The "Carol Davila" University of Medicine and Pharmacy, 050474 Bucharest, Romania; cristian.scheau@umfcd.ro (C.S.); costin.caruntu@gmail.com (C.C.)
2 Department of Radiology and Medical Imaging, "Foisor" Clinical Hospital of Orthopaedics, Traumatology and Osteoarticular TB, 021382 Bucharest, Romania
3 Department of Embryology and Microbiology, Faculty of Dentistry, The "Carol Davila" University of Medicine and Pharmacy, 050474 Bucharest, Romania
4 Department of Dermatology, "Prof. N.C. Paulescu" National Institute of Diabetes, Nutrition and Metabolic Diseases, 011233 Bucharest, Romania
* Correspondence: andreea.didilescu@umfcd.ro

Numerous therapies for a multitude of pathologies have reached their limits [1]. Although disease management and medical care are standardized, we must acknowledge that each patient is different, with varied responses to the disease and the cure [2]. Moreover, for many diseases, the treatment depends on the ability of the medical system to provide donor organs, the availability of which is highly limited [3]. Some patients do not respond well to non-targeted treatments, whether for cancer or in cases where low-specificity drugs are utilized [4]. Thus, it is essential to identify options for specific biocompatible transporters with high fidelity for certain affected areas. These are only a few of the major problems for which the accelerated development of biomaterials and manufacturing technologies in recent years has brought promising solutions [5,6].

One area where many biomaterials have shown excellent results is orthopedics. However, the 3D printing of these materials poses challenges regarding degradation over time and compatibility with the human body, especially at the level of the graft–real tissue interface [7]. Enthusiastic research conducted using viable cells in combination with biomaterials has already tested the mechanical stability and bioactive properties of these materials, yielding great results in this field [8].

In their comprehensive review, Timofticiuc et al. explained how the properties of 3D-bioprinted constructs can spare patients from limb amputation [9]. Surgical teams with a strong vascular microsurgery background have perfectly integrated full or partial cell-laden biomaterial-based bones as replacements for bones that were candidates for amputation due to severe defects. Full bone grafts employed in minor patients and the designs used for optimally anchoring the 3D-bioprinted constructs with the surrounding tissues constitute some of the true innovations. Newly developed biomaterials situated in the testing area either in vitro or in animal models, the printing techniques used, and a summary of their physical and chemical properties are also presented in this review paper [9].

Designing large bone grafts is a challenging task, mainly because of the poor blood supply, which limits the exchange of metabolites and the supply of oxygen and nutrients [10,11]. Integrating viable cells into the grafts offers great advantages regarding their biocompatibility but also creates residues, which accumulate and precipitate the development of a cytotoxic microenvironment in the absence of proper blood flow [12]. A potential solution to this issue is designing pre-vascularized grafts, a method exemplified by Buranawat et al. in their research on maxillofacial reconstruction [13]. The team designed a porous calcium metaphosphate scaffold in which a co-culture containing endothelial cells and human alveolar osteoblasts was introduced. Creating porous structures is essential for cell development, especially in bone structures, where osteointegration, osteoconductivity, and angiogenesis are critical for graft sustainability [14,15]. The pores created in this study ranged from 80 to 100 μm and were optimal for cell development, which resulted in optimal intrinsic VEGF-release (10,455.6 pg/mL), the main factor for angiogenesis. Furthermore, a scaffold with rapid biodegradability was created using calcium metaphosphate, a bioactive ceramic that retains large quantities of water. This property, although potentially affecting the mechanical strength of the grafts, allows enhanced tissue integration and cell viability. Hence, a pre-vascularized graft was obtained, thus overcoming a major drawback of large bone grafts [13].

Some orthopedic grafts are designed in a way that prioritizes elasticity rather than mechanical strength [16]. In the realm of adult-acquired flatfoot deformities, a spring ligament (SL) injury requires the replacement of a ligament with a synthetic graft, which should be bioactive and possess essential mechanical properties, such as elasticity and stress resistance [17]. In their research, Nieto et al. designed an SL graft made of polycaprolactone (PCL) and type-B gelatin enhanced with graphene oxide. The graft was tested in vitro to demonstrate its bioactive properties and later studied in silico regarding its biomechanical behavior. PCL and gelatin were chosen for their known biocompatibility and optimal wettability as well as their ability to promote cell adhesion and proliferation for better in situ integration. To create a ligament structure, a fiber-like structure was obtained using electrospinning. However, the nanofibers resulting from using this technique lacked mechanical strength, an issue addressed by adding nanocomposites such as graphene oxide. Finding the optimal fiber concentration and orientation is essential for a precise ligament equivalent. In this study, the optimal Young's Modulus of 240 MPa was achieved with a 2% graphene oxide concentration in a twisted yarn configuration of the ligament graft [17].

There are also cases where the mechanical properties of biomaterials are not as relevant to a given task as they are for the majority of the pathologies for which they are used. A good example is provided in the study by Tabanella et al., who designed a collagen scaffold for tissue augmentation. The aesthetic aspect of a repair is a major concern in the realm of oral defects, and mucosal height plays a crucial role in this regard [18]. In a comparison between porcine-cross-linked collagen and a traditional approach for vertical augmentation of the oral mucosa, the former was demonstrated to be an aesthetic solution and statistically correlated with an enhanced height of the keratinized mucosa [19].

Another major issue in bone healing pertains to the low estrogen levels in menopausal women, who have high osseous tissue catabolism and pose difficulties in the restauration of peri-implant bone defects [20]. Duarte et al. managed to design a scaffold made of deproteinized bovine bone with genistein via sonification to mimic the local, peri-dental effects of estrogen and tested it in ovariectomized rats. Genistein is a phytoestrogen that can act on estrogen receptors in the surrounding bone, activating osteoblast differentiation [21]. To further test bone production and implant integration, the removal torque was calculated, and the genistein-loaded scaffold presented the highest value, 5.4 Ncm, as well as the highest bone volume/tissue volume compared to the test group, wherein no estrogen equivalents were used [20].

In the last decade, a new branch of industry rapidly developed alongside new biomaterials and methods for better integration. Finding new technologies with which to transform biomaterials from micro- to nano-dimensions and using them as carriers or coatings constitute new and exciting directions for research in the field of 3D printing and biomaterials [22,23]. Boyuklieva et al. developed microspheres made of nanocomposites for use as drug carriers [24]. Substances with very short biological half-lives require higher serum concentrations for long and effective responses, but these high concentrations may cause severe adverse reactions. Thus, by creating microspheres composed of PCL nanoparticles and controlling the pH levels, good vectors exhibiting tropism to hard-penetrating tissues were designed, and the effects of the drug were preserved, while the side effects were not [24].

Kaupbayeva et al.'s study helps us to further understand how biomaterials can be used as vectors not only for drugs but also in gene editing [25]. CRISPR/Cas9 is a gene-editing technique that presents many drawbacks, especially with respect to the intriguing area of genetic defects [26]. This comprehensive review presents the methods and tools used to create carriers, such as vectors, biomaterials, synthetic approaches, and physical methods. The technologies and techniques were reviewed and efficiently categorized in order to clarify the possibilities that have been discovered so far, highlighting the vast advantages that biomaterials can bring to the medical realm [25].

Another example of a nanoparticle application is presented in the research conducted by Melchor-Moncada et al., where a coating of titanium oxide nanoparticles was used to improve the stability and antibacterial activity of serratiopeptidases [27]. Serratiopeptidase is a natural bacterial enzymatic compound and an innovative alternative to antibiotics [28]. However, its low solubility, heightened sensitivity to temperature and pH variations, and self-cleavage tendency are some of the traits hindering its large-scale usage in the context of antibiotic resistance [28]. However, in the cited paper, the research team managed to achieve enzyme immobilization through bioconjugation with titanium oxide nanoparticles, increasing stability and doubling antibacterial activity, especially against *E. coli* [27].

Magnesium alloys also present good biocompatibility and may be used as implants. However, they are highly corrosive and do not perform well under dynamic stress [29]. Saqib et al. used plasma electrolytic oxidation to create an anodic layer on top of a magnesium alloy while also coating it with biopolymers, granting it excellent performance under dynamic stress without signs of corrosion [30]. However, the coatings eventually degraded, and the added layer disappeared almost completely after approximately 30 days, returning the implant to its original corrosion rate. These results are promising, especially for the few cases where stents are constructed from magnesium alloys, but further studies must be conducted to improve the survival rates of the implants and develop additional applications for these metal alloys [30].

Biomaterials also present numerous advantages in cancer research and treatment. The paper by Knight et al. highlights the piezoelectric properties of nanomaterials and how said properties can be used to efficiently treat glioblastoma, with reduced side effects [31]. Many novel treatments for glioblastoma involve the use of electric fields to target cancerous cells, but such methods carry a risk of serious burns [32]. By introducing nanomaterials to the cancer site and applying a mechanical force such as ultrasound, biomaterials can exhibit piezoelectric properties and generate a local electric field that stops the tumoral cells from proliferating [31]. In this review, a classification of all the organic or inorganic nanomaterials that can exhibit these properties is presented, highlighting the technologies used and their properties in combating tumoral cells [31].

Biomaterials can also be used in research on tumoral cell activity. Building 3D models that mimic the microenvironments of different cancers is a novel approach to gaining further insight into the development and behavior of tumor cells. Evangelista et al. presented the techniques and models used in this direction for head-and-neck squamous cell carcinoma [33]. They also highlighted how the mechanical properties of these 3D-printed models translate the behaviors of tumoral cells. Stiffness, elasticity, and dynamic behavior are some of the properties that influence tumor growth, metastasis, and treatment response.

Furthermore, understanding the type of mechanical environment required by cancer cells can contribute to conceptualizing a treatment. Altering cell tension, hydrostatic pressure, mechanical strength, Young's modulus, or viscosity could play a role in the therapeutic approach [33].

The data presented in the latest studies demonstrate that the field of biomaterials is rapidly developing, with excellent results in numerous medical areas. Future research will be able to translate more characteristics of organs and tissues into scaffolds or other biomaterial constructs in order to mimic human structures and functionality to a greater extent. Furthermore, as biomaterials are incorporated into modern therapies, current treatments will likely improve, with better targeting and efficiency, while risks associated with human errors will be progressively mitigated.

**Author Contributions:** Conceptualization, C.S., A.C.D. and C.C.; writing—original draft preparation, C.S., A.C.D. and C.C.; writing—review and editing, C.S., A.C.D. and C.C. All authors have read and agreed to the published version of the manuscript.

**Funding:** This research received no external funding.

**Data Availability Statement:** Not applicable.

**Conflicts of Interest:** The authors declare no conflicts of interest.

## References

1. Jammalamadaka, U.; Tappa, K. Recent Advances in Biomaterials for 3D Printing and Tissue Engineering. *J. Funct. Biomater.* **2018**, *9*, 22. [CrossRef] [PubMed]
2. Yon, C.J.; Choi, B.C.; Lee, J.M.; Lee, S.W. Personalized 3D-Printed Prostheses for Bone Defect Reconstruction After Tumor Resection in the Foot and Ankle. *J. Funct. Biomater.* **2025**, *16*, 62. [CrossRef]
3. Chapman, J. Moving Boundaries for Improving Organ Transplant Availability. *Exp. Clin. Transplant.* **2024**, *22*, 7–11. [CrossRef]
4. Zhou, Y.; Tao, L.; Qiu, J.; Xu, J.; Yang, X.; Zhang, Y.; Tian, X.; Guan, X.; Cen, X.; Zhao, Y. Tumor biomarkers for diagnosis, prognosis and targeted therapy. *Signal Transduct. Target. Ther.* **2024**, *9*, 132. [CrossRef]
5. Scheau, C.; Didilescu, A.C.; Caruntu, C. Innovative Biomaterials: The Cornerstone of Next-Generation Medical Solutions. *J. Funct. Biomater.* **2024**, *15*, 218. [CrossRef]
6. Todd, E.A.; Mirsky, N.A.; Silva, B.L.G.; Shinde, A.R.; Arakelians, A.R.L.; Nayak, V.V.; Marcantonio, R.A.C.; Gupta, N.; Witek, L.; Coelho, P.G. Functional Scaffolds for Bone Tissue Regeneration: A Comprehensive Review of Materials, Methods, and Future Directions. *J. Funct. Biomater.* **2024**, *15*, 280. [CrossRef] [PubMed]
7. Timofticiuc, I.-A.; Călinescu, O.; Iftime, A.; Dragosloveanu, S.; Caruntu, A.; Scheau, A.-E.; Badarau, I.A.; Didilescu, A.C.; Caruntu, C.; Scheau, C. Biomaterials adapted to VAT photopolymerization in 3D printing: Characteristics and medical applications. *J. Funct. Biomater.* **2023**, *15*, 7. [CrossRef]
8. Sousa, A.C.; Alvites, R.; Lopes, B.; Sousa, P.; Moreira, A.; Coelho, A.; Santos, J.D.; Atayde, L.; Alves, N.; Maurício, A.C. Three-Dimensional Printing/Bioprinting and Cellular Therapies for Regenerative Medicine: Current Advances. *J. Funct. Biomater.* **2025**, *16*, 28. [CrossRef] [PubMed]
9. Timofticiuc, I.-A.; Dragosloveanu, S.; Caruntu, A.; Scheau, A.-E.; Badarau, I.A.; Garofil, N.D.; Didilescu, A.C.; Caruntu, C.; Scheau, C. 3D Bioprinting in Limb Salvage Surgery. *J. Funct. Biomater.* **2024**, *15*, 383. [CrossRef]
10. Choi, J.; Lee, E.J.; Jang, W.B.; Kwon, S.M. Development of Biocompatible 3D-Printed Artificial Blood Vessels through Multidimensional Approaches. *J. Funct. Biomater.* **2023**, *14*, 497. [CrossRef]
11. Dragosloveanu, S.; Capitanu, B.S.; Moise, M.N.; Vulpe, D.E.; Josanu, R.; Gherghe, M.E.; Preda, E.M.; Cergan, R.; Scheau, C. Restoring Hip Symmetry and Its Impact on Outcomes: A Case Series on Megaprosthesis Use in Non-Oncological Patients with Complications After Total Hip Arthroplasty. *Symmetry* **2025**, *17*, 322. [CrossRef]
12. Wong, S.K.; Yee, M.M.F.; Chin, K.Y.; Ima-Nirwana, S. A Review of the Application of Natural and Synthetic Scaffolds in Bone Regeneration. *J. Funct. Biomater.* **2023**, *14*, 286. [CrossRef]
13. Buranawat, B.; Shaalan, A.; Garna, D.F.; Di Silvio, L. Development of Prevascularized Synthetic Block Graft for Maxillofacial Reconstruction. *J. Funct. Biomater.* **2025**, *16*, 18. [CrossRef] [PubMed]
14. Pudełko-Prażuch, I.; Balasubramanian, M.; Ganesan, S.M.; Marecik, S.; Walczak, K.; Pielichowska, K.; Chatterjee, S.; Kandaswamy, R.; Pamuła, E. Characterization and In Vitro Evaluation of Porous Polymer-Blended Scaffolds Functionalized with Tricalcium Phosphate. *J. Funct. Biomater.* **2024**, *15*, 57. [CrossRef] [PubMed]

15. Durán Hernández, O.; Baumer, V.; Marrero, G.; Karumanchi, S.; Prawel, D. Fabrication and Characterization of Highly Porous Gyroid Scaffolds Composed of Deproteinized Bone Mineral. *J. Funct. Biomater.* **2025**, *16*, 119. [CrossRef]
16. Cecuda-Adamczewska, V.; Romanik-Chruścielewska, A.; Kosowska, K.; Sokołowska, I.; Łukasiewicz, N.; Korycka, P.; Florys-Jankowska, K.; Zakrzewska, A.; Wszoła, M.; Klak, M. Elasticity Modification of Biomaterials Used in 3D Printing with an Elastin-Silk-like Recombinant Protein. *J. Funct. Biomater.* **2024**, *15*, 141. [CrossRef]
17. Nieto, S.; Gantiva-Díaz, M.; Hoyos, M.A.; Montoya, Y.; Cruz, J.C.; Cifuentes-De la Portilla, C. Advancing Adult-Acquired Flatfoot Deformity Treatment: Enhanced Biomechanical Support Through Graphene Oxide-Integrated Bioengineered Grafts Tested In Silico. *J. Funct. Biomater.* **2024**, *15*, 335. [CrossRef]
18. Monje, A.; González-Martín, O.; Ávila-Ortiz, G. Impact of peri-implant soft tissue characteristics on health and esthetics. *J. Esthet. Restor. Dent.* **2023**, *35*, 183–196. [CrossRef]
19. Tabanella, G.; Viale, M. Porcine Cross-Linked Collagen Matrix for Peri-Implant Vertical Soft Tissue Augmentation: A Randomized Prospective Observational Study. *J. Funct. Biomater.* **2024**, *15*, 261. [CrossRef]
20. Duarte, N.D.; Mulinari-Santos, G.; Batista, F.R.d.S.; Gomes, M.B.; Monteiro, N.G.; Silva, A.C.E.d.; Gruber, R.; Lisboa-Filho, P.N.; Gomes-Ferreira, P.H.S.; Okamoto, R. Sonification of Deproteinized Bovine Bone Functionalized with Genistein Enhances Bone Repair in Peri-Implant Bone Defects in Ovariectomized Rats. *J. Funct. Biomater.* **2024**, *15*, 328. [CrossRef]
21. Skrajnowska, D.; Bielecki, W.; Szterk, A.; Ofiara, K.; Bobrowska-Korczak, B. Genistein Supplementation and Bone Health in Breast Cancer in Rats. *Nutrients* **2024**, *16*, 912. [CrossRef]
22. Zhu, H.; Kuang, H.; Huang, X.; Li, X.; Zhao, R.; Shang, G.; Wang, Z.; Liao, Y.; He, J.; Li, D. 3D printing of drug delivery systems enhanced with micro/nano-technology. *Adv. Drug Deliv. Rev.* **2025**, *216*, 115479. [CrossRef]
23. Anyachor, C.P.; Orish, C.N.; Ezejiofor, A.N.; Cirovic, A.; Cirovic, A.; Dooka, B.D.; Ezealisiji, K.; Orisakwe, O.E. Silica nanoparticles (SiNPs) derived from melon seed husk ameliorate Ni/Al mixture-mediated cognitive impairment in rats. *J. Med. Life* **2024**, *17*, 856–867. [CrossRef] [PubMed]
24. Boyuklieva, R.; Katsarov, P.; Zagorchev, P.; Abarova, S.; Hristozova, A.; Pilicheva, B. Development of Nanocomposite Microspheres for Nasal Administration of Deferiprone in Neurodegenerative Disorders. *J. Funct. Biomater.* **2024**, *15*, 329. [CrossRef] [PubMed]
25. Kaupbayeva, B.; Tsoy, A.; Safarova, Y.; Nurmagambetova, A.; Murata, H.; Matyjaszewski, K.; Askarova, S. Unlocking Genome Editing: Advances and Obstacles in CRISPR/Cas Delivery Technologies. *J. Funct. Biomater.* **2024**, *15*, 324. [CrossRef] [PubMed]
26. Shumega, A.R.; Pavlov, Y.I.; Chirinskaite, A.V.; Rubel, A.A.; Inge-Vechtomov, S.G.; Stepchenkova, E.I. CRISPR/Cas9 as a Mutagenic Factor. *Int. J. Mol. Sci.* **2024**, *25*, 823. [CrossRef]
27. Melchor-Moncada, J.J.; Vasquez-Giraldo, S.; Zuluaga-Vélez, A.; Orozco, L.M.; Veloza, L.A.; Sepúlveda-Arias, J.C. Bioconjugation of Serratiopeptidase with Titanium Oxide Nanoparticles: Improving Stability and Antibacterial Properties. *J. Funct. Biomater.* **2024**, *15*, 300. [CrossRef]
28. Nair, S.R.; C, S.D. Serratiopeptidase: An integrated View of Multifaceted Therapeutic Enzyme. *Biomolecules* **2022**, *12*, 1468. [CrossRef]
29. Dragosloveanu, Ş.; Cotor, D.C.; Dragosloveanu, C.D.M.; Stoian, C.; Stoica, C.I. Preclinical study analysis of massive magnesium alloy graft for calcaneal fractures. *Exp. Ther. Med.* **2021**, *22*, 731. [CrossRef]
30. Saqib, M.; Kremmer, K.; Opitz, J.; Schneider, M.; Beshchasna, N. Evaluation of the Degradation Properties of Plasma Electrolytically Oxidized Mg Alloy AZ31 Using Fluid Dynamic Accelerated Tests for Biodegradable Implants. *J. Funct. Biomater.* **2024**, *15*, 366. [CrossRef]
31. Knight, Z.; Ruiz, A.; Elies, J. Piezoelectric Nanomaterials for Cancer Therapy: Current Research and Future Perspectives on Glioblastoma. *J. Funct. Biomater.* **2025**, *16*, 114. [CrossRef] [PubMed]
32. Valerius, A.R.; Webb, L.M.; Thomsen, A.; Lehrer, E.J.; Breen, W.G.; Campian, J.L.; Riviere-Cazaux, C.; Burns, T.C.; Sener, U. Review of Novel Surgical, Radiation, and Systemic Therapies and Clinical Trials in Glioblastoma. *Int. J. Mol. Sci.* **2024**, *25*, 10570. [CrossRef] [PubMed]
33. Evangelista, A.; Scocozza, F.; Conti, M.; Auricchio, F.; Conti, B.; Dorati, R.; Genta, I.; Benazzo, M.; Pisani, S. Exploring Mechanical Features of 3D Head and Neck Cancer Models. *J. Funct. Biomater.* **2025**, *16*, 74. [CrossRef] [PubMed]

Journal of
*Functional Biomaterials*

MDPI

*Article*

# Porcine Cross-Linked Collagen Matrix for Peri-Implant Vertical Soft Tissue Augmentation: A Randomized Prospective Observational Study

**Giorgio Tabanella [1,*] and Massimiliano Viale [2]**

1 O.R.E.C.—Oral Reconstruction and Education Center, Via Rovereto 6, 00198 Rome, Italy
2 Institute for Complex Systems—CNR, P.le Aldo Moro 2, 00185 Rome, Italy; massimiliano.viale@gmail.com
* Correspondence: gtabanella@gmail.com; Tel.: +39-06-8424-0686

**Abstract:** The mucosa height has always been of interest in modern implant dentistry to obtain biomimetic results. Papilla height, mucosa scalloping, and free mucosal margin level are crucial to achieve "pink aesthetics". The aim of this study was to investigate the vertical increase in the peri-implant soft tissues with a porcine cross-linked collagen matrix (Geistlich Fibro-Gide®). **Methods:** A total of 60 patients were divided into the following three groups: Group 1—patients who received porcine cross-linked collagen matrix for vertical soft tissue augmentation and a cover screw combined with a coronally advanced flap (CAF); Group 2—patients who received the collagen matrix combined with a healing abutment and CAF; Group 3 (control group)—patients who received a traditional surgical approach based on crestal incision and no collagen matrix as well as no CAF. **Results:** The average horizontal tissue thickness growth after 3 months was more effective for Group 1 (1.35 ± 1.23 mm) compared to Group 2 (0.85 ± 0.67 mm) and the control group (0.20 ± 0.41 mm). The average tissue height growth was 1.05 ± 1.39 mm for Group 1, 0.32 ± 1.28 mm for Group 2, and −0.05 ± 0.39 mm for the control group. Finally, the average increase in the band of keratinized mucosa was 0.60 ± 1.23 mm for Group 1, −0.60 ± 0.94 mm for Group 2, and 0.45 ± 0.60 mm for the control group. **Conclusions:** The combination of the CAF, porcine cross-linked collagen matrix, and cover screw resulted in better clinical results compared to Group 2 and 3.

**Keywords:** peri-implant mucosa; emergence profile; soft tissue augmentation; vertical soft tissue augmentation; horizontal soft tissue augmentation; papilla regeneration; 3D soft tissue augmentation; periodontal plastic surgery; mucosa phenotype boosting; collagen matrix; papilla regeneration

## 1. Introduction

The peri-implant mucosa plays a critical role in the success and longevity of endosseous dental implants [1]. This specialized tissue interface between the implant and the surrounding oral environment not only facilitates osseointegration but also helps in maintaining the health and stability of the implant over time [2–5]. The condition of the peri-implant mucosa, including its thickness, quality, and vascularity significantly influences the success of dental implant treatment [4]. A thick and healthy peri-implant mucosa provides better support for the peri-implant soft tissues, minimizing the risk of complications such as bone loss, mucosal recession and implant exposure [5].

However, if it is true that the horizontal thickness of the peri-implant mucosa significantly affects the biomechanical behavior, biological response, and aesthetic outcome of endosseous dental implants, very little has been reported in the scientific literature about the significance of the vertical thickness as well as the mucosa height [3,6–8]. The vertical thickness of the mucosa is the measurement from the implant platform to the mucosa facing the oral cavity before the uncovery of the implant, whereas the mucosa height is the distance, after implant uncovery, from the implant platform to the free mucosal margin, which is the vertical dimension of the connective tissue, the junctional epithelium, and the sulcus above the implant platform. Both measurements are correlated to each other and very close in dimensions.

Accordingly, the vertical dimension of the peri-implant mucosa represents the transmucosal compartment directly in contact with the emergence profile [9] of the definitive restoration. This transitional zone between the implant crown and the surrounding soft tissues plays a crucial role to influence both the aesthetics and longevity of dental implants [9]. In fact, the emergence profile directly affects the visual appearance of the implant-supported restoration; it contributes to the stability and health of the peri-implant soft tissues, minimizing the risk of soft tissue recession, inflammation, and the loss of attachment and, finally, it significantly influences patient satisfaction and quality of life following implant treatment [9].

Several techniques have been proposed to horizontally augment the peri-implant mucosa [10–14] to create an ideal soft tissue environment for implant placement. However, few papers have reported techniques to increase the vertical thickness of the mucosa around dental implants [9,15]. In fact, whereas horizontal mucosa augmentation has been considered more relevant because of its capabilities to reduce peri-implant bone loss, vertical soft tissue augmentation has mainly been related to "pink aesthetics" and considered to be of less importance. Although Thoma et al. [9] introduced the application of biomaterials to increase the mucosa height and Verardi et al. [15] suggested the use of biomaterial in contact with the implant head, no other studies have compared the use of biomaterials in conjunction with coronally advanced flap and the use of cover screws or healing abutment.

The aim of this study was thus to investigate a novel approach to increase the vertical thickness of the peri-implant mucosa with a porcine cross-linked collagen matrix (Geistlich Fibro-Gide®) combined with a coronally advanced flap (CAF) and a cover screw or a healing abutment versus the traditional approach with no soft tissue grafting and no CAF management.

## 2. Materials and Methods

This randomized prospective clinical study included 60 patients who received single endosseous dental implants. Patients were divided into the following three different groups based on the type of surgical technique utilized at second stage surgery: Group 1—patients who received porcine cross-linked collagen matrix for vertical soft tissue augmentation and a cover screw combined with a coronally advanced flap; Group 2—patients who received collagen matrix combined with a healing abutment and CAF; and Group 3 (control group)—patients who received a traditional surgical approach based on crestal incision and no collagen matrix as well as no CAF. The healing abutment used in Group 2 was 3 mm in height in order to clearly show a clinical evident difference compared to Group 1 (collagen matrix combined with cover screw and CAF).

All clinical procedures were performed in full compliance with the Declaration of Helsinki, and the subsequent revisions (Fortaleza 2013) and study protocol were approved by the Ethical Committee Lazio 1 (Prot. N. 1396/CE Lazio 1).

All patients were consecutively enrolled and assigned to a group based on a randomization software (random.org). A random generator software assigned each patient to a specific group after having specified the total patient number of patients and the numbers of patients for each group.

Before enrolling the patients, they were asked to sign the informed consent and informed about the therapeutic alternatives.

The inclusion criteria were as follows: (1) need for an implant-supported single-crown restoration; (2) >21 years of age; (3) any type of definitive abutment; (4) single cemented or screw-retained definitive restorations; and (5) mono-edentulism. The exclusion criteria included the following: (1) any systemic disorder or medication known to alter bone metabolism; (2) infection of the implant site; (3) probing depth > 4 mm at natural teeth; (4) inadequate oral hygiene; (5) pregnancy: (6) lactation; and (7) uncontrolled medical conditions such as diabetes mellitus. Sample size calculation was based on comparable clinical studies [16].

At the second-stage surgery, an incision was executed in the middle of the crest and the following measurements were performed by one examiner (G.T.) at each implant site which was considered as a statistical unit: (1) the height of the keratinized tissue from the mucogingival junction to the free mucosal margin through a periodontal probe (Hu-Friedy® Color-Coded Single-End Unc Probe 1-15, Chicago, IL, USA) on the medial aspect of the implant; (2) the thickness of the mucosa which was measured with a caliper (Hu-Friedy® Castroviejo Caliper, Chicago, IL, USA), considering the medial aspect of implant platform as a point of reference; (3) the height of the mucosa which was measured with the same periodontal probe from the medial aspect of the implant platform to the free mucosal margin. Each implant was previously inserted at the same level of the crestal bone in order to avoid false measurements related to the depth of insertion. Probe measurements were rounded off to the nearest millimeter. Before each second-stage surgery, the site was scanned using an intraoral scanner (iTero Elements Plus Series®, Align Technology, Inc., San Jose, CA, USA)) in order to obtain multiple stl files to analyze the mucosa 3D augmentation at 1, 3, and 12 months after the periodontal plastic surgery. The overlapping of the stl files allowed us to analyze the maturation, migration, thickening, or recession of the soft tissue over a period of 12 months.

### 2.1. Surgical Techniques

In Group 1, a crestal incision was executed in combination with two vertical releasing incisions in order to properly advance the flap in a coronal position (Figures 1–3). The collagen matrix was then positioned on the cover screw and microsutures were performed to secure the flap in a coronal position as well as allowing a first intention healing of the mucosa. The collagen matrix was not fixated with pins, screws, or periosteal sutures since the pressure related to the microsuturing was enough to avoid a shifting of the matrix. In Group 2, the same surgical approach was used, except for the fact that a healing abutment was screwed onto the implant platform (Figures 4–6). In the control group (Group 3), only a crestal incision was performed to get access to the implant platform without CAF and collagen matrix.

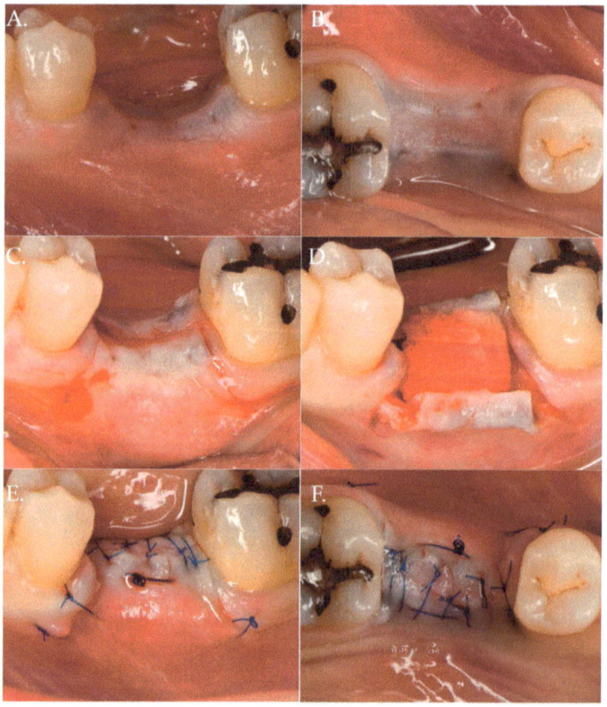


**Figure 1.** Clinical case related to 1 of the 20 patients of Group 1 patients who received Geistlich Fibro-Gide® combined with a cover screw and CAF. The pre-op (Frame **A**,**B**) clinical view shows a vertical and horizontal

deficiency of the soft tissue. A crestal incision, combined with two vertical releasing incisions (Frame **C**), was executed to access the implant platform. (Frame **D**) shows the collagen matrix of 5 mm of thickness positioned crestally. Micro 6-0 polypropylene sutures (Frame **E**,**F**) were executed to precisely close the wound allowing a primary intention healing of the coronally positioned flap.

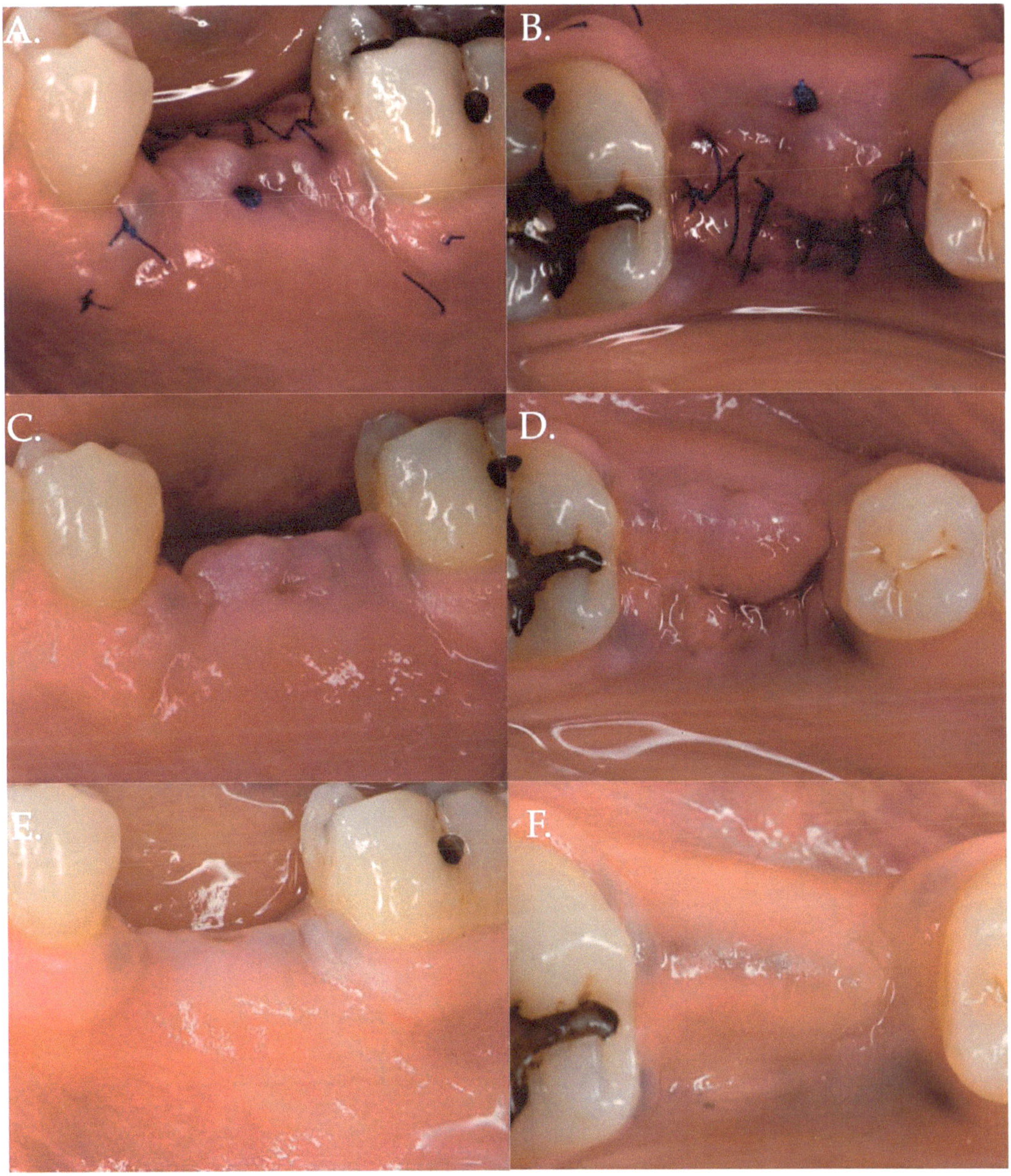


**Figure 2.** Post-operative healing after Geistlich Fibro-Gide® combined with cover screw and CAF: 1 week (Frame **A**,**B**), 2 weeks (Frame **C**,**D**), and 3 months post-op (Frame **E**,**F**).

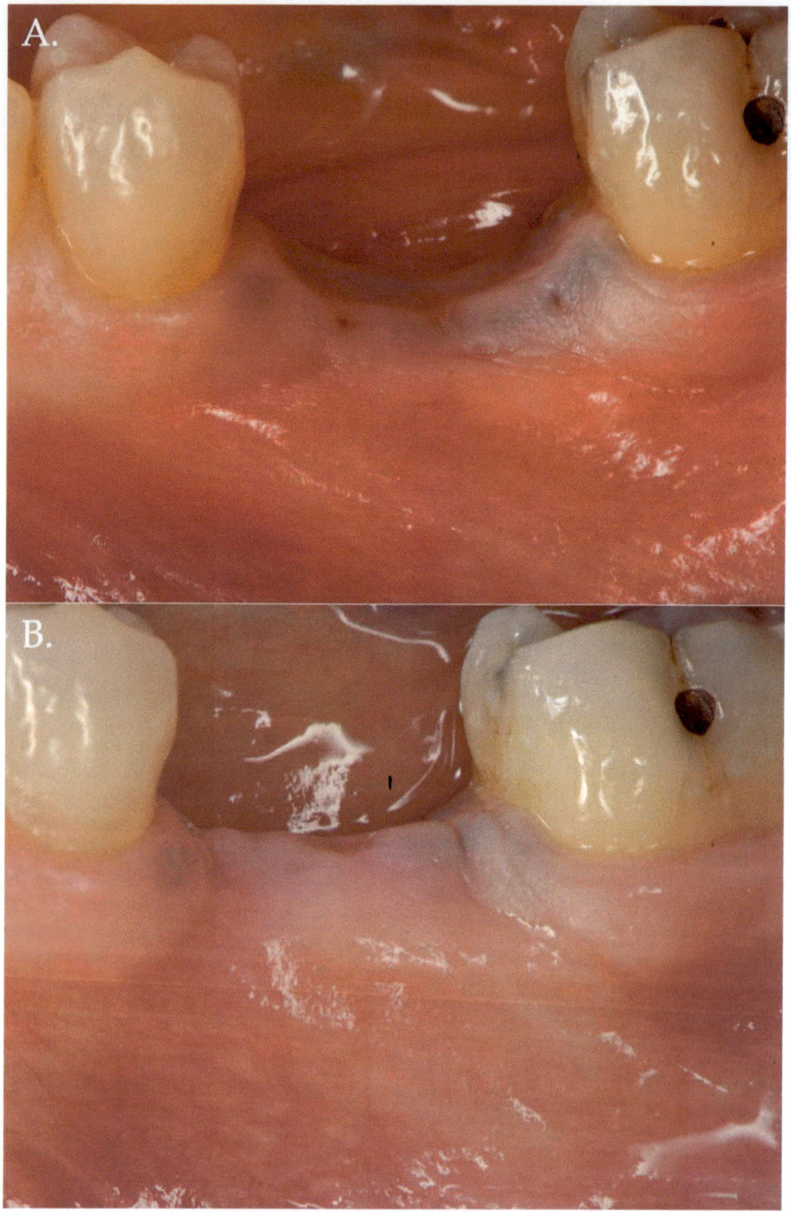


**Figure 3.** Before (Frame **A**) and after (Frame **B**) Geistlich Fibro-Gide® combined with a cover screw and CAF. The post-operative clinical picture shows a significant improvement in the "pink aesthetics" in the vertical dimension.

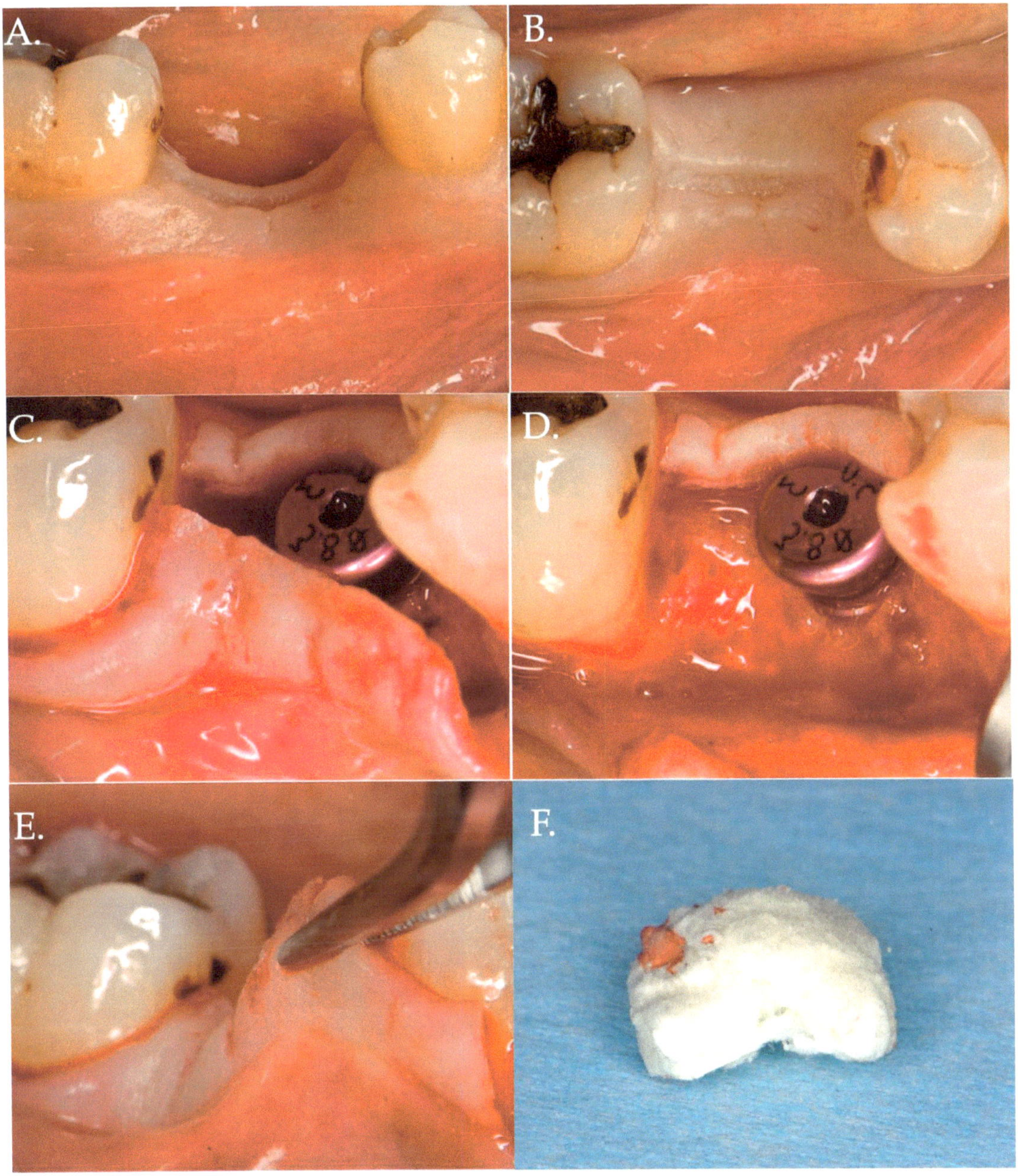


**Figure 4.** Surgical steps of a patient of Group 2—porcine cross-linked collagen matrix for vertical soft tissue augmentation and a healing abutment combined with a coronally advanced flap (CAF). The pre-surgical pictures demonstrate vertical and horizontal deficiency of the mucosa (Frame **A**,**B**). A full thickness flap is raised to get access to the implant platform and position a healing abutment of 3 mm height (Frame **C**,**D**). The flap is then released to obtain the necessary advancement (Frame **E**) and a collagen matrix of 5 mm in thickness is positioned above the healing abutment (Frame **F**).

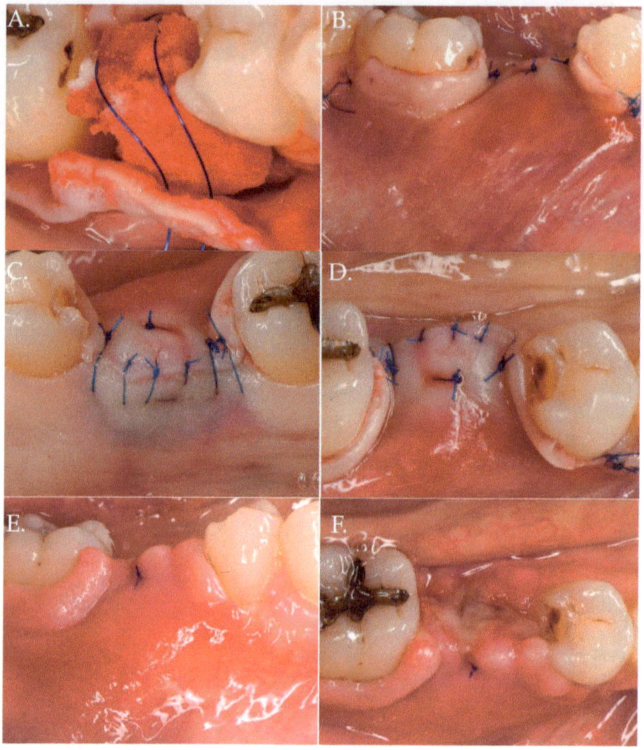


**Figure 5.** The collagen matrix is positioned coronally to the healing abutment and secured with 6.0 polypropylene sutures (Frame **A**). The CAF is secured coronally (Frame **B**) and microsutures (Frame **C**,**D**) maintain in position the flap. The clinical aspect after 1 week (Frame **E**,**F**) is demonstrating a delayed healing. This delay was very likely due to the excessive stretching of the advanced flap of more than 8 mm (5 mm matrix thickness + 3 mm healing abutment) compared to the bony crest.

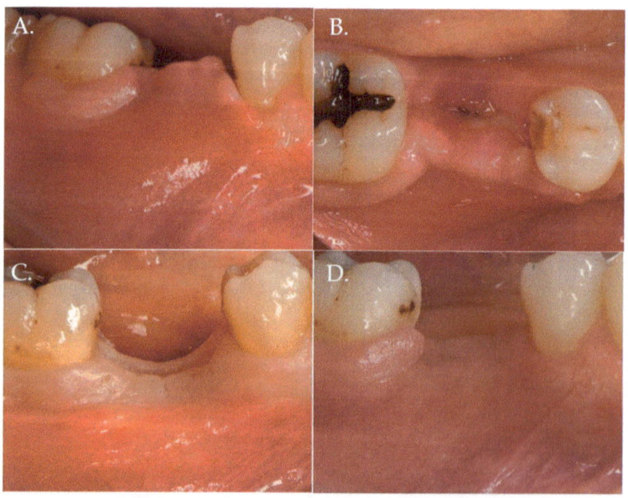


**Figure 6.** Healing after 2 weeks (Frame **A**,**B**) and 3 months (Frame **C**,**D**): The result is a significant improvement in the vertical "pink aesthetics".

### 2.2. Stl Files Measurements

An intraoral scanner (iTero Elements Plus Series®) was used to scan each patient at each time point: 0, 1, 3, and 12 months after mucogingival plastic surgery. The iTero software (Plus Computing Unit 2.8.15.70 ) was able to precisely measure the increase or decrease in the mucosa volume by overlapping the stl files. The software was also able to provide a difference in color to better visualize the 3D mucosa changes (Figures 7 and 8).

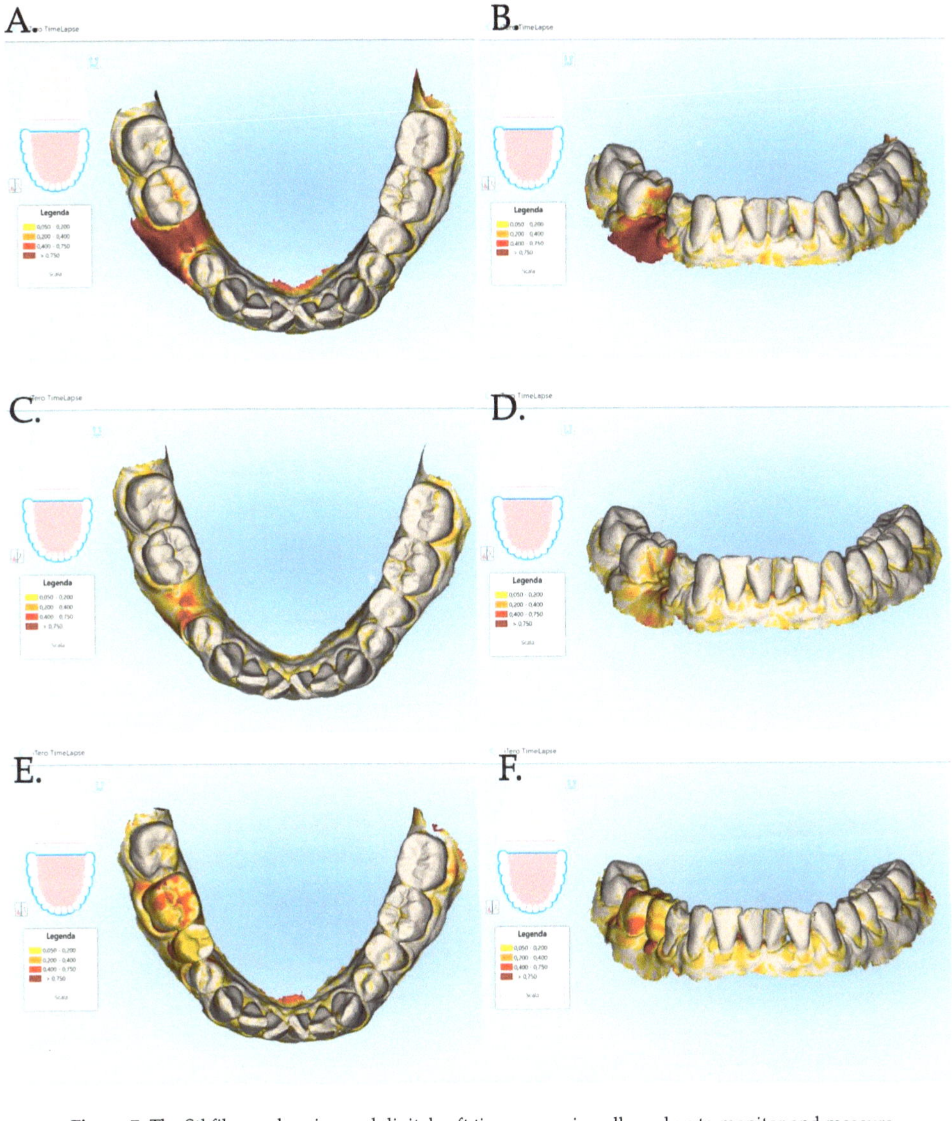


**Figure 7.** The Stl file overlapping and digital soft tissue mapping allowed us to monitor and measure the volume changes of the achieved results after 1 month (**A**,**B**), between 0 and 3 months (**C**,**D**), between and 0 and 12 months (**E**,**F**). A patient of Group 1 is reported in the digital reconstructions.

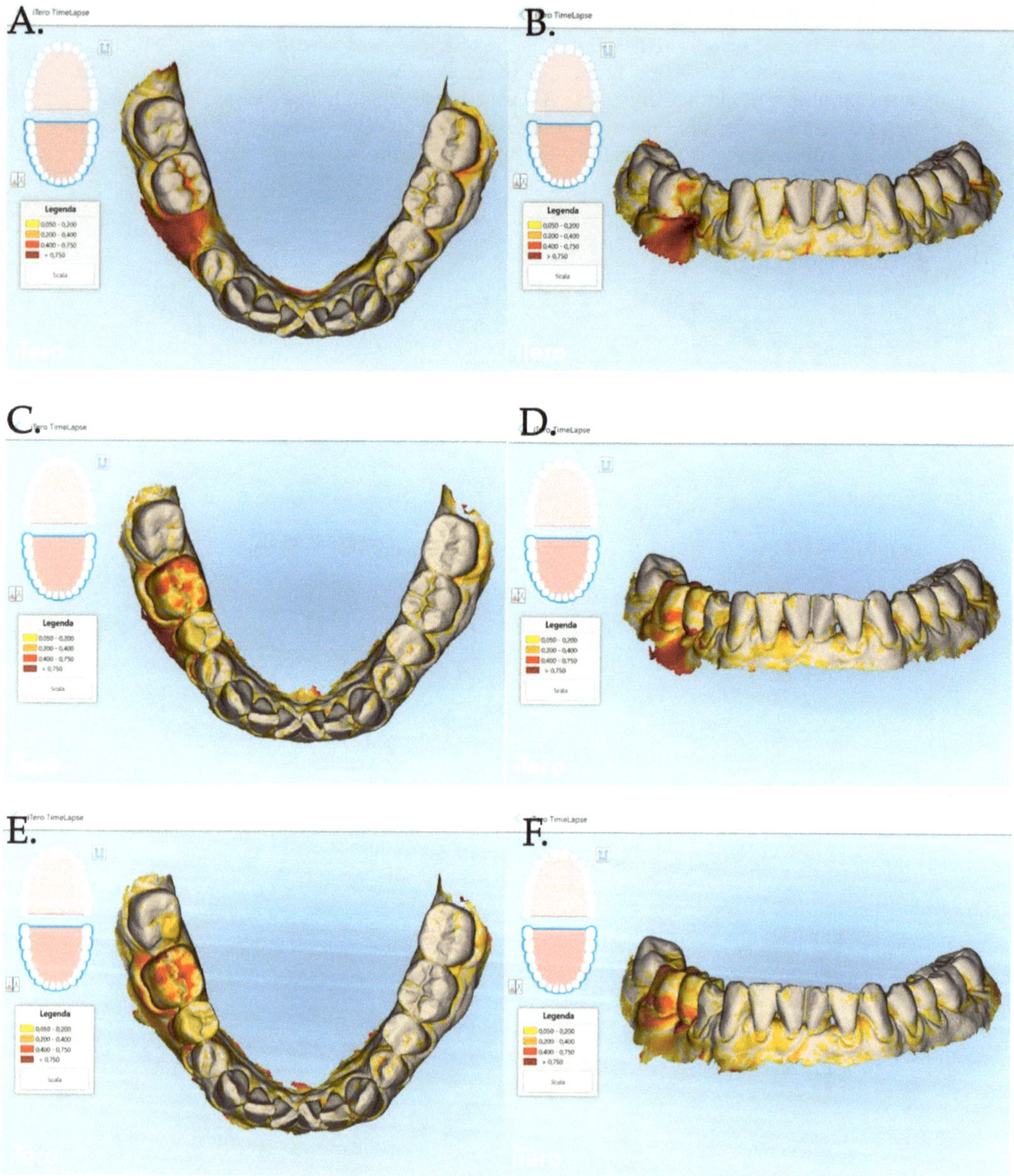


**Figure 8.** Stl files analyses between 1 and 3 months post muco-gingival plastic surgery (**A**,**B**), 1 and 12 months (**C**,**D**) and 3 and 12 months (**E**,**F**). The same patient of Figure 7 is reported in the above digital reconstruction.

## 3. Statistical Analysis—Spearman's Rank

For the same patients, the effect of the clinical evolution was evaluated by looking at an index that summarized the progress of mucosal strengthening one year after the mucogingival plastic surgery—Spearman's rank correlation index. The Stl files were produced before soft tissue augmentation and at 1, 3, and 12 months after second-stage surgery to measure the horizontal and vertical regeneration of the mucosa.

In order to evaluate the mucosa volume augmentation, Spearman's rank correlation coefficient of the pair series $X_i$, $Y_i$ was used. Spearman's index is worth +1 if there is a correlation (grows or have the same value with increasing) and −1 if there is an anti-correlation (decreases with increasing) regardless of if it is linear or not. Spearman's index of $y = e^x$ sampling (certainly a very increasing function for $x > 0$) is always 1.

## 4. Results

A total of 60 (28 females and 32 males) patients were included in the study. Patients ranged between 22 and 72 years of age and 10 patients were smokers.

For each patient, the area of interest was observed by overlapping the stl files at the time of surgery and at 1, 3, and 12 months after the mucosa management in order to analyze the augmentation as well as the creeping (vertical mucosa movement), thickening, and stabilization of the obtained results. The stl files overlapping allowed us to evaluate the 3D soft tissue augmentation that includes the simultaneous horizontal and vertical augmentation.

The height and the thickness of the mucosa as well as the band of keratinized tissue were measured at the time of surgery and after 3 months in order to evaluate its direct growth correlated to the surgical technique which was used to increase the phenotype's thickness and volume. The 60 patients were divided into the following three groups of 20 patients each based on the type of surgery they underwent: green (Group 1) for the cover screw combined with CAF and collagen matrix, red (Group 2) for healing abutment combined with CAF and collagen matrix, blue (Group 3) for the control group for which we performed a crestal incision. Figure 9 is clearly showing that the group treated with "Cover Screw Implant combined with CAF and collagen matrix" (green) had a more favorable evolution compared to the other two groups such as the one treated with "Healing Abutment Implant combined with CAF and collagen matrix" (red) and the control group (blue).

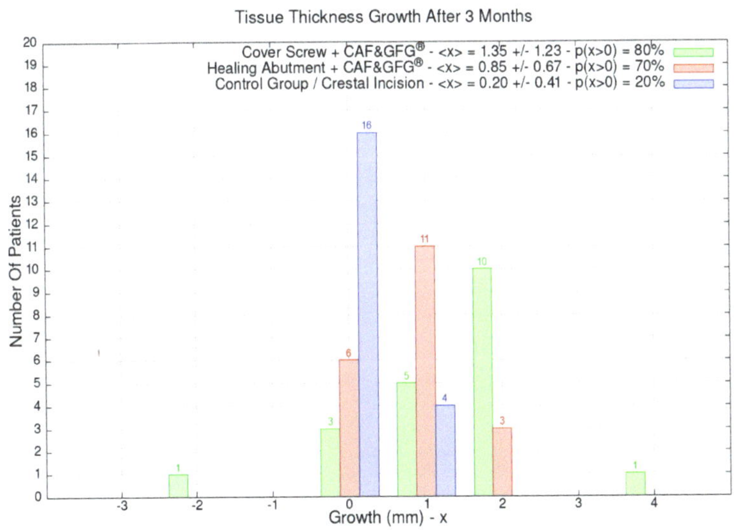


**Figure 9.** *Cont.*

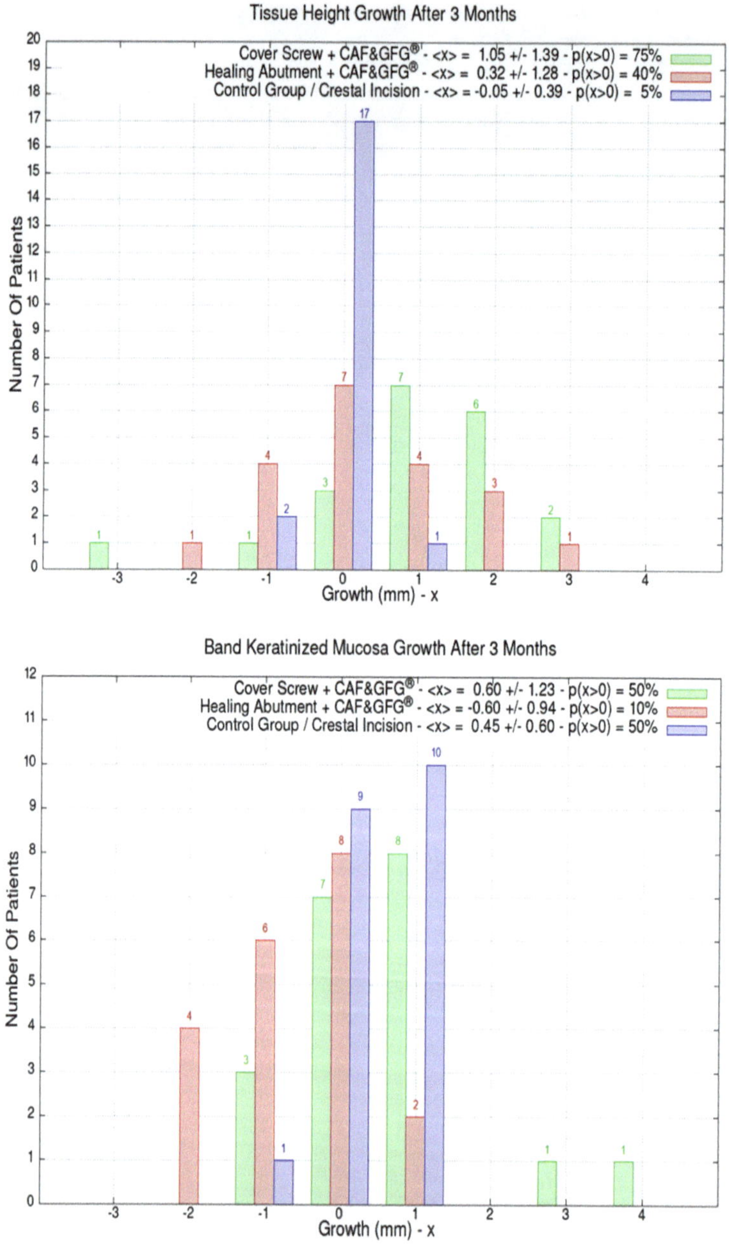


**Figure 9.** Mucosa thickness, height, and keratinized tissue changes 3 months after mucogingival plastic surgery. Divided by groups, the number of patients is shown as a function of the millimeters of growth or decrease. In the plot keys, the average growth value <x> and the percentage of patients p(x > 0) who have had a strictly positive evolution are reported. It is evident that the group treated with the "Cover Screw Implant combined with CAF and collagen matrix" (green) had a better evolution compared to both the one treated with the "Healing Abutment Implant combined with CAF and collagen matrix" (red) and the control one (blue) for which we performed a crestal incision only.

The average horizontal tissue thickness growth after 3 months was more effective for Group 1 (1.35 ± 1.23 mm) compared to Group 2 (0.85 ± 0.67 mm) and the control group (0.20 ± 0.41 mm). The average tissue height growth was 1.05 ± 1.39 mm for Group 1, 0.32 ± 1.28 mm for Group 2, and −0.05 ± 0.39 mm for the control group. Finally, the average increase in the band of keratinized mucosa was 0.60 ± 1.23 mm for Group 1, −0.60 ± 0.94 mm for Group 2, and 0.45 ± 0.60 mm for the control group. Group 1 resulted in better clinical results compared to Group 2 and 3 (Figure 9).

The data related to the Stl file analysis are reported in Figure 10. The continuous boosting of and improvement in the mucosa are also evident in this data analysis (Figure 11). In particular, the greater effectiveness of the "Cover Screw Implant combined with CAF and collagen matrix" is concrete but less prominent than the tissue growth shown in Figure 9. Interestingly, after 1 year, the control group (blue) had a slightly better evolution than the one treated with the "Healing Abutment Implant combined with CAF and collagen matrix" (red).

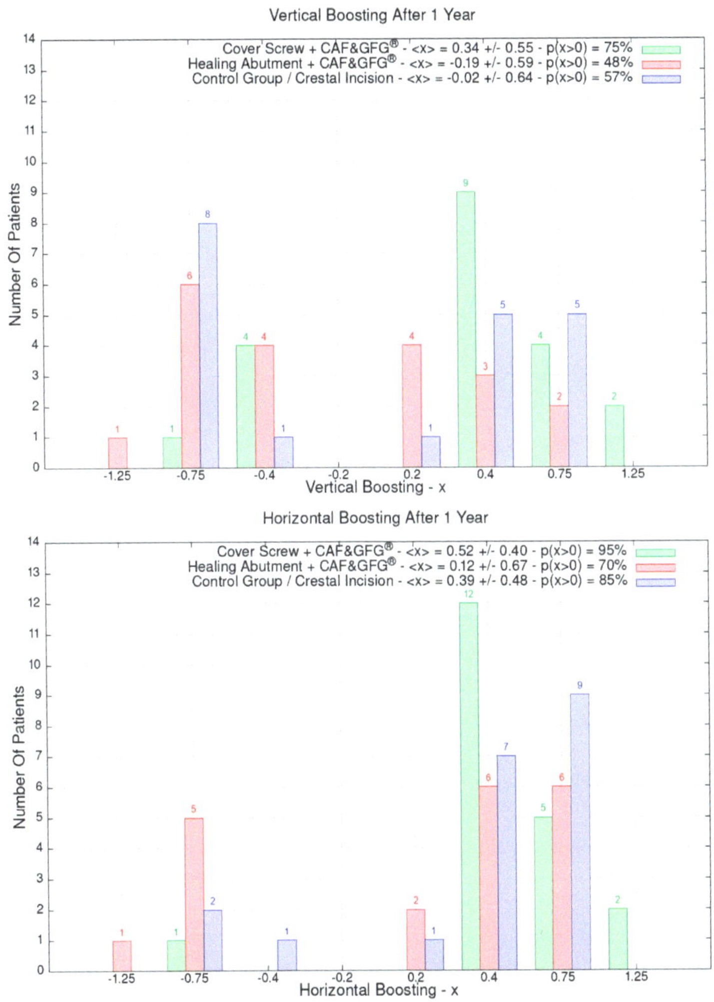


**Figure 10.** Vertical and horizontal boosting 1 year after surgery. As for Figure 1, divided by groups, the number of patients is reported as a function of boosting. In the plot keys, the average boosting <x> and the percentage of patients p(x > 0) who have had a strictly positive boosting are presented.

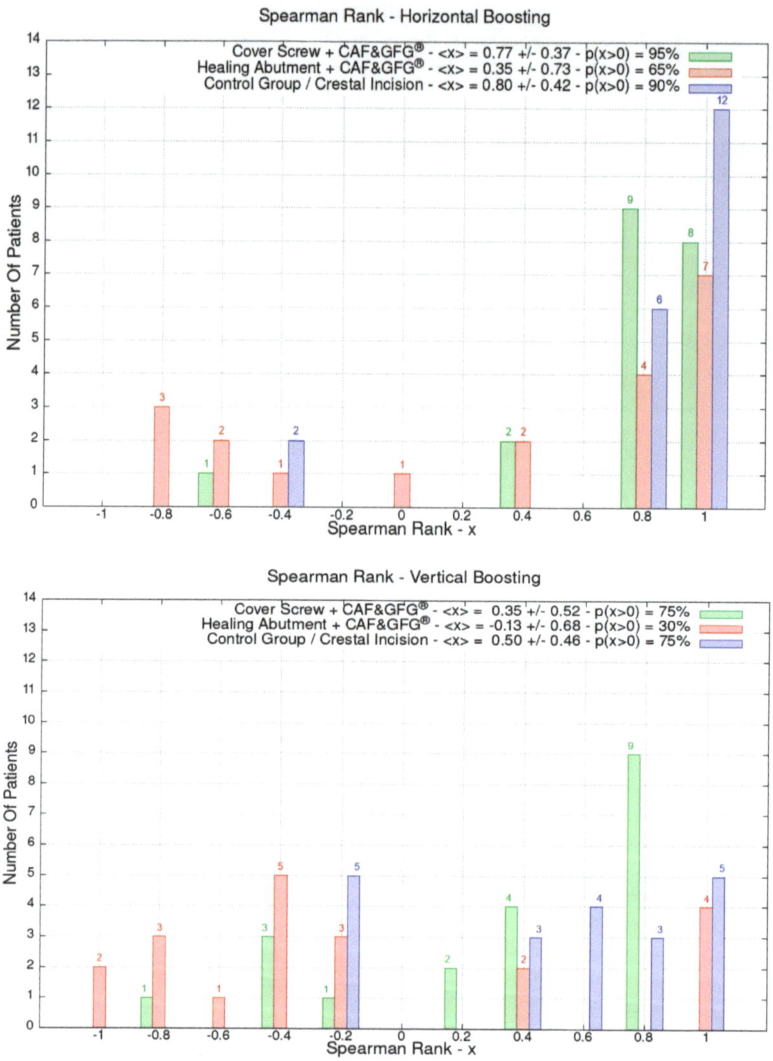


**Figure 11.** The vertical and horizontal augmentation is described using Spearman's rank. The values close to 1 represent the highest performing results. The vertical and soft tissue augmentation is significantly higher when the cover screw was used and when a coronally positioned flap was combined with collagen matrix.

## 5. Discussion

The emergence of dental implants as a reliable treatment modality for replacing missing teeth has revolutionized the field of implant dentistry. However, achieving optimal aesthetic outcomes with dental implants, particularly in the anterior maxilla, remains a challenge due to the complex interplay of hard and soft tissue dynamics. Soft tissue augmentation techniques have emerged as valuable tools for enhancing peri-implant soft tissue volume and contour, thereby improving the aesthetic outcomes and long-term implant stability. This stability is crucial for maintaining implant health and preventing complications such as peri-implant mucositis and peri-implantitis, which can compromise the longevity of the implant. The "pink aesthetics" must match with the "white aesthetics" so that the patients' aesthetic outcomes and natural-looking restorations blend with their existing dentition. Furthermore, a well-designed emergence profile contributes to a confident smile, improved self-esteem, and overall satisfaction with the implant-supported restoration. Scientifically, the thickness of the peri-implant mucosa influences the biomechanical and biological responses at the implant interface, impacting osseointegration and long-term stability. In particular, the importance of the peri-implant mucosa is related to the following:

- Biomechanical Stability: The thickness of the peri-implant mucosa provides mechanical support to the soft tissue, distributing occlusal forces evenly and reducing stress concentration around the implant–abutment complex [17]. Thicker mucosa can better resist mechanical trauma and prevent soft tissue recession, thereby preserving the integrity of the peri-implant soft tissues [18,19].
- Biological Response: Thicker peri-implant mucosa enhances the blood supply and vascularity, promoting optimal wound healing and tissue adaptation to the implant surface. Adequate vascularization facilitates nutrient and oxygen delivery to the surrounding tissues, fostering cellular proliferation and collagen deposition, which are essential for osseointegration and soft tissue integration [17,20,21].
- Aesthetic Outcome: The thickness of the peri-implant mucosa directly influences the [22] stability and contour of the peri-implant soft tissues, which are critical for achieving optimal aesthetic outcomes. Thicker mucosa provides better support for the papillae and gingival architecture, minimizing the risk of mucosal recession and ensuring harmonious gingival contours around the implant restoration [4,5,23,24].
- Implant Emergence Profile: The soft tissue thickness influences the emergence profile of the implant restoration, which determines the transition zone between the implant crown and the surrounding soft tissues. A thicker mucosa allows for better emergence profile management, resulting in a more natural-looking and harmonious integration of the restoration with the gingival architecture [25,26]. Similarly, the implant crown volume and its angulation of no more than 30° compared to the long axis of the implant may be responsible for an excessive compression of the achieved mucosa volume. Both parameters, mucosa and crown volume, may influence the final aesthetic and functional outcome.

Although, the vertical soft tissue thickness of the mucosa around endosseous dental implants may play a critical role in ensuring implant success, stability, and aesthetics, the scientific literature underscores the significance of vertical soft tissue thickness in various aspects of implant dentistry, including biomechanics, biological response, and aesthetic outcome. In our study, we reported two different approaches to vertically augment the peri-implant mucosa. The use of cross-linked collagen matrices is becoming more popular due to less invasive surgical procedures and results which are comparable with those achieved with connective tissue grafts [22,27–29]. The results of our study clearly demonstrated a substantial positive evolution, on average and in percentage, for patients treated with the cover screw combined with CAF and collagen matrix and a negative evolution, also compared to the control group, for patients treated with the healing abutment combined with the CAF and collagen matrix. The low effectiveness of the healing abutment combined with the CAF and collagen matrix is evident, but this could be related to the excessive stretching of the mucosa to completely cover the standard concave healing abutment of 3 mm. If it is considered that the thickness of the collagen matrix utilized in this study was 5 mm, a CAF of more than 8 mm would have been executed to completely cover the healing abutment. This procedure could have led to an excessive coronal repositioning of the flap and an evident low blood supply. In order to properly study the mucosa, all implants were placed crestally so that the depth of insertion could not influence the mucosa height and the biologic width reformation. We also reported that the soft tissue augmentation that was achieved was vertical and horizontal thus allowing us to obtain a simultaneous good quality and quantity of the peri-implant mucosa to face the emergence profile as well as the oral cavity. Compared to the other surgical techniques [30–32] that have been proposed to improve the peri-implant mucosa, our approach was minimally invasive and asymptomatic thus allowing us to achieve not only horizontal thickness but also an increase in the band of keratinized mucosa as well as a higher mucosa dimension facing the definitive restoration. Furthermore, the stl file analyses demonstrated the continuous volume increase, creeping (soft tissue growth in areas where inaccessible spaces were either intentionally created or naturally present), and stability of the achieved mucosa volume for the follow-up period of 12 months.

In summary, excessive stress of the mucosa during a coronally repositioned flap should be avoided but, at the same time, it is not advisable to still perform the traditional approach based on crestal incision at the time of uncovery since this could lead to a poor quality and quantity of the mucosa.

This study also showed how this simplified technique could be of help to switch from a thin to a thick phenotype thus potentially reducing the risk of complication in implant dentistry. However, the potential limitations of the study may be related to the reduced number of statistical units, the short period of follow-up, and the surgical technique which may be operator dependent. Furthermore, all measurements were taken by only one examiner (G.T.) thus being a limitation of this study. However, all measurements were executed as described in previous publications [6,11]. At the same time, we believe the strength of the study is the statistical analysis performed by the second author (M.V.). In fact, the blinding of the statistician in this study is an established approach to minimize the risk of performance and detection bias.

Finally, it is the authors' opinion that digital technology should be used to monitor implant health over a long period of time. Digital soft tissue mapping had already been proposed in the previous publications [22,33]; however, the increasing importance of proper communication with patients, along with the potential legal issues, as well as the need to share information with other colleagues will definitely increase the use of this technology. In fact, digital soft tissue monitoring would allow for easy access to recorded data and shared information. The proposed protocol to monitor implant health would be minimally invasive compared to peri-apical radiographs and probing. Furthermore, the first approach would monitor only the peri-implant bone level. Similarly, the periodontal probing would disrupt the delicate adhesion of the peri-implant mucosa onto the abutment interface. On the patient side, it takes the communication to a visual level, allowing patients to see the differences which are often difficult to understand when talking about changes of a few millimeters.

Clinicians should carefully consider augmenting the peri-implant mucosa with atraumatic plastic surgery. The results of this study clearly demonstrated the excellent outcome to improve the quality and quantity of the vertical mucosa thickness when a coronally advanced flap was used in conjunction with a collagen matrix and a cover screw. The vertical soft tissue thickness of the mucosa around endosseous dental implants is a crucial determinant of implant success, stability, and aesthetics. Clinicians should consider this parameter during treatment planning and prosthetic design to optimize outcomes and patient satisfaction. Advancements in biomaterials, surgical techniques, and regenerative therapies will continue to expand the armamentarium of vertical soft tissue augmentation in implant dentistry. Future research efforts should focus on optimizing treatment protocols, exploring innovative biomaterials, and investigating the role of tissue engineering approaches in enhancing peri-implant soft tissue volume and contour. The results of this study show how new biomaterials can be of importance in soft tissue regeneration when combined with the proper surgical approach. In particular, the technique we described clearly allows us to improve the quality of the mucosa with a minimally invasive and biomimetic approach, simultaneously resulting in low morbidity with the implant placement or at second-stage surgery. The direct clinical application may be the immediate and simplified 3D soft tissue augmentation as well as the reduction in surgical interventions. Finally, the vertical positioning of the mucosa which has always been critical and difficult to reach may be significantly improved when the collagen matrix is used in combination with a cover screw and a coronally positioned flap. Ultimately, this approach may add an extra tool to significantly improve biomimetic results in the anterior maxilla such as papilla height, mucosa scalloping, and free mucosal margin levels.

## 6. Conclusions

The results of this study support the use of mucogingival plastic surgery to increase the volume as well as improve the quality of the peri-implant mucosa. In particular, among the different surgical techniques that have been proposed, the coronally advanced flap combined with porcine cross-linked collagen matrix and a cover screw resulted in more thickness, vertical soft tissue height, and an adequate band of keratinized tissue.

**Author Contributions:** G.T. was responsible for study design, soft tissue grafting and data collection. M.V. was responsible for statistical analysis. All authors have read and agreed to the published version of the manuscript.

**Funding:** This research received external funding from GeistlichPharma, grant number PHFB 04783022 2019.

**Institutional Review Board Statement:** The study was conducted in accordance with the Declaration of Helsinki and approved by the Institutional Review Board Ethical Committee Lazio 1 (Prot. N. 1396/CE Lazio 1).

**Informed Consent Statement:** Informed consent was obtained from all subjects involved in the study.

**Data Availability Statement:** The original contributions presented in the study are included in the article, further inquiries can be directed to the corresponding author.

**Acknowledgments:** The author would like to express his gratitude to Jessica Volo and Karin Ianniciello for their amazing work in helping collect the data as well as providing pro bono surgeries to patients in need of implant treatment. The author would like also to thank Mus Erkan who has been of crucial support to make this complex clinical trial possible.

**Conflicts of Interest:** The authors declare no conflicts of interest since all the clinical data were evaluated by an independent researcher (M.V.). Furthermore, the funders had no role in the design of the study; in the collection, analyses, or interpretation of data; in the writing of the manuscript; or in the decision to publish the results.

## References

1. Lang, N.P.; Berglundh, T. Working Group 4 of Seventh European Workshop on Periodontology. Periimplant diseases: Where are we now?—Consensus of the Seventh European Workshop on Periodontology. *J. Clin. Periodontol.* **2011**, *38* (Suppl. 11), 178–181. [CrossRef] [PubMed]
2. Araujo, M.G.; Lindhe, J. Peri-implant health. *J. Periodontol.* **2018**, *89* (Suppl. 1), S249–S256. [CrossRef]
3. Tabanella, G. The buccal pedicle flap technique for periimplant soft tissue boosting. *Int. J. Esthet. Dent.* **2019**, *14*, 18. [PubMed]
4. Jung, R.E.; Pjetursson, B.E.; Glauser, R.; Zembic, A.; Zwahlen, M.; Lang, N.P. A systematic review of the 5-year survival and complication rates of implant-supported single crowns. *Clin. Oral Implants Res.* **2008**, *19*, 119–130. [CrossRef] [PubMed]
5. Linkevicius, T.; Apse, P.; Grybauskas, S.; Puisys, A. The influence of soft tissue thickness on crestal bone changes around implants: A 1-year prospective controlled clinical trial. *Int. J. Oral Maxillofac. Implants* **2009**, *24*, 712–719. [PubMed]
6. Tabanella, G. Busccal Pedicle Flap Technique Combined with Porcine Collagen Matrix for Volumetric Augmentation of Peri-Implant Mucosa. *Clin. Adv. Periodontics* **2022**, *12*, 5–11. [CrossRef]
7. Chou, C.; Mo, J.; Si, M.; Gu, Y.; Du, J.; Zhang, Z.; Lai, H. Papilla alteration in different gingival biotypes at single implant-supported restoration in anterior maxilla. *Shanghai Kou Qiang Yi Xue* **2012**, *21*, 541–545.
8. Tavelli, L.; Zucchelli, G.; Wang, H.-L.; Barootchi, S. Soft-Tissue Reconstruction at Anterior Implant Sites with Soft-Tissue Dehiscences. *Compend. Contin. Educ. Dent.* **2023**, *44*, 378–383, quiz 384.
9. Thoma, D.S.; Mühlemann, S.; Jung, R.E. Critical soft-tissue dimensions with dental implants and treatment concepts. *Periodontology 2000* **2014**, *66*, 106–118. [CrossRef]
10. Misch, C.E.; Perel, M.L.; Wang, H.-L.; Sammartino, G.; Galindo-Moreno, P.; Trisi, P.; Steigmann, M.; Rebaudi, A.; Palti, A.; Pikos, M.A.; et al. Implant success, survival, and failure: The International Congress of Oral Implantologists (ICOI) Pisa Consensus Conference. *Implant Dent.* **2008**, *17*, 5–15. [CrossRef] [PubMed]
11. Tabanella, G.; Viale, M. The influence of mucosa thickness and quality on single implant tissue stability: A prospective controlled clinical trial. *Int. J. Periodontics Restor. Dent.* **2021**, *41*, e93–e101. [CrossRef] [PubMed]
12. Thoma, D.S.; Zeltner, M.; Hilbe, M.; Hämmerle, C.H.F.; Hüsler, J.; Jung, R.E. Randomized controlled clinical study evaluating effectiveness and safety of a volume-stable collagen matrix compared to autogenous connective tissue grafts for soft tissue augmentation at implant sites. *J. Clin. Periodontol.* **2016**, *43*, 874–885. [CrossRef] [PubMed]
13. Zeltner, M.; Jung, R.E.; Hämmerle, C.H.F.; Hüsler, J.; Thoma, D.S. Randomized controlled clinical study comparing a volume-stable collagen matrix to autogenous connective tissue grafts for soft tissue augmentation at implant sites: Linear volumetric soft tissue changes up to 3 months. *J. Clin. Periodontol.* **2017**, *44*, 446–453. [CrossRef] [PubMed]

14. Silverstein, L.H.; Kurtzman, D.; Garnick, J.J.; Trager, P.S.; Waters, P.K. Connective tissue grafting for improved implant esthetics: Clinical technique. *Implant Dent.* **1994**, *3*, 231–234. [CrossRef] [PubMed]
15. Verardi, S.; Orsini, M.; Lombardi, T.; Ausenda, F.; Testori, T.; Pulici, A.; Oreglia, F.; Valente, N.A.; Stacchi, C. Comparison between two different techniques for peri-implant soft tissue augmentation: Porcine dermal matrix graft versus tenting screw. *J. Periodontol.* **2020**, *91*, 1011–1017. [CrossRef]
16. Cairo, F.; Barbato, L.; Tonelli, P.; Batalocco, G.; Pagavino, G.; Nieri, M. Xenogeneic collagen matrix versus connective tissue graft for buccal soft tissue augmentation at implant site. A randomized, controlled clinical trial. *J. Clin. Periodontol.* **2017**, *44*, 769–776. [CrossRef]
17. Buser, D.; Weber, H.P.; Donath, K.; Fiorellini, J.P.; Paquette, D.W.; Williams, R.C. Soft tissue reactions to non-submerged unloaded titanium implants in beagle dogs. *J. Periodontol.* **1992**, *63*, 225–235. [CrossRef]
18. Koh, R.U.; Oh, T.-J.; Rudek, I.; Neiva, G.F.; Misch, C.E.; Rothman, E.D.; Wang, H.L. Hard and soft tissue changes after crestal and subcrestal immediate implant placement. *J. Periodontol.* **2011**, *82*, 1112–1120. [CrossRef]
19. Cochran, D.L.; Mau, L.P.; Higginbottom, F.L.; Wilson, T.G.; Bosshardt, D.D.; Schoolfield, J.; Jones, A.A. Soft and hard tissue histologic dimensions around dental implants in the canine restored with smaller-diameter abutments: A paradigm shift in peri-implant biology. *Int. J. Oral Maxillofac. Implants* **2013**, *28*, 494–502. [CrossRef] [PubMed]
20. Buser, D.; Ingimarsson, S.; Dula, K.; Lussi, A.; Hirt, H.P.; Belser, U.C. Long-term stability of osseointegrated implants in augmented bone: A 5-year prospective study in partially edentulous patients. *Int. J. Periodontics Restor. Dent.* **2002**, *22*, 109–117.
21. Avila-Ortiz, G.; Elangovan, S.; Kramer, K.W.O.; Blanchette, D.; Dawson, D.V. Effect of alveolar ridge preservation after tooth extraction: A systematic review and meta-analysis. *J. Dent. Res.* **2014**, *93*, 950–958. [CrossRef] [PubMed]
22. Tabanella, G. Buccal Pedicle Flap Combined with Porcine Collagen Matrix: A Follow-Up of 2 Years on 40 Consecutive Cases. *Clin. Adv. Periodontics* **2022**, *12*, 80–87. [CrossRef]
23. Fu, J.-H.; Yeh, C.-Y.; Chan, H.-L.; Tatarakis, N.; Leong, D.J.M.; Wang, H.-L. Tissue biotype and its relation to the underlying bone morphology. *J. Periodontol.* **2010**, *81*, 569–574. [CrossRef] [PubMed]
24. Linkevicius, T.; Apse, P.; Grybauskas, S.; Puisys, A. Influence of thin mucosal tissues on crestal bone stability around implants with platform switching: A 1-year pilot study. *J. Oral Maxillofac. Surg.* **2010**, *68*, 2272–2277. [CrossRef]
25. Abrahamsson, I.; Berglundh, T.; Linder, E.; Lang, N.P.; Lindhe, J. Early bone formation adjacent to rough and turned endosseous implant surfaces. An experimental study in the dog. *Clin. Oral Implants Res.* **2004**, *15*, 381–392. [CrossRef] [PubMed]
26. Linkevicius, T.; Puisys, A.; Steigmann, M.; Vindasiute, E.; Linkeviciene, L. Influence of Vertical Soft Tissue Thickness on Crestal Bone Changes Around Implants with Platform Switching: A Comparative Clinical Study. *Clin. Implant Dent. Relat. Res.* **2015**, *17*, 1228–1236. [CrossRef]
27. Artzi, Z.; Vered, M.; Maymon-Gil, T.; Renert, U.; Netanely, E.; Thoma, D.S. Stromal cells associated with soft tissue augmentation by a volume stable collagen matrix (VCMX) are predominated by anti-inflammatory/reparative macrophages. *Int. J. Periodontics Restor. Dent.* **2023**. [CrossRef]
28. Song, Y.W.; Kim, S.; Waller, T.; Cha, J.-K.; Cho, S.-W.; Jung, U.-W.; Thoma, D.S. Soft tissue substitutes to increase gingival thickness: Histologic and volumetric analyses in dogs. *J. Clin. Periodontol.* **2019**, *46*, 96–104. [CrossRef]
29. Thoma, D.S.; Sancho-Puchades, M.; Ettlin, D.A.; Hämmerle, C.H.F.; Jung, R.E. Impact of a collagen matrix on early healing, aesthetics and patient morbidity in oral mucosal wounds—A randomized study in humans. *J. Clin. Periodontol.* **2012**, *39*, 157–165. [CrossRef]
30. Oh, S.-L.; Shahami, S.; Bernal-Cepeda, L.J.; Fu, Y.; Chung, M.-K. Therapeutic effectiveness of keratinized mucosa augmentation for functioning dental implants: A systematic review and meta-analysis. *J. Prosthodont. Res.* **2024**, JPR_D_24_00002. [CrossRef]
31. Kuebler, A.; Noelken, R. The influence of connective tissue grafting on the reconstruction of a missing facial bone wall using immediate implant placement and simultaneous bone reconstruction: A retrospective long-term cohort study. *Int. J. Implant Dent.* **2024**, *10*, 25. [CrossRef] [PubMed]
32. Giannelli, M.; Pinzani, M.; Lorenzini, L.; Fossi, T.; Bani, D. Soft tissue augmentation around dental implants by a new laser-aided pouch roll technique.Volumetric and clinical evaluation after 1-year. *J. Oral Implantol.* **2024**, *50*, 153–159. [CrossRef] [PubMed]
33. Tabanella, G. A New Method to Monitor Long-Term Tissue Stability and Pink Esthetics around Endosseous Dental Implants: Ultrafast Optical Sectioning Technique for 3D Soft Tissue Mapping. *EC Dent. Sci.* **2019**, *18*, 1–12.

Journal of *Functional Biomaterials*

MDPI

*Article*

# Bioconjugation of Serratiopeptidase with Titanium Oxide Nanoparticles: Improving Stability and Antibacterial Properties

**Jhon Jairo Melchor-Moncada [1], Santiago Vasquez-Giraldo [1], Augusto Zuluaga-Vélez [1], Lina Marcela Orozco [2], Luz Angela Veloza [2] and Juan Carlos Sepúlveda-Arias [1,*]**

1 Grupo Infección e Inmunidad, Departamento de Ciencias Básicas, Facultad de Ciencias de la Salud, Universidad Tecnológica de Pereira, Pereira 660003, Colombia; jjmelchor@utp.edu.co (J.J.M.-M.); santivg17@utp.edu.co (S.V.-G.); azuluagav@utp.edu.co (A.Z.-V.)

2 Grupo Polifenoles, Facultad de Tecnología, Escuela de Tecnología Química, Universidad Tecnológica de Pereira, Pereira 660003, Colombia; marcely@utp.edu.co (L.M.O.); lveloza@utp.edu.co (L.A.V.)

* Correspondence: jcsepulv@utp.edu.co (J.C.S.-A.)

**Abstract:** Antimicrobial resistance (AMR) poses a significant global health threat, necessitating the development of novel antibacterial strategies. Serratiopeptidase (SP), a metalloprotease produced by bacteria such as *Serratia marcescens*, has gained attention not only for its anti-inflammatory properties but also for its potential antibacterial activity. However, its protein nature makes it susceptible to pH changes and self-proteolysis, limiting its effectiveness. This study aimed to increase both the enzymatic stability and antibacterial activity of serratiopeptidase through immobilization on titanium oxide nanoparticles ($TiO_2$-NPs), leveraging the biocompatibility and stability of these nanomaterials. Commercial $TiO_2$-NPs were characterized using TGA/DTG, FT-IR, UV–Vis, and XRD analyses, and their biocompatibility was assessed through cytotoxicity studies. Serratiopeptidase was produced via fermentation using the C8 isolate of *Serratia marcescens* obtained from the intestine of *Bombyx mori* L., purified chromatographically, and immobilized on carboxylated nanoparticles via EDC/NHS coupling at various pH conditions. The optimal enzymatic activity was achieved by using pH 5.1 for nanoparticle activation and pH 5.5 for enzyme coupling. The resulting bioconjugate demonstrated stable proteolytic activity at 25 °C for 48 h. Immobilization was confirmed by FT-IR spectroscopy, and the Michaelis–Menten kinetics were determined. Notably, the bioconjugate exhibited two-fold greater antibacterial activity against *E. coli* than the free enzyme or $TiO_2$-NPs at 1000 μg/mL. This study successfully developed a serratiopeptidase–$TiO_2$ bioconjugate with enhanced enzymatic stability and antibacterial properties. The improved antibacterial activity of the immobilized enzyme presents a promising approach for developing new tools to combat antimicrobial resistance, with potential applications in healthcare, food safety, and environmental protection.

**Keywords:** serratiopeptidase; titanium oxide; nanoparticles; antibacterial agent; bioconjugate

## 1. Introduction

Antimicrobial resistance (AMR) has emerged as one of the most important global health challenges of the 21st century. The World Health Organization has declared AMR one of the top ten global public health threats facing humanity [1]. By 2050, AMR is estimated to cause 10 million deaths annually, resulting in a cumulative cost of up to USD 100 trillion to the global economy [2].

The rapid emergence of multidrug-resistant bacteria, coupled with a decline in the discovery of new antibiotics, has created an urgent need for innovative antibacterial strategies [3–5]. This crisis has prompted researchers to investigate alternative approaches, including the examination of proteolytic enzymes [6].

Serratiopeptidase (SP), also known as serralysin or serrapeptase, is a bacterial extracellular serine protease that has garnered attention for its anti-inflammatory and potential antimicrobial properties [7–9]. With a molecular weight of approximately 50 kDa and containing $Ca^{2+}$ and $Zn^{2+}$ cofactors [10], SP is produced by various bacteria, including *Serratia marcescens*.

SP encounters various obstacles, including its low solubility, sensitivity to changes in temperature and pH, and tendency to undergo self-cleavage, all of which may have a detrimental impact on its catalytic efficiency and therapeutic potential [11,12]. To address these limitations, enzyme immobilization has emerged as a promising strategy to increase stability under various physiological and environmental conditions [13].

Covalent binding is an immobilization method that provides several advantages, such as remarkable stability, preserved properties over time, and the possibility of enzyme recovery and reuse [14]. Notably, compared with alternative methods, immobilized enzyme-based antimicrobial agents have a lower tendency to induce resistance, as revealed by previous studies [15,16].

Titanium oxide nanoparticles ($TiO_2$-NPs) have gained significant interest as support structures for enzyme immobilization because of their biocompatibility, ease of fabrication, and large surface area [17]. However, $TiO_2$-NPs require functionalization, such as carboxylation, to enable covalent binding with enzymes [18]. The EDC/NHS (1-ethyl-3-(3-dimethylaminopropyl) carbodiimide and N-hydroxysuccinimide) coupling strategy has proven effective for immobilizing macromolecules, forming stable amide bonds between carboxyl and amino groups [19,20].

The objective of this study was to evaluate the stability of serratiopeptidase (SP) covalently bonded to carboxyl-modified $TiO_2$ nanoparticles. This approach was proposed to improve the antibacterial activity of the enzyme, which could lead to the development of new therapeutic strategies to combat antimicrobial resistance. The formation of bioconjugates is expected to pave the way for groundbreaking therapeutic solutions to address growing health issues.

## 2. Materials and Methods

### 2.1. Materials

The study materials were obtained from commercial providers. Titanium oxide nanoparticles (a mixture of rutile and anatase, nanopowder < 100 nm, product number 634,662, batch number MKCB9913), chloroacetic acid, casein from bovine milk (Bioreagent), and N-hydroxysuccinimide sodium (NHS, >97.0%) were purchased from Sigma-Aldrich (Sigma Chemical Co, Saint Louis, MO, USA). Hydroxylamine hydrochloride and 1-ethyl-3-(3-dimethylaminopropyl) carbodiimide hydrochloride (EDC) were acquired from Thermo Scientific (Thermo Fisher Scientific, Waltham, MA, USA).

### 2.2. $TiO_2$-NP Characterization

The stability of the nanoparticles was investigated using thermogravimetric analysis (TGA). The analysis was performed on an SDT-650 instrument under a nitrogen atmosphere. The temperature was increased from room temperature to 800 °C at a rate of 10 °C/min. To characterize the thermal decomposition process further, the first derivative curves of the mass percentage with respect to temperature (DTG) were calculated from the TGA data.

Fourier-transform infrared spectroscopy (FT-IR) was employed to identify functional groups via a Cary 630 FTIR instrument (Agilent Technologies Inc., Santa Clara, CA, USA) equipped with a diamond-tipped attenuated total reflectance (ATR) accessory. The spectra were acquired with a resolution of 4 $cm^{-1}$ in the range of 4000–400 $cm^{-1}$, and 32 scans were used for background correction. Additionally, UV–Visible spectroscopy was performed using a Thermo Scientific MULTISKAN GO spectrophotometer to analyze nanoparticle dispersions (1 mg/mL) in the wavelength range of 200–800 nm, utilizing a quartz cell. This analysis allowed for the determination of surface plasmons. The optical bandgap was estimated through the application of the Tauc plot method [21] (Table 1).

The crystal structure information of the samples was obtained using a CubiX PRO (X'Pert PRO) X-ray diffraction system (Malvern Panalytical Ltd, Almelo, The Netherlands) with Cu K$\alpha$ radiation ($\lambda$ = 1.5406 Å). Measurements were taken in the 2$\theta$ range of 2° to 90° with a scan step time of 17.15 s and a step size of 0.02°. The samples were analyzed with the X'Pert HighScore Plus software Version 5.1, and the crystallite size was calculated. Morphology and size were analyzed by transmission electron microscopy (TEM).

**Table 1.** Equations and constants for optical bandgap determination via Tauc plot analysis.

| | **Tauc Equation** $(\alpha \times h \times v)^{\gamma} = A \times (hv - Eg)$ | **Units** |
|---|---|---|
| A | Absorbance | a.u |
| $\alpha$ | Absorption coefficient $= 2.302 \times A$ | $cm^{-1}$ |
| h | Planck's constant $= 4.135 \times 10^{-15}$ | eV.s |
| c | Speed of light $= 3 \times 10^{8} m/s$ | m/s |
| v | Frequency $= \frac{c}{wavelength}$ | $s^{-1}$ |
| $\gamma$ | For direct electronic transitions, it takes a value of 2; for indirect transitions, it is 1/2. | a.u |
| Eg | *Band gap* | eV |

### 2.3. *Biocompatibility of $TiO_2$-NPs*

#### 2.3.1. Cell Culture

Adherent fibroblasts (HFF-1) obtained from the American Type Culture Collection (ATCC) were used. These cells were cultured in Dulbecco's modified Eagle's medium (DMEM) supplemented with 2.5 µg/mL amphotericin, 1% PSN (5 mg/mL penicillin, 5 mg/mL streptomycin, and 10 mg/mL neomycin), 1% 100 mM sodium pyruvate, and 10% heat-inactivated fetal bovine serum. The cells were maintained in an incubator at 37 °C and 5% $CO_2$.

#### 2.3.2. Preparation of $TiO_2$ Nanomaterial Suspensions

The initial suspensions of previously autoclave-sterilized nanoparticles were prepared in a supplemented DMEM containing glycerol (at a ratio of 1000 parts DMEM to 10 parts glycerol by volume) and stirred at 1500 rpm for 20 h. The concentration of the nanoparticles was prepared using serial dilutions (3000, 2500, 2000, 1500, 1000, 500, and 250 µg/mL).

#### 2.3.3. HFF-1 Cell Viability

In each well, 10,000 HFF-1 cells were added to the supplemented DMEM and incubated for 24 h under standard conditions. The nanoparticle suspensions were subsequently added for 48 h and 72 h. HFF-1 cells in DMEM supplemented with glycerol (1000:10) were used as the negative control, while 200 µL of doxorubicin at 25 µg/mL and 12.5 µg/mL served as positive controls for both 48 h and 72 h incubations. DMEM culture medium (200 µL) was used as the blank control, and titanium oxide nanoparticle suspensions without cells (200 µL) were used as sample blanks at different concentrations. After incubation, the medium was removed, and the cells were washed with 1× PBS. The cells were subsequently incubated with 200 µL of 0.5 mg/mL MTT solution for 4 h at 37 °C with 5% $CO_2$. Afterward, the supernatant was removed, and 100 µL of DMSO was added to dissolve the formazan crystals formed. The absorbance was measured at a wavelength of 570 nm with a reference wavelength correction at 630 nm via a Thermo Scientific MULTISKAN GO plate spectrophotometer.

### 2.4. *Production and Purification of Serratiopeptidase*

A strain of *Serratia marcescens* C8 isolated from the intestine of a Colombian silkworm hybrid was utilized for serratiopeptidase production. The bacterium was inoculated at a 0.5 McFarland scale. The culture medium consisted of casein (0.5% *w*/*v*), yeast extract

(0.1% $w/v$), soybean oil (0.3% $v/v$), $(NH_4)_2HPO_4$ (0.5% $w/v$), KCl (0.05% $w/v$), NaCl (0.1% $w/v$), $CaCl_2 \cdot 2H_2O$ (0.02% $w/v$), $MgSO_4 \cdot 7H_2O$ (0.02% $w/v$), and $ZnCl_2$ (0.01% $w/v$). Fermentation was carried out at 26 °C and 180 rpm for 36 h. After fermentation, the mixture was centrifuged at 4 °C and 15,500× $g$ for 30 min. The supernatant was filtered through 0.45 μm and 0.22 μm membranes and concentrated via a 10 kDa ultrafiltration membrane. The bacteria-free concentrate was subsequently purified via a weak anion exchange column (Bio-Scale Mini Macro-Prep DEAE, Bio-Rad, Hercules, CA, USA). The fraction exhibiting proteolytic activity was further concentrated using ultrafiltration at 10 kDa. Purification was finalized through molecular exclusion chromatography (ENrich SEC 70, Bio-Rad, Hercules, CA, USA) at a flow of 1 mL/min [10] and monitored at 280 nm. The pure serratiopeptidase fraction was identified via molecular weight analysis using SEC and SDS-PAGE. Additionally, proteolytic activity, protein concentration, and specific activity were determined. This purified enzyme (SP) was employed in immobilization assays.

### 2.5. Proteolytic Activity and Total Protein Assay

The proteolytic activity was assessed following the method reported by Vélez et al. [10]. Azocasein served as the substrate in 25 mM Tris-HCl buffer containing 1 mM $CaCl_2$ at pH 8.0. The reaction proceeded at 37 °C for 10 min, followed by inactivation with trichloroacetic acid and supernatant collection via centrifugation. An aliquot of the supernatant was mixed with sodium hydroxide, and the absorbance was measured at 440 nm. One unit of proteolytic activity (U) was defined as the amount of enzyme that catalyzed the release of one microgram of substrate per minute under standard pH and temperature conditions. The total protein concentration was determined using the Bradford commercial assay (Bio-Rad Protein Assay, Hercules, CA, USA).

### 2.6. Immobilization of the Serratiopeptidase Enzyme on Titanium Oxide Nanoparticles ($TiO_2$/SP)

The carboxylation of $TiO_2$-NPs followed the methodology reported by Rajaeian et al. with modifications [22]. In a stainless steel autoclave, 65 mg of $TiO_2$-NPs were combined with 10 mL of deionized water. The mixture was stirred for 30 min and then sonicated for another 30 min. Subsequently, 80 mg of chloroacetic acid was added, the mixture was stirred for 5 min, and the autoclave was sealed and heated in an oven at 100 °C for 7 h. After cooling, the $TiO_2$-NPs were filtered and washed with deionized water until a neutral pH was reached. Finally, the $TiO_2$-NPs were lyophilized for future applications.

For the activation of the nanoparticles, 1 mg of carboxylated $TiO_2$-NPs was weighed and resuspended in 250 μL of 100 mM phosphoric acid/monosodium phosphate at pH 2.6, or MES (2-(N-morpholino)ethanesulfonic acid) at pH 5.1, or sodium phosphate at pH 7.6. All buffers contained 500 mM NaCl. Subsequently, 50 μL of an EDC/NHS solution at a final concentration of 2 mM/5 mM was added, and the mixture was stirred for 2 h at room temperature. The reaction was quenched with 10 μL of β-mercaptoethanol. Ultrafiltration was then performed using a 3 kDa filter. The SP coupling was carried out one and two units above the enzyme's isoelectric point. The nanoparticles were washed three times with 25 mM MES buffer containing 1 mM $CaCl_2$ at pH 5.5 or 6.7. The $TiO_2$-NPs were mixed with 0.2 mg of SP in 800 μL of 25 mM MES buffer with 1 mM $CaCl_2$ and 500 mM NaCl at pH 5.5 and stirred at 4 °C for 12 h. The coupling process was repeated at pH 6.7. Finally, the reaction with hydroxylamine at a final concentration of 10 mM was carried out. Subsequently, ultrafiltration was performed using a 3 kDa filter. Afterward, the nanoparticles were washed three times with 25 mM Tris-HCl buffer containing 1 mM $CaCl_2$ at pH 8.0 and stored in 300 μL of buffer. This process yielded the bioconjugate ($TiO_2$/SP).

### 2.7. Characterization of the Bioconjugate $TiO_2$/SP

The secondary structure of both free and immobilized serratiopeptidase enzyme was analyzed via FT-IR with an ATR cell, covering the range from 4000 to 400 cm$^{-1}$, with 16 scans per sample. The amide I band (1700–1600 cm$^{-1}$) was isolated for structural analysis.

Baseline correction and band deconvolution of the amide I bands were subsequently performed for both enzyme forms [23,24].

The average particle size and zeta potential were measured using dynamic light scattering (DLS) (Malvern Instruments Ltd., Model ZSU3100). The samples were dispersed in distilled water at a concentration of 0.5% *w*/*v*. A 1 mL sample solution was placed in a cuvette and equilibrated at room temperature for 1 min. Measurements were taken for each sample group three times, with 16 scanning cycles per measurement.

The thermal stability of the bioconjugate ($TiO_2$/SP) was assessed at 4 °C, 25 °C, and 37 °C for 48 h at pH 7.4. Proteolytic activity was measured every 6 h and expressed as a percentage of the relative activity.

Michaelis-Menten parameters were determined by measuring the proteolytic activity of SP and $TiO_2$/SP using azocasein at different concentrations (0.04 mM to 2.11 mM). The enzymatic activity was evaluated under optimal conditions of pH 6 and 50 °C as previously determined by Vélez et al. [10]. The $K_m$ and $V_{max}$ values were obtained from Lineweaver-Burk plots.

### 2.8. Antibacterial Activity of the Bioconjugate $TiO_2$/SP

*Escherichia coli* strain NCTC 9001(ATCC, Manassas, VI, USA) was used to evaluate the antibacterial capacity of covalently immobilized serratiopeptidase on titanium oxide nanoparticles ($TiO_2$/SP), titanium oxide nanoparticles ($TiO_2$), and free serratiopeptidase (SP). The experiment included kanamycin (50 µg/mL) as a positive control and untreated *E. coli* as a negative control. The samples were incubated at 37 °C, and measurements were taken each hour at 600 nm for 24 h in a 96-well plate.

### 2.9. Statistical Analysis

The results are presented as the mean ± standard deviation from the tests. Each experiment was conducted in triplicate. Data analysis and graphical representation were carried out using OriginPro 9 and GraphPad Prism 7.0 software. To evaluate the significant differences in enzyme immobilization and antimicrobial activity, a one-way analysis of variance (ANOVA) was performed with Tukey's post hoc test. Differences were considered significant when $p < 0.05$.

## 3. Results and Discussion

### 3.1. Characterization of Titanium Oxide Nanoparticles ($TiO_2$-NPs)

Figure 1a shows the results of thermogravimetric analysis (TGA), and the first derivative of the TGA curve of the titanium oxide nanoparticles. This TGA curve illustrates the thermal behavior of titanium dioxide ($TiO_2$) nanoparticles over a temperature range of room temperature to 800 °C (solid black line). Two distinct mass losses were observed with respect to temperature (gray shaded boxes labeled 1 and 2).

The initial steep decline of 2.84% occurs between room temperature and approximately 150 °C. This is likely due to the evaporation of physisorbed water and volatile surface-bound species. A second, more gradual weight loss of 2.42% is observed between approximately 150 and 300 °C. This may be attributed to the desorption of chemisorbed water molecules or the decomposition of surface hydroxyl groups [25]. Above 300 °C, the weight loss rate decreases significantly, indicating increased thermal stability of the $TiO_2$ nanoparticles at elevated temperatures. According to some studies [26], alkaline hydrothermal synthesis in the presence of a titanium source promotes the formation of sodium titanium nanostructures. The thermogram obtained was similar to that reported by Ramanath Prabhu and colleagues when evaluating pure $TiO_2$ nanopowder [27].

The derivative thermogravimetric (DTG) curve (dashed blue line in Figure 1a) corroborates these observations, showing two distinct peaks corresponding to the primary weight loss events. The first peak, centered at approximately 100 °C, is sharper and more intense, whereas the second peak, occurring between 200 °C and 300 °C, is broader and less pronounced. The total weight loss at 800 °C was approximately 6.5%, suggesting relatively high purity of the $TiO_2$ nanoparticles with minimal organic contaminants or surface modifiers.

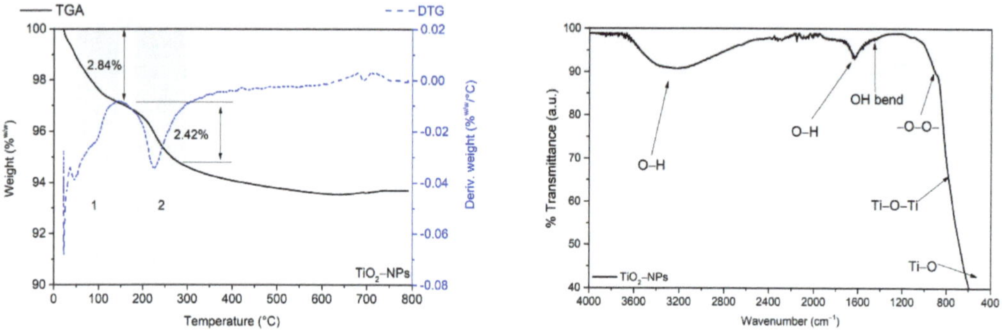


(a) (b)

**Figure 1.** (**a**) Thermogravimetric and derivative thermogravimetric analysis of the $TiO_2$ nanoparticles and (**b**) FT-IR spectrum of the $TiO_2$ nanoparticles in the ATR cell.

In the FT-IR spectrum of the $TiO_2$-NPs (Figure 1b), a vibrational band in the 3000–3750 $cm^{-1}$ region is observed, which is attributed to the stretching vibrations of both the O-H group bonds on the nanomaterial surface and the water present in the sample. Additionally, the presence of the -OH group can be confirmed by weak in-plane and out-of-plane bending absorptions at 1340 and 896 $cm^{-1}$, respectively. The O-H of water was confirmed from the band at 1632 $cm^{-1}$, corresponding to the scissoring bending vibration of water, indicating the presence of water molecules on the nanoparticle surface, either as extra or intramolecular moisture, as discussed in the TGA [28,29].

It has been reported that Ti–O and Ti–O–Ti vibrations are observed in the region from 1000 to 400 $cm^{-1}$. Specifically, a band near 460 $cm^{-1}$ is linked to the Ti-O bond in the anatase phase, whereas a band at 730 $cm^{-1}$ is associated with Ti-O-Ti vibrations. Furthermore, the band between 900 and 800 $cm^{-1}$ may be related to peroxo groups. This feature can account for the second mass loss observed in TGA, along with intramolecular water. Therefore, the presence of hydroxyl groups and metal-oxygen interactions suggest that the material corresponds to titanium oxide [30,31].

On the other hand, UV–Vis spectroscopic analysis and Tauc plot treatment provide valuable insights into the optical properties of titanium dioxide nanoparticles. The UV–Vis absorption spectrum (inset of Figure 2a) reveals a distinct absorption peak at 334 nm, which can be attributed to the surface plasmon resonance (SPR) of the $TiO_2$ nanoparticles. This finding aligns with several studies in the literature, which suggest that the UV absorption edge of titanium oxide nanoparticles is influenced by particle size [31–34]. Jiménez et al. demonstrated that titanium oxide nanoparticles (with an anatase structure) of 19 nm exhibited an absorption band at a wavelength of 357 nm, whereas microparticles of 1.60 μm had a band at 391 nm [33]. However, this SPR wavelength is redshifted compared with the previously reported value of 315 nm for titanium oxide [30]. This shift could be due to the presence of rutile, which generally has a lower bandgap or a higher absorption band than anatase does, as well as possible interactions between the two phases [35,36].

The main graph in Figure 2a shows the Tauc plot, which was derived from the UV–Vis data to determine the optical bandgap of the material. The x-axis represents the photon energy (eV), whereas the y-axis represents $(\alpha h\nu)^2$, where $\alpha$ is the absorption coefficient and $h\nu$ is the photon energy [21]. The linear extrapolation of the absorption edge to the x-axis yields a bandgap energy of 3.21 eV for the $TiO_2$ nanoparticles. This bandgap value of 3.21 eV is consistent with previous literature reports [30,37]. Additionally, on the basis of the Brus model equation [29,31,34], a particle size value of 2.60 nm was estimated via the determined bandgap value and the average bandgap values of bulk anatase and rutile (3.20 eV and 3.0 eV, respectively) [33,35,36,38], suggesting that the nanoparticles maintain the characteristic electronic structure of $TiO_2$.

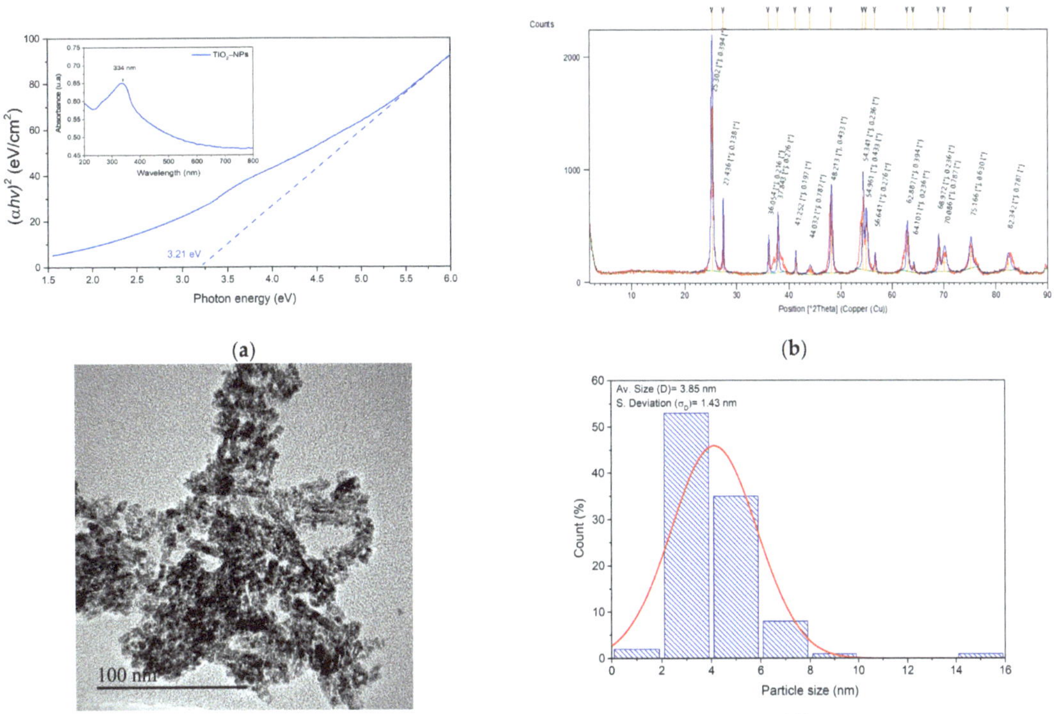


(**a**)

(**b**)

(**c**)

(**d**)

**Figure 2.** (**a**) Absorption spectrum in the UV–Vis range (inside the figure) and Tauc plot (outside the figure); (**b**) X-ray diffraction (XRD) pattern; (**c**) TEM (transmission electron microscopy) analysis; and (**d**) particle size distribution by TEM of titanium oxide nanoparticles.

Further analysis, such as X-ray diffraction (XRD), was used to correlate the observed optical properties with the crystalline structure of the $TiO_2$ nanoparticles. In Figure 2b (Table S1), the XRD pattern exhibits characteristic peaks corresponding to rutile (reference code: 96-900-7433) and anatase (reference code: 96-900-9087) $TiO_2$ structures. The presence of sharp, well-defined peaks indicates good crystallinity of the sample [34]. The analysis performed using the X'Pert HighScore Plus software yielded a crystallite size of 29.72 nm, suggesting nanocrystalline $TiO_2$ particles (Table S2) [29]. This nanoparticulate size is important because the material has a relatively large surface area [31], which is directly related to the amount of enzyme that can be immobilized. Additionally, the value obtained by UV–Vis spectroscopy is relatively small, which could serve as a basis for determining the crystallite size. Moreover, the phase identification scores of 86 for rutile and 79 for anatase indicate high confidence in the presence of both polymorphs, with rutile being slightly more dominant. The phase contents were obtained from the following formula [29]: $\%W_R = 1/(1 + 0.8(I_A/I_R)) \times 100$ and $\%W_A = (1 - W_R) \times 100$, where $W_R$ and $W_A$ represent the contents of rutile and anatase, respectively, and $I_A$ and $I_R$ denote the diffraction intensities of anatase (101) at 25.30° and rutile (110) at 27.43°, respectively. The phase content was found to be 30.70% rutile and 69.30% anatase. These XRD data, combined with the crystallite size and phase scores, suggest a well-crystallized, nanostructured $TiO_2$ material with a mixture of rutile and anatase phases.

On the other hand, transmission electron microscopy (TEM) analysis of $TiO_2$ particles (Figure 2c) reveals clusters of nanoparticles with irregular shapes and an average size of 3.85 nm ± 1.43 nm (Figure 2d), corresponding to the primary particle size. This observation is consistent with the product's lot specifications, which report a particle size distribution below 100 nm. However, the particles predominantly form aggregates or agglomerates. Leynen et al. reported a size of 21 nm by TEM for a mixture of anatase and rutile; however, they also observed that the particles were agglomerated on the EM grid [39]. A similar behavior was reported by Mohd for biosynthesized zinc oxide nanoparticles [40].

### 3.2. Biocompatibility of Titanium Oxide Nanoparticles

The cytotoxicity of titanium dioxide nanoparticles ($TiO_2$-NPs) was evaluated in HFF-1 cells (Figure 3). The results demonstrated that $TiO_2$-NPs exhibited minimal toxicity, with cell viability remaining above 80% across a concentration range of 250–2500 µg/mL at both 48 and 72 h of exposure. These findings are consistent with those of previous studies. Romoser et al. reported a low cytotoxicity of $TiO_2$-NPs (25 nm) in human dermal fibroblasts [41]. Feng et al. reported a decrease in viability of approximately 18% at a $TiO_2$-NP concentration of 200 µg/mL [42]. Another study reported an $IC_{50}$ value of 168.9 µg/mL for $TiO_2$-NPs in nontransformed normal human fibroblasts (GM07492). Interestingly, the same study reported no significant cytotoxic effects up to 100 µg/mL in A549 cancer cell lines after 24 h of exposure [43]. Our data indicated slightly lower cytotoxicity at comparable concentrations, which may be attributed to variations in cell type or nanoparticle characteristics. The observed cytotoxicity patterns could be related to time-dependent cellular internalization. Research has shown that NP accumulation, predominantly in the cytoplasm, can induce ultrastructural changes and rupture the cell membrane, leading to cell death. Longer exposure times typically result in increased internalization, consequently reducing cell viability or increasing cytotoxicity [44]. This finding aligns with the results obtained for the positive control, doxorubicin (DOXO), which showed significant time-dependent cytotoxicity in various cell lines [45].

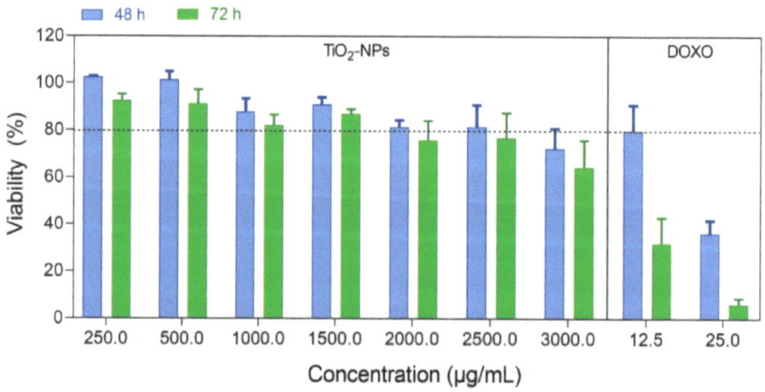


**Figure 3.** Effect of $TiO_2$ nanoparticles on the viability of HFF-1 human fibroblasts after 48 h and 72 h of exposure. The dashed line indicates the level of 80% viability.

Generally, as the concentration of nanoparticles increases, their cytotoxicity tends to increase due to their greater surface area, which promotes better interactions between the nanomaterial and cells. This relationship between concentration and cytotoxicity has been well documented in previous studies [46]. The biocompatibility demonstrated by these nanoparticles, as evidenced by their low cytotoxicity, suggests their potential for various biomedical applications. By using these nanomaterials to improve the properties of serratiopeptidase, we aim to develop more effective and stable therapeutic agents. This approach of using biocompatible nanoparticles to enhance enzyme properties represents a promising direction in nanomedicine, potentially leading to improved treatments and diagnostic tools.

### 3.3. Production and Purification of Serratiopeptidase (SP)

The production kinetics of serratiopeptidase (SP) from the *Serratia marcescens* C8 isolate demonstrated a typical growth-associated pattern of enzyme production (Figure 4a). The graph illustrates a lag phase in the first 10 h, followed by a rapid increase in proteolytic activity, reaching its peak at approximately 36 h of fermentation. The maximum SP production, quantified at 2540 U/mL proteolytic activity, was achieved under optimal conditions of 36 h fermentation time, pH 7, and a temperature of 26 °C. These parameters align well with previously reported conditions for *Serratia marcescens* fermentation, suggesting that the C8 isolate behaves similarly to other strains of this species in terms of SP production [10,47–50]. After peak production was reached at 36 h, a gradual decline in proteolytic activity was observed. This decrease could be attributed to various factors, such as nutrient depletion, accumulation of metabolic byproducts, or potential proteolytic degradation of the enzyme itself [51,52]. The shape of the production curve suggests that optimization of fermentation time is crucial for maximizing the SP yield. Extended fermentation beyond the 36 h mark may not be beneficial and could lead to reduced enzyme activity or increased production costs without corresponding increases in yield.

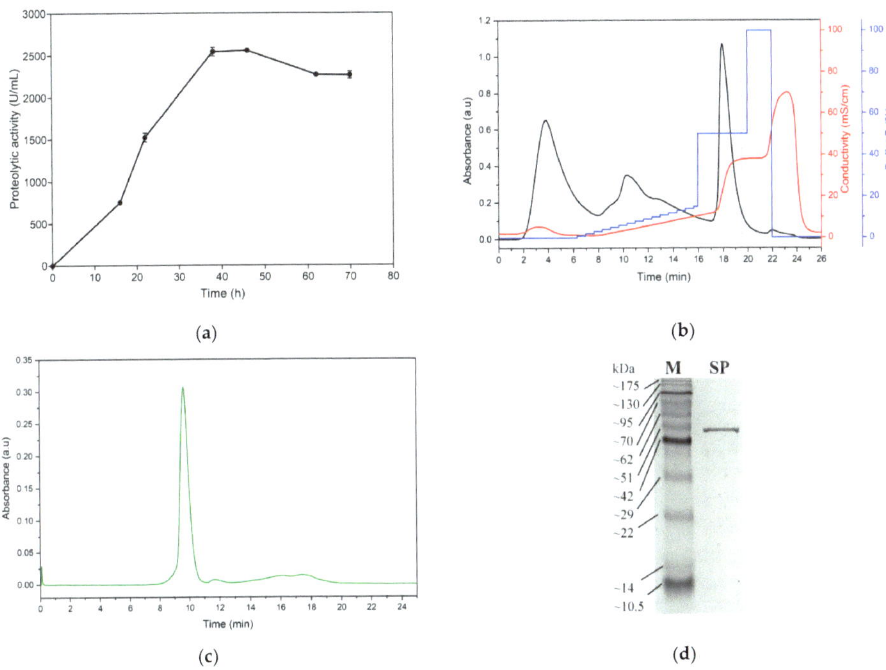


**Figure 4.** (**a**) Production kinetics of serratiopeptidase (SP) from the *Serratia marcescens* C8 isolate; enzyme purification; (**b**) chromatographic profile of weak anion exchange for the ultrafiltered supernatant from fermentation with *Serratia marcescens* (buffer B: 25 mM Tris-HCl + 1 mM $CaCl_2$, pH 8.0); (**c**) size exclusion chromatography (SEC) profile of the active fraction from weak anion exchange; and (**d**) SDS-PAGE gel. M: molecular weight marker; SP: serratiopeptidase.

The chromatographic profile of weak anion exchange for the ultrafiltered supernatant revealed an efficient purification process for SP (Figure 4b). The chromatogram displays multiple peaks, indicating the separation of different protein components. The peak of interest, enclosed in the gray box, represents the proteolytically active fraction, which eluted at 17.93 min. This peak coincides with a significant increase in conductivity, ranging from 12.90 to 37.4 mS/cm, indicating the elution of SP in response to the applied salt gradient. The elution of SP at this specific point suggests that the enzyme has a net negative charge at pH 8.0, allowing its interaction with the weak anion exchange resin. The use of a buffer containing 1 M sodium chloride at pH 8.0 for elution is consistent with typical conditions for serratiopeptidase purification reported in the literature [10]. Ultrafiltration with a 10 kDa cut-off prior to chromatography is particularly relevant, as SP has a reported molecular weight of approximately 45–60 kDa. This step not only concentrated the enzyme but also effectively removed low-molecular-weight impurities and salts, thereby increasing the efficacy of the subsequent chromatographic separation [53,54]. The combination of ultrafiltration and weak anion exchange chromatography has proven to be an effective approach for SP purification. The active fraction was concentrated by ultrafiltration and evaluated using size-exclusion chromatography (SEC) at 1 mL/min (Figure 4c). The fraction obtained by SEC (gray box) was used for immobilization assays. The sharp, symmetrical shape of the SP elution peak indicates good resolution and separation from other proteins, suggesting a high degree of purity for the obtained enzyme. The purified enzyme exhibited a specific activity of 31,873.76 ± 2240.81 U/mg, a relative molecular mass of 50.35 ± 0.11 kDa determined by SDS-PAGE (Figure 4d), and 51.35 ± 0.67 kDa determined by SEC (Figure S1). These results are comparable to those reported by Koul et al., who reported a value of 51.3 kDa for serratiopeptidase produced from *S. marcescens* MES-4, with a specific activity of 13,030 U/mg [51]. Additionally, Doshi et al. reported an approximate molecular weight of 50 kDa for recombinant serratiopeptidase, with a specific activity of 8382 U/mg [55]. The purification method demonstrates good resolution and selectivity, as evidenced by the distinct peak in the chromatogram, suggesting its potential for achieving high-purity SP preparations suitable for immobilization on titanium oxide nanoparticles.

### 3.4. Immobilization of the Serratiopeptidase Enzyme on Titanium Oxide Nanoparticles ($TiO_2$/SP)

Figure 5 illustrates the step-by-step process of serratiopeptidase (SP) immobilization on titanium oxide nanoparticles via the EDC/NHS strategy. This method involves three main stages: carboxylation, activation, and coupling. The process begins with the modification of the $TiO_2$-NP surface. Chloroacetic acid is used to introduce carboxyl groups onto the nanoparticle surface. The carboxylated $TiO_2$-NPs are then activated via the combination of 1-ethyl-3-(3-dimethylaminopropyl)carbodiimide (EDC) and N-hydroxysuccinimide (NHS). EDC acts as a coupling agent that activates the carboxyl groups, whereas NHS creates a stable reactive intermediate. In the final step, SP is introduced to the activated nanoparticles. The amine groups of SP react with the activated carboxyl groups on the nanoparticle surface, forming stable amide bonds. This results in the covalent immobilization of SP onto the $TiO_2$-NPs ($TiO_2$/SP). The use of EDC/NHS chemistry for protein immobilization is well established because of its efficiency and the stability of the resulting covalent bonds [30,31].

The carboxylation of $TiO_2$-NPs and the pH-dependent activity of immobilized serratiopeptidase (SP) were investigated, as shown in Figure 6. The ATR FT-IR spectrum (Figure 6a) confirmed the successful carboxylation of the $TiO_2$-NPs. Pure $TiO_2$-NPs exhibit a band at 3250 $cm^{-1}$, attributed to -OH stretching vibrations of adsorbed water, corroborated by a band at 1636 $cm^{-1}$ due to O-H bending (Figure 1b) [30].

In contrast, carboxylated nanoparticles show distinctive stretching vibrations at ~1636 $cm^{-1}$ and 1370 $cm^{-1}$, which are associated with C=O and C-O bonds, respectively, indicating successful carboxylation. The increase in the intensity of the hydroxyl group bands in the carboxylated material is consistent with the presence of carboxylic acids. A faint band at 2930 $cm^{-1}$, likely due to C–H bond vibrations from chloroacetic acid residues, and a band at ~1093 $cm^{-1}$, attributed to Ti–O–C bond bending vibrations, further confirm the carboxylation process [22,53].

The pH-dependent specific activity of the SPs immobilized on the carboxylated $TiO_2$-NPs is illustrated in Figure 6b. This graph shows the effects of activation (A) and coupling (C) buffer pH on the specific activity of the enzyme. The highest specific activity (2698 ± 147.07 U/mg NP · mg immobilized protein) was achieved with an activation buffer pH of 5.1 and a coupling buffer pH of 5.5. Notably, SP immobilization was successful across various pH combinations, demonstrating the versatility of the method. The Shapiro–Wilk test revealed a normal distribution of the data, with a $p$-value of 0.4757. The one-way ANOVA analysis yielded an F-value of 16.28 and a $p$-value of 0.0020 (less than 0.05), suggesting statistically significant variations in the specific activity of immobilized serratiopeptidase across different pH groups. Tukey's multiple comparison test results (Figure 6b) showed no significant differences within the pH 5.5 groups for coupling or within the pH 6.7 group. However, a notable difference was observed between the coupling pH of 5.5 and 6.7, particularly with A-5.1/C.5.5 ($p$-value $\leq$ 0.01). These findings indicate that pH is a crucial factor influencing the proteolytic activity of immobilized serratiopeptidase. The optimal pH range (5.1–5.5) aligns closely with the reported isoelectric point of SP, suggesting that this pH range facilitates effective coupling while preserving enzymatic activity [56]. Both the activation and coupling buffer pH significantly impact the resulting specific activity, highlighting the importance of pH optimization in the immobilization process. The optimal pH range (4.5–7.5) for EDC/NHS activation aligns with previous reports, validating the experimental approach [57–59]. These findings indicate that pH plays a crucial role in both the activation of carboxylated nanoparticles and their subsequent coupling with SP. The optimal conditions likely strike a balance between effective EDC/NHS chemistry and favorable enzyme conformation. This pH range, which is close to the isoelectric point of SP [10,60], minimizes electrostatic repulsion, potentially facilitating more efficient coupling [61]. In conclusion, this study provides valuable insights for optimizing the immobilization of SP on $TiO_2$-NPs. The successful carboxylation of $TiO_2$-NPs and identification of the optimal pH conditions for enzyme immobilization have contributed to the development of enhanced biocatalytic systems.

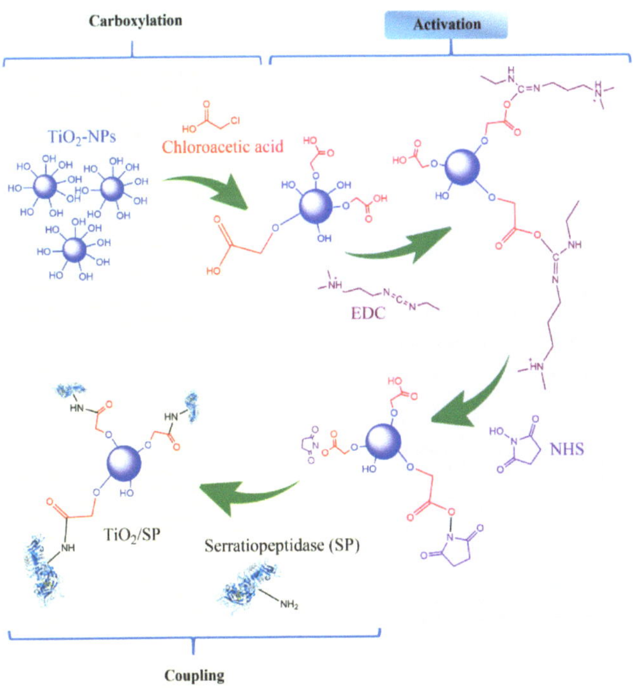


**Figure 5.** Scheme of SP immobilization reactions on carboxylated $TiO_2$-NPs via the EDC/NHS strategy.

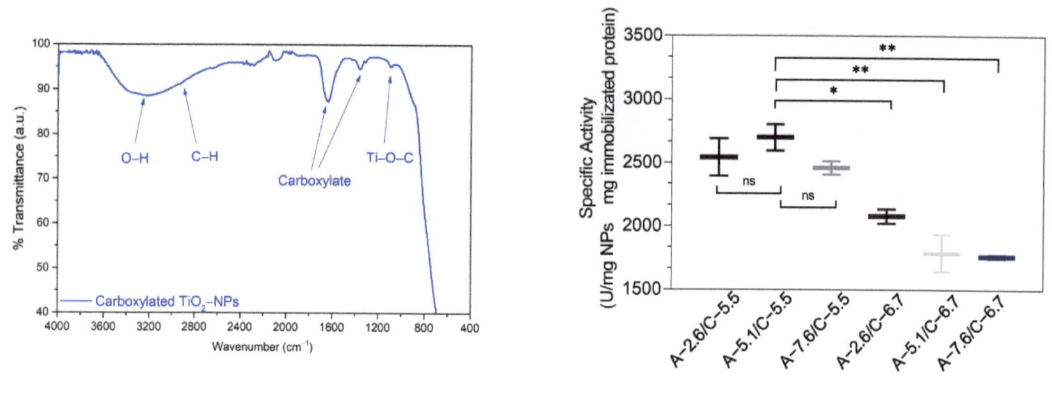


(a) (b)

**Figure 6.** (**a**) FT-IR spectrum of carboxylated $TiO_2$ nanoparticles in the ATR cell and (**b**) pH-dependent specific activity of serratiopeptidase immobilized on carboxylated $TiO_2$ nanoparticles: effects of activation (A) and coupling (C) buffer pH. ns: not significant, * $p \leq 0.05$, ** $p \leq 0.01$.

### 3.5. Characterization of $TiO_2$/SP

To elucidate the decrease in proteolytic activity during immobilization, an analysis of the secondary structure of the SP enzyme was conducted via Fourier-transform infrared spectroscopy (FT-IR) with an ATR cell. Spectra were recorded from 4000 to 400 $cm^{-1}$, with 16 scans per sample. The amide I band (1700–1600 $cm^{-1}$) was extracted for structural analysis, followed by baseline correction and deconvolution of the constituent bands [23].

Figure 7a presents the FT-IR spectra of free SP and the bioconjugate ($TiO_2$/SP) recorded in the ATR cell, confirming successful SP immobilization. The spectra exhibit characteristic bands corresponding to C=O, C-N, and N-H stretching and bending vibrations, specifically amide I, amide II, and amide III, for both the nanoparticles and bioconjugate. Vibrations of the N–H and O–H bonds were observed at 3400–3050 $cm^{-1}$, indicating the presence of immobilized SP on the nanostructured support. These findings align with those reported by Kumar et al., who observed similar bands at 3400 $cm^{-1}$ and in the range of 1648 $cm^{-1}$–1545 $cm^{-1}$ when performing immobilization through amino functionalization [62]. Additionally, studies on lipases immobilized on carboxylated $Fe_3O_4$ nanoparticles have reported comparable bands in their FT-IR spectra [63,64].

Figure 7b,c illustrate the changes in the secondary structure of SP upon immobilization on titanium oxide nanoparticles activated with EDC/NHS. The deconvoluted amide I bands reveal shifts in the proportions of different secondary structural elements, suggesting conformational changes in the enzyme upon immobilization (Figure 7d). The most notable alterations included a substantial decrease in the α-helical content (from 42.45% to 18.33%) and a marked increase in the β-turn content (from 11.46% to 27.45%). Interestingly, both parallel and antiparallel β-sheet structures remained relatively unchanged, whereas nonorganized regions presented a moderate increase (from 9.75% to 17.75%). These structural modifications suggest a complex reorganization of the enzyme upon immobilization, potentially affecting its catalytic properties [65].

However, some degree of structural change is often inevitable during immobilization, and the retained activity may still be sufficient [66]. The significant loss of the α-helical structure may compromise the enzyme's active site geometry and substrate binding capability, likely leading to decreased proteolytic activity [67]. Conversely, the increase in β-turns could contribute to a more rigid overall structure, possibly enhancing the stability against denaturation [68]. The unexpected increase in nonorganized regions hints at partial unfolding or increased flexibility in certain areas, which may have mixed effects on enzyme function and stability. Despite these changes, the preservation of β-sheet content indicates that some core structural elements remain intact, potentially allowing the enzyme to retain a degree of its native functionality [67]. These structural alterations collectively suggest a trade-off between the catalytic activity and stability of the immobilized enzyme, warranting further investigation into its kinetic parameters and long-term stability under various conditions.

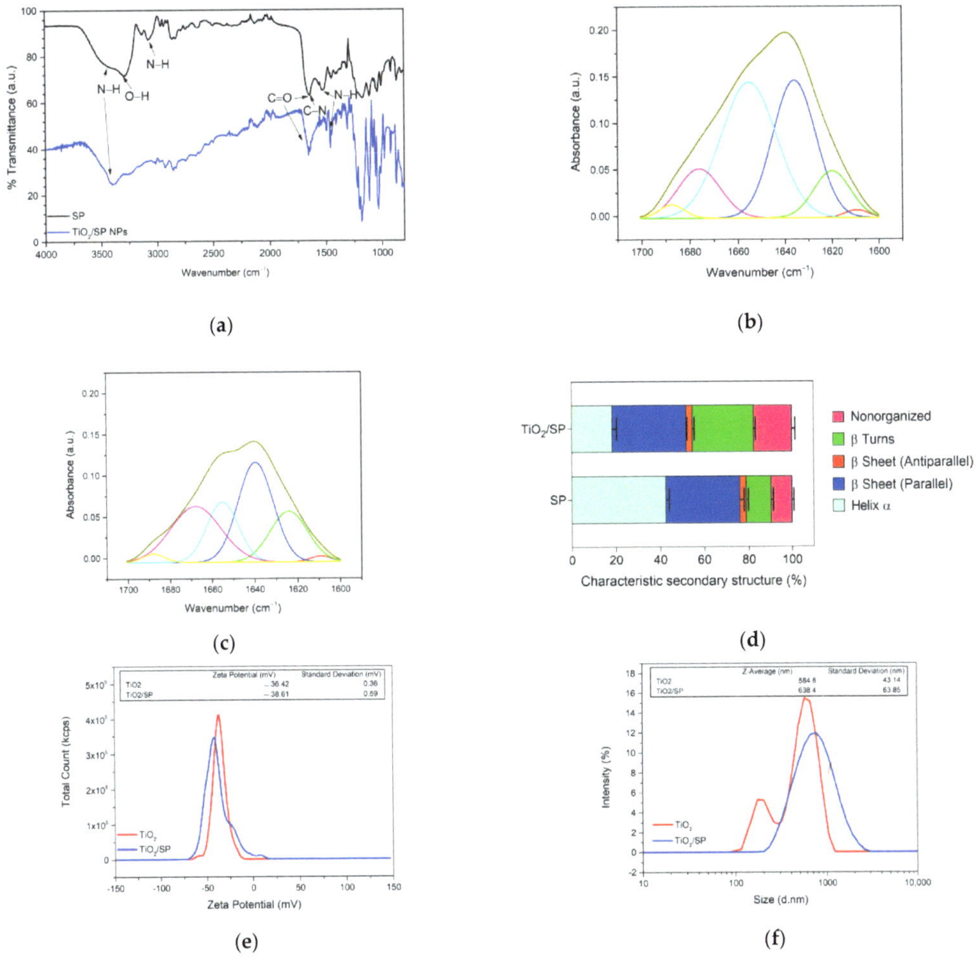


**Figure 7.** Structural analysis of serratiopeptidase and $TiO_2$/SP bioconjugate: (**a**) FT-IR spectra; amide I deconvolution of (**b**) serratiopeptidase and (**c**) bioconjugate; the colors of the lines in subfigures (**b**,**c**) represent the secondary structure; (**d**) secondary structure comparison; (**e**) zeta potential; and (**f**) DLS of $TiO_2$ and $TiO_2$/SP bioconjugate.

The titanium dioxide nanoparticles exhibit a zeta potential of $-36.42 \pm 0.36$ mV, as shown in Figure 7e. This value suggests that the material is moderately stable in aqueous solution [69], and the negative charge indicates that the nanoparticles are at a pH above the isoelectric point [70], meaning the surface carries a net negative charge. This property is critical for drug delivery, as the cell surface is negatively charged due to the presence of numerous anions, allowing positively charged particles to be rapidly taken up, potentially causing severe side effects and toxicity [71]. Therefore, nanoparticles with a negative surface charge could offer controlled adsorption. However, the size range obtained from dynamic light scattering measurements of the nanoparticles (Figure 7f) differs from that determined by TEM. This difference arises because TEM measures the primary particle size, whereas DLS quantifies the hydrodynamic diameter. This phenomenon has been observed in both titanium dioxide and zinc oxide nanoparticles, where the hydrodynamic size is consistently larger than the size measured by TEM [39,40,70,72,73]. As a result, in solution, the particles tend to form aggregates, leading to an increase in the hydrodynamic size of the titanium dioxide nanoparticles.

The zeta potential curve for $TiO_2$/SP is slightly broader than that of $TiO_2$ (Figure 7e), which may indicate greater variability in surface charge, possibly due to non-uniform functionalization and the presence of the enzyme. Additionally, since the immobilization was performed at pH 5.5, both the serratiopeptidase enzyme and the nanoparticles are above their isoelectric points [10]. Therefore, the surface charge of the bioconjugate is expected to be negative, as confirmed by the zeta potential measurement, which shifts from −36.42 mV for $TiO_2$ to −38.61 mV for $TiO_2$/SP. This change suggests a surface modification of the nanoparticles, consistent with enzyme immobilization. Moreover, the immobilization is further supported by the increase in the bioconjugate's hydrodynamic size compared to $TiO_2$ (Figure 7f). However, the DLS curve for the bioconjugate exhibits greater variability in size distribution, as reflected by a larger standard deviation. This increase in hydrodynamic size has also been observed during the immobilization of bovine serum albumin on ZnO via EDC/NHS coupling chemistry [72].

Thermostability assessments at 37 °C (Figure 8a) demonstrated a significant increase in enzyme stability upon immobilization. After 12 h, free SP lost 38.23% ± 0.14% of its activity, whereas $TiO_2$/SP maintained 101.66% ± 7.04% of its initial activity. This trend persisted over 48 h, with $TiO_2$/SP losing only 36.39% of its activity compared with 60.69% for free SP. The improved thermostability aligns with the observed increase in β-turns, which likely contributes to a more rigid and stable enzyme conformation. Moreover, the loss of proteolytic activity is a natural process when the enzyme is at work temperature [48,74,75].

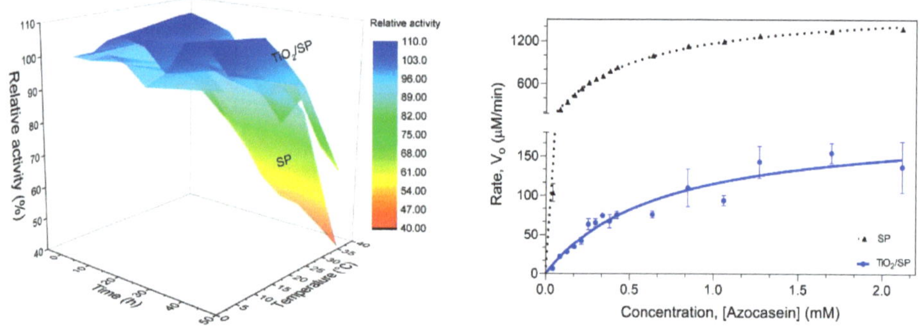


(a) (b)

**Figure 8.** (**a**) Thermostability assessment of SP and $TiO_2$/SP at various temperatures and (**b**) Michaelis-Menten kinetics of free and immobilized serratiopeptidases on titanium oxide supports.

Michaelis-Menten kinetic analysis (Figure 8b) revealed interesting changes in enzyme behavior upon immobilization. The $K_m$ value increased slightly from 0.4727 mM (free SP) to 0.6812 mM ($TiO_2$/SP), suggesting a minor reduction in substrate affinity. More notably, the $V_{max}$ decreased dramatically from 1723 µM/min (free SP) to 193.7 µM/min ($TiO_2$/SP), indicating a significant reduction in the enzyme's maximum catalytic rate when immobilized. The observed kinetic changes correlate with the structural modifications. The substantial decrease in $V_{max}$, coupled with the slight increase in $K_m$, aligns with the significant loss of α-helical content observed in the structural analysis. This conformational change likely impacts the active site geometry, reducing the catalytic efficiency [76]. The increase in β-turns and nonorganized regions may create a more compact structure that, while stabilizing the enzyme, could hinder substrate access to the active site, explaining the reduced $V_{max}$. These findings collectively suggest a trade-off between enhanced stability and reduced catalytic activity upon immobilization of serratiopeptidase on $TiO_2$ nanoparticles. Structural rigidification improves the thermal resistance but constrains the conformational flexibility necessary for optimal catalysis. Despite the lower catalytic efficiency, the significantly improved stability of $TiO_2$/SP suggests potential advantages for long-term applications, such as antimicrobial activity.

*E. coli* bacteria were used to determine the minimum inhibitory concentration of the serratiopeptidase covalently immobilized on titanium oxide nanoparticles ($TiO_2$/SP), titanium oxide nanoparticles ($TiO_2$), and free serratiopeptidase. The incubation was carried out at 37 °C, and measurements were taken every hour at 600 nm for 24 h. As shown in Figure 9a–c, at concentrations of 1000 µg/mL, 500 µg/mL, and 250 µg/mL, the immobilized enzyme and the titanium oxide nanoparticles inhibited bacterial growth. This can be attributed to the antimicrobial properties of the titanium oxide nanoparticles [77]. To assess the behavior of the $TiO_2$/SP bioconjugate at 1000 µg/mL concentration across 6, 12, and 24 h intervals, an ANOVA was performed. The findings revealed that the $TiO_2$/SP bioconjugate displayed a statistically significant difference ($p < 0.0001$) when compared to the unmodified SP and $TiO_2$ systems. Comparable outcomes were noted at 12 and 24 h, with the $TiO_2$/SP bioconjugate showing a significant difference with $TiO_2$ ($p < 0.01$). Furthermore, after 24 h, the $TiO_2$/SP bioconjugate exhibited a significant difference ($p < 0.0004$) compared to the negative control, an effect not observed with free SP and $TiO_2$. In particular, a greater effect was observed with the immobilized serratiopeptidase than with the nanoparticles alone. These findings demonstrate the potential of serratiopeptidase immobilized on titanium oxide nanoparticles as an antibacterial agent against *E. coli*.

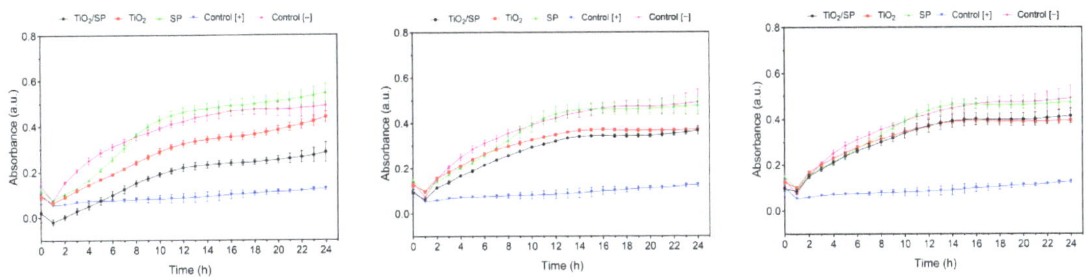


(a) (b) (c)

**Figure 9.** Determination of the minimum inhibitory concentration (MIC) against *E. coli* at 37 °C, measured at 600 nm, for $TiO_2$/SP bioconjugates, $TiO_2$ nanoparticles, serratiopeptidase (SP), kanamycin (positive control, 32 µg/mL), and no treatment (negative control) at concentrations of (**a**) 1000 µg/mL, (**b**) 500 µg/mL, and (**c**) 250 µg/mL.

Additionally, the minimum inhibitory concentration (50%) for $TiO_2$/SP was 857.8 µg/mL. This was determined via the logarithm of the concentrations versus the maximum absorbance obtained at 24 h, which was normalized with respect to the controls.

The bioconjugation process alters the enzyme structure and catalytic properties but also results in significant antibacterial activity. Figure 9a–c show the minimum inhibitory concentration (MIC) for *E. coli* at 37 °C, which was measured at 600 nm over 24 h. At concentrations of 1000 µg/mL, 500 µg/mL, and 250 µg/mL, both $TiO_2$/SP and $TiO_2$ nanoparticles inhibited *E. coli* growth, with $TiO_2$/SP exhibiting a more pronounced effect ($p$-value < 0.0001). The enhanced antibacterial efficacy of $TiO_2$/SP over both free SP and $TiO_2$ nanoparticles suggests a synergistic action resulting from the immobilization process. This synergy may arise from the structural changes observed in the enzyme upon immobilization, combined with the intrinsic antimicrobial properties of the $TiO_2$ nanoparticles. Quantitative analysis revealed that the minimum inhibitory concentration ($MIC_{50}$) for $TiO_2$/SP against *E. coli* was 857.8 μg/mL, as determined by plotting the logarithm of concentrations against the maximum absorbance at 24 h, normalized to controls. These findings complement our earlier observations on the structural and kinetic changes in SP upon immobilization. While the catalytic efficiency ($V_{max}$) of the enzyme decreased after immobilization, the bioconjugate exhibited enhanced thermostability and significant antibacterial activity. This multifaceted improvement in enzyme properties illustrates the potential of enzyme immobilization techniques in the development of advanced biomaterials.

Purnima et al. demonstrated that levofloxacin, when combined with serratiopeptidase, has synergistic antimicrobial and anti-biofilm activities [78]. Previous studies have shown that immobilizing serratiopeptidase on magnetite nanoparticles enhances drug permeation through membranes in vitro and significantly improves the anti-inflammatory response in carrageenan-induced paw edema in rats, even at much lower doses compared to free enzyme treatments [62]. Additionally, serratiopeptidase immobilized on cellulose nanofibers using the polyethyleneimine method demonstrated a higher inhibition of biofilm formation against *P. aeruginosa* and *S. aureus* [79]. This suggests that immobilization not only increases proteolytic activity but also enhances anti-biofilm properties. Similarly, Hanieh et al. reported that encapsulating serratiopeptidase within hyaluronic acid–lysine nanogels improves its stability under varying environmental conditions and increases enzymatic efficiency [80]. In this context, the improved antibacterial activity of the $TiO_2$/SP bioconjugate observed in our study may result from the accumulation of the bioconjugate on bacterial cell surfaces, which prolongs enzyme–bacteria interactions and disrupts protein synthesis critical for bacterial invasion [80–82]. Furthermore, the inherent antibacterial properties of titanium oxide have been demonstrated in pathogenic *Escherichia coli* strains isolated from clinical samples, supporting the potential dual action of the $TiO_2$/SP bioconjugate [83]. The enhanced ability of $TiO_2$/SP to inhibit bacterial growth highlights the importance of enzyme modification for the development of innovative antimicrobial therapies.

The antibacterial properties of $TiO_2$/SP, combined with its improved thermal stability, open new possibilities for applications in various fields. Potential areas of application include biomedical devices, where the bioconjugate could create self-sterilizing surfaces on medical implants or instruments; water treatment systems, leveraging its ability to inhibit *E. coli* growth; food packaging [84], where its antibacterial nature could extend food shelf-life; and wound healing [85], where the combination of proteolytic activity and antibacterial properties could aid in both wound debridement and infection prevention.

## 4. Conclusions

This study demonstrated the successful enhancement of serratiopeptidase (SP) through its immobilization on biocompatible titanium oxide nanoparticles ($TiO_2$-NPs), aligning with our aim to develop a more stable and effective therapeutic agent. The purification of SP from *Serratia marcescens* and its subsequent covalent immobilization on carboxylated $TiO_2$-NPs via the EDC/NHS strategy resulted in a bioconjugate ($TiO_2$/SP) with significantly improved properties. The $TiO_2$/SP bioconjugate exhibited remarkable thermal stability, retaining 63.61% of its initial activity after 48 h at 37 °C, whereas only 39.31% of the free enzyme was stable. This enhanced stability, confirmed through FT-IR analysis and kinetic studies, suggests a longer shelf-life and improved cost-effectiveness for potential large-scale production. Notably, the immobilized enzyme demonstrated significant antibacterial activity against *Escherichia coli*, surpassing the effects of both free SP and $TiO_2$-NPs alone. The synergistic effect of the antibacterial properties, coupled with the biocompatibility and low toxicity of $TiO_2$-NPs, presents new opportunities for biomedical applications. Although a reduction in catalytic efficiency was observed, the gains in stability and antibacterial properties presented a favorable trade-off, highlighting the multifunctional nature of the bioconjugate. The structural changes induced by immobilization, particularly the α-helical content and β-turns, provide insights into the mechanism underlying these enhanced properties. This study underscores the potential of enzyme immobilization strategies for creating advanced biomaterials with diverse functionalities. The use of biocompatible $TiO_2$-NPs as a support not only enhances the stability and bacterial efficacy of SP but also ensures its potential for safe therapeutic use.

**Supplementary Materials:** The following supporting information can be downloaded at https://www.mdpi.com/article/10.3390/jfb15100300/s1, Figure S1: Calibration curve for determination of relative molecular mass by SEC. As standards, conalbumin, chicken ovalbumin, soybean trypsin inhibitor, and equine myoglobin were used; Table S1: XRD data peak list for $TiO_2$; Table S2: Calculated crystallite sizes of titanium oxide nanoparticles via the Scherrer calculator in X'Pert HighScore Plus software (mean crystallite size: 29.72 nm).

**Author Contributions:** Conceptualization, J.J.M.-M., J.C.S.-A., A.Z.-V., S.V.-G., L.M.O. and L.A.V.; methodology, J.J.M.-M., J.C.S.-A., A.Z.-V. and L.A.V.; validation, J.J.M.-M., A.Z.-V. and S.V.-G.; formal analysis, J.J.M.-M., J.C.S.-A., A.Z.-V., L.M.O. and L.A.V.; investigation, J.J.M.-M. and S.V.-G.; resources, L.A.V., J.C.S.-A., L.M.O. and A.Z.-V.; data curation, L.A.V., J.C.S.-A. and A.Z.-V.; writing—original draft preparation, J.J.M.-M., A.Z.-V., S.V.-G. and L.M.O.; writing—review and editing, J.C.S.-A. and L.A.V.; visualization, J.J.M.-M., A.Z.-V., S.V.-G. and L.A.V.; supervision, J.C.S.-A. and L.A.V.; project administration, J.C.S.-A. and L.A.V.; funding acquisition, J.C.S.-A. and L.A.V. All authors have read and agreed to the published version of the manuscript.

**Funding:** This study was funded by Universidad Tecnológica de Pereira (grants 5-20-5, 5-23-1, and JI5—21-3) and Minciencias (grant 111084468129, contract 391–2020). J.J.M.-M. acknowledges Minciencias (909–2021) for a PhD student assistantship.

**Data Availability Statement:** The original contributions presented in this study are included in the article/Supplementary Materials. Further inquiries can be directed to the corresponding author.

**Acknowledgments:** The authors express their gratitude to Enrique Aguilar for providing the silkworm.

**Conflicts of Interest:** The authors declare that they have no conflicts of interest. The funders had no role in the design of this study; in the collection, analyses, or interpretation of the data; in the writing of the manuscript; or in the decision to publish the results.

## References

1. Murray, C.J.; Ikuta, K.S.; Sharara, F.; Swetschinski, L.; Robles Aguilar, G.; Gray, A.; Han, C.; Bisignano, C.; Rao, P.; Wool, E.; et al. Global Burden of Bacterial Antimicrobial Resistance in 2019: A Systematic Analysis. *Lancet* **2022**, *399*, 629–655. [CrossRef] [PubMed]
2. Thompson, K. *Vaccines Could Avert Half a Million Deaths Associated with Anti-Microbial Resistance a Year*; WHO: Geneva, Switzerland, 2023.
3. Chinemerem Nwobodo, D.; Ugwu, M.C.; Oliseloke Anie, C.; Al-Ouqaili, M.T.S.; Chinedu Ikem, J.; Victor Chigozie, U.; Saki, M. Antibiotic Resistance: The Challenges and Some Emerging Strategies for Tackling a Global Menace. *J. Clin. Lab. Anal.* **2022**, *36*, e24655. [CrossRef] [PubMed]
4. Iskandar, K.; Murugaiyan, J.; Halat, D.H.; El Hage, S.; Chibabhai, V.; Adukkadukkam, S.; Roques, C.; Molinier, L.; Salameh, P.; Van Dongen, M. Antibiotic Discovery and Resistance: The Chase and the Race. *Antibiotics* **2022**, *11*, 182. [CrossRef] [PubMed]
5. Muteeb, G.; Rehman, M.T.; Shahwan, M.; Aatif, M. Origin of Antibiotics and Antibiotic Resistance, and Their Impacts on Drug Development: A Narrative Review. *Pharmaceuticals* **2023**, *16*, 1615. [CrossRef] [PubMed]
6. Tonoyan, L.; Montagner, D.; Friel, R.; O'Flaherty, V. Antimicrobials Offered from Nature: Peroxidase-Catalyzed Systems and Their Mimics. *Biochem. Pharmacol.* **2020**, *182*, 114281. [CrossRef]
7. Nair, S.R.; C, S.D. Serratiopeptidase: An Integrated View of Multifaceted Therapeutic Enzyme. *Biomolecules* **2022**, *12*, 1468. [CrossRef]
8. Sharma, C.; Jha, N.K.; Meeran, M.F.N.; Patil, C.R.; Goyal, S.N.; Ojha, S. Serratiopeptidase, A Serine Protease Anti-Inflammatory, Fibrinolytic, and Mucolytic Drug, Can Be a Useful Adjuvant for Management in COVID-19. *Front. Pharmacol.* **2021**, *12*, 603997. [CrossRef]
9. Artini, M.; Vrenna, G.; Trecca, M.; Tuccio Guarna Assanti, V.; Fiscarelli, E.V.; Papa, R.; Selan, L. Serratiopeptidase Affects the Physiology of Pseudomonas Aeruginosa Isolates from Cystic Fibrosis Patients. *Int. J. Mol. Sci.* **2022**, *23*, 12645. [CrossRef]
10. Vélez-Gómez, J.M.; Melchor-Moncada, J.J.; Veloza, L.A.; Sepúlveda-Arias, J.C. Purification and Characterization of a Metalloprotease Produced by the C8 Isolate of Serratia Marcescens Using Silkworm Pupae or Casein as a Protein Source. *Int. J. Biol. Macromol.* **2019**, *135*, 97–105. [CrossRef]
11. Jadhav, S.B.; Shah, N.; Rathi, A.; Rathi, V.; Rathi, A. Serratiopeptidase: Insights into the Therapeutic Applications. *Biotechnol. Rep.* **2020**, *28*, e00544. [CrossRef]
12. Hosseinzadeh, S.A.; Valizadeh, V.; Rouhani, M.; Mirkazemi, S.; Azizi, M.; Norouzian, D.; Ahangari Cohan, R. Novel Serratiopeptidase Exhibits Different Affinities to the Substrates and Inhibitors. *Chem. Biol. Drug Des.* **2022**, *100*, 553–563. [CrossRef] [PubMed]

13. Bié, J.; Sepodes, B.; Fernandes, P.C.B.; Ribeiro, M.H.L. Enzyme Immobilization and Co-Immobilization: Main Framework, Advances and Some Applications. *Processes* **2022**, *10*, 494. [CrossRef]
14. Guisan, J.M.; Fernandez-Lorente, G.; Rocha-Martin, J.; Moreno-Gamero, D. Enzyme Immobilization Strategies for the Design of Robust and Efficient Biocatalysts. *Curr. Opin. Green Sustain. Chem.* **2022**, *35*, 100593. [CrossRef]
15. Zhou, C.; Wang, Q.; Jiang, J.; Gao, L. Nanozybiotics: Nanozyme-Based Antibacterials against Bacterial Resistance. *Antibiotics* **2022**, *11*, 390. [CrossRef] [PubMed]
16. Thallinger, B.; Prasetyo, E.N.; Nyanhongo, G.S.; Guebitz, G.M. Antimicrobial Enzymes: An Emerging Strategy to Fight Microbes and Microbial Biofilms. *Biotechnol. J.* **2013**, *8*, 97–109. [CrossRef]
17. Ziental, D.; Czarczynska-Goslinska, B.; Mlynarczyk, D.T.; Glowacka-Sobotta, A.; Stanisz, B.; Goslinski, T.; Sobotta, L. Titanium Dioxide Nanoparticles-Prospects and Applications in Medicine. *Nanomaterials* **2020**, *10*, 387. [CrossRef]
18. Hasanzadeh Kafshgari, M.; Goldmann, W.H. Insights into Theranostic Properties of Titanium Dioxide for Nanomedicine. *Nanomicro Lett.* **2020**, *12*, 22. [CrossRef]
19. Tang, Z.; He, H.; Zhu, L.; Liu, Z.; Yang, J.; Qin, G.; Wu, J.; Tang, Y.; Zhang, D.; Chen, Q.; et al. A General Protein Unfolding-Chemical Coupling Strategy for Pure Protein Hydrogels with Mechanically Strong and Multifunctional Properties. *Adv. Sci.* **2022**, *9*, 2102557. [CrossRef]
20. Wickramathilaka, M.P.; Tao, B.Y. Characterization of Covalent Crosslinking Strategies for Synthesizing DNA-Based Bioconjugates. *J. Biol. Eng.* **2019**, *13*, 63. [CrossRef]
21. Haryński, Ł.; Olejnik, A.; Grochowska, K.; Siuzdak, K. A Facile Method for Tauc Exponent and Corresponding Electronic Transitions Determination in Semiconductors Directly from UV–Vis Spectroscopy Data. *Opt. Mater.* **2022**, *127*, 112205. [CrossRef]
22. Rajaeian, B.; Heitz, A.; Tade, M.O.; Liu, S. Improved Separation and Antifouling Performance of PVA Thin Film Nanocomposite Membranes Incorporated with Carboxylated $TiO_2$ Nanoparticles. *J. Membr. Sci.* **2015**, *485*, 48–59. [CrossRef]
23. Srour, B.; Bruechert, S.; Andrade, S.L.A.; Hellwing, P. Secondary Structure Determination by Means of ATR-FTIR Spectroscopy. *Methods Mol. Biol.* **2017**, *1635*, 195–203. [PubMed]
24. Zuluaga-Vélez, A.; Toro-Acevedo, C.A.; Quintero-Martinez, A.; Melchor-Moncada, J.J.; Pedraza-Ordoñez, F.; Aguilar-Fernández, E.; Sepúlveda-Arias, J.C. Performance of Colombian Silk Fibroin Hydrogels for Hyaline Cartilage Tissue Engineering. *J. Funct. Biomater.* **2022**, *13*, 297. [CrossRef] [PubMed]
25. Kong, H.; Song, J.; Jang, J. Photocatalytic Antibacterial Capabilities of $TiO_2$−Biocidal Polymer Nanocomposites Synthesized by a Surface-Initiated Photopolymerization. *Environ. Sci. Technol.* **2010**, *44*, 5672–5676. [CrossRef]
26. Kolaei, M.; Tayebi, M.; Masoumi, Z.; Tayyebi, A.; Lee, B.K. Optimal Growth of Sodium Titanate Nanoflower on $TiO_2$ Thin Film for the Fabrication of a Novel $Ti/TiO_2/Na_2Ti_3O_7$ Photoanode with Excellent Stability. *J. Alloys Compd.* **2022**, *913*, 165337. [CrossRef]
27. Prabhu, R.; Jeevananda, T.; Mohan, N. Spectral and Thermal Studies on Polyaniline-Titanium Dioxide Nanocomposites by Inverted Emulsion Techniques. *Mater. Today Proc.* **2019**, *27*, 2164–2168. [CrossRef]
28. Wei, J.; Zhao, L.; Peng, S.; Shi, J.; Liu, Z.; Wen, W. Wettability of Urea-Doped $TiO_2$ Nanoparticles and Their High Electrorheological Effects. *J. Solgel Sci. Technol.* **2008**, *47*, 311–315. [CrossRef]
29. Kathiravan, A.; Renganathan, R. Photosensitization of Colloidal $TiO_2$ Nanoparticles with Phycocyanin Pigment. *J. Colloid Interface Sci.* **2009**, *335*, 196–202. [CrossRef]
30. Mobeen Amanulla, A.; Sundaram, R. Green Synthesis of $TiO_2$ Nanoparticles Using Orange Peel Extract for Antibacterial, Cytotoxicity and Humidity Sensor Applications. *Mater. Today Proc.* **2019**, *8*, 323–331. [CrossRef]
31. Valsaraj, P.V. Divyarthana. Structural, Optical and Antimicrobial Properties of Green Synthesized Cerium Oxide Nanoparticles. In *AIP Conference Proceedings*; AIP Publishing: Melville, NY, USA, 2019; Volume 2162.
32. Mendonça, C.D.; Khan, S.U.; Rahemi, V.; Verbruggen, S.W.; Machado, S.A.S.; De Wael, K. Surface Plasmon Resonance-Induced Visible Light Photocatalytic $TiO_2$ Modified with AuNPs for the Quantification of Hydroquinone. *Electrochim. Acta* **2021**, *389*, 138734. [CrossRef]
33. Reinosa, J.J.; Leret, P.; Álvarez-Docio, C.M.; Del Campo, A.; Fernández, J.F. Enhancement of UV Absorption Behavior in ZnO-$TiO_2$ composites. *Bol. Soc. Esp. Ceram. Vidr.* **2016**, *55*, 55–62. [CrossRef]
34. Lin, H.; Huang, C.P.; Li, W.; Ni, C.; Shah, S.I.; Tseng, Y.H. Size Dependency of Nanocrystalline $TiO_2$ on Its Optical Property and Photocatalytic Reactivity Exemplified by 2-Chlorophenol. *Appl. Catal. B* **2006**, *68*, 1–11. [CrossRef]
35. Nosaka, Y.; Nosaka, A.Y. Reconsideration of Intrinsic Band Alignments within Anatase and Rutile $TiO_2$. *J. Phys. Chem. Lett.* **2016**, *7*, 431–434. [CrossRef] [PubMed]
36. Scanlon, D.O.; Dunnill, C.W.; Buckeridge, J.; Shevlin, S.A.; Logsdail, A.J.; Woodley, S.M.; Catlow, C.R.A.; Powell, M.J.; Palgrave, R.G.; Parkin, I.P.; et al. Band Alignment of Rutile and Anatase $TiO_2$. *Nat. Mater.* **2013**, *12*, 798–801. [CrossRef] [PubMed]
37. Dhivya Pushpa, M.; Sanclemente Crespo, M.; Cristopher, M.M.; Karthick, P.; Sridharan, M.; Sanjeeviraja, C.; Jeyadheepan, K. Influence of Pyrolytic Temperature on Optoelectronic Properties and the Energy Harvesting Applications of High Pressure $TiO_2$ Thin Films. *Vacuum* **2019**, *161*, 81–91. [CrossRef]
38. Ko, K.C.; Bromley, S.T.; Lee, J.Y.; Illas, F. Size-Dependent Level Alignment between Rutile and Anatase $TiO_2$ Nanoparticles: Implications for Photocatalysis. *J. Phys. Chem. Lett.* **2017**, *8*, 5593–5598. [CrossRef]
39. Leynen, N.; Tytgat, J.S.; Bijnens, K.; Jaenen, V.; Verleysen, E.; Artois, T.; Van Belleghem, F.; Saenen, N.D.; Smeets, K. Assessing the in Vivo Toxicity of Titanium Dioxide Nanoparticles in Schmidtea Mediterranea: Uptake Pathways and (Neuro)Developmental Outcomes. *Aquat. Toxicol.* **2024**, *270*, 106895. [CrossRef]

40. Mohd Yusof, H.; Abdul Rahman, N.A.; Mohamad, R.; Zaidan, U.H.; Samsudin, A.A. Biosynthesis of Zinc Oxide Nanoparticles by Cell-Biomass and Supernatant of Lactobacillus Plantarum TA4 and Its Antibacterial and Biocompatibility Properties. *Sci. Rep.* **2020**, *10*, 19996. [CrossRef]
41. Romoser, A.A.; Figueroa, D.E.; Sooresh, A.; Scribner, K.; Chen, P.L.; Porter, W.; Criscitiello, M.F.; Sayes, C.M. Distinct Immunomodulatory Effects of a Panel of Nanomaterials in Human Dermal Fibroblasts. *Toxicol. Lett.* **2012**, *210*, 293–301. [CrossRef]
42. Feng, X.; Zhang, S.; Lou, X. Controlling Silica Coating Thickness on $TiO_2$ Nanoparticles for Effective Photodynamic Therapy. *Colloids Surf. B Biointerfaces* **2013**, *107*, 220–226. [CrossRef]
43. Franchi, L.P.; Manshian, B.B.; de Souza, T.A.J.; Soenen, S.J.; Matsubara, E.Y.; Rosolen, J.M.; Takahashi, C.S. Cyto- and Genotoxic Effects of Metallic Nanoparticles in Untransformed Human Fibroblast. *Toxicology In Vitro* **2015**, *29*, 1319–1331. [CrossRef] [PubMed]
44. Jain, A.K.; Senapati, V.A.; Singh, D.; Dubey, K.; Maurya, R.; Pandey, A.K. Impact of Anatase Titanium Dioxide Nanoparticles on Mutagenic and Genotoxic Response in Chinese Hamster Lung Fibroblast Cells (V-79): The Role of Cellular Uptake. *Food Chem. Toxicol.* **2017**, *105*, 127–139. [CrossRef] [PubMed]
45. Kovrlija, I.; Pańczyszyn, E.; Demir, O.; Laizane, M.; Corazzari, M.; Locs, J.; Loca, D. Doxorubicin Loaded Octacalcium Phosphate Particles as Controlled Release Drug Delivery Systems: Physico-Chemical Characterization, in Vitro Drug Release and Evaluation of Cell Death Pathway. *Int. J. Pharm.* **2024**, *653*, 123932. [CrossRef] [PubMed]
46. Gea, M.; Bonetta, S.; Iannarelli, L.; Giovannozzi, A.M.; Maurino, V.; Bonetta, S.; Hodoroaba, V.D.; Armato, C.; Rossi, A.M.; Schilirò, T. Shape-Engineered Titanium Dioxide Nanoparticles (TiO 2 -NPs): Cytotoxicity and Genotoxicity in Bronchial Epithelial Cells. *Food Chem. Toxicol.* **2019**, *127*, 89–100. [CrossRef] [PubMed]
47. Bhargavi, P.L.; Prakasham, R.S. Agro-Industrial Wastes Utilization for the Generation of Fibrinolytic Metalloprotease by Serratia Marcescens RSPB11. *Biocatal. Agric. Biotechnol.* **2017**, *9*, 201–208. [CrossRef]
48. Kim, H.S.; Golyshin, P.N.; Timmis, K.N. Characterization and Role of a Metalloprotease Induced by Chitin in *Serratia* sp. KCK. *J. Ind. Microbiol. Biotechnol.* **2007**, *34*, 715–721. [CrossRef]
49. Bach, E.; Sant'Anna, V.; Daroit, D.J.; Corrêa, A.P.F.; Segalin, J.; Brandelli, A. Production, One-Step Purification, and Characterization of a Keratinolytic Protease from Serratia Marcescens P3. *Process Biochem.* **2012**, *47*, 2455–2462. [CrossRef]
50. Badhe, R.V.; Nanda, R.K.; Kulkarni, M.B.; Bhujbal, M.N.; Patil, P.S.; Badhe, S.R. Media Optimization Studies for Serratiopeptidase Production from Serratia Marcescens ATCC 13880. *Hindustan Antibiot. Bull.* **2009**, *51*, 17–23.
51. Koul, D.; Chander, D.; Manhas, R.S.; Hossain, M.M.; Dar, M.J.; Chaubey, A. Purification, Functional Characterization and Enhanced Production of Serratiopeptidase from Serratia Marcescens MES-4: An Endophyte Isolated from Morus Rubra. *J. Biotechnol.* **2024**, *387*, 58–68. [CrossRef]
52. Melchor-Moncada, J.J.; García-Barco, A.; Zuluaga-Vélez, A.; Veloza, L.A.; Sepúlveda-Arias, J.C. Scale-Up of the Fermentation Process for the Production and Purification of Serratiopeptidase Using Silkworm Pupae as a Substrate. *Methods Protoc.* **2024**, *7*, 19. [CrossRef]
53. Bohdziewicz, J. Ultrafiltration of Technical Amylolytic Enyzymes. *Process Biochem.* **1996**, *31*, 185–191. [CrossRef]
54. Schratter, P. Purification and Concentration by Ultrafiltration. In *Protein Purification Protocols*; Humana Press: Totowa, NJ, USA, 2004; Volume 244, pp. 101–116.
55. Doshi, P.; Dantroliya, S.; Modi, A.; Shukla, A.; Patel, D.; Joshi, C.; Joshi, M. Enhanced Production Process of Recombinant Mature Serratiopeptidase in Escherichia Coli Using Fed-Batch Culture by Self-Proteolytic Activity of Fusion Protein. *Fermentation* **2022**, *8*, 307. [CrossRef]
56. Yaashikaa, P.R.; Devi, M.K.; Kumar, P.S. Advances in the Application of Immobilized Enzyme for the Remediation of Hazardous Pollutant: A Review. *Chemosphere* **2022**, *299*, 134390. [CrossRef] [PubMed]
57. Raghav, R.; Srivastava, S. Immobilization Strategy for Enhancing Sensitivity of Immunosensors: L-Asparagine-AuNPs as a Promising Alternative of EDC-NHS Activated Citrate-AuNPs for Antibody Immobilization. *Biosens. Bioelectron.* **2016**, *78*, 396–403. [CrossRef] [PubMed]
58. Xia, N.; Xing, Y.; Wang, G.; Feng, Q.; Chen, Q.; Feng, H.; Sun, X.; Liu, L. Probing of EDC/NHSS-Mediated Covalent Coupling Reaction by the Immobilization of Electrochemically Active Biomolecules. *Int. J. Electrochem. Sci.* **2013**, *8*, 2459–2467. [CrossRef]
59. Kazenwadel, F.; Wagner, H.; Rapp, B.E.; Franzreb, M. Optimization of Enzyme Immobilization on Magnetic Microparticles Using 1-Ethyl-3-(3-Dimethylaminopropyl)Carbodiimide (EDC) as a Crosslinking Agent. *Anal. Methods* **2015**, *7*, 10291–10298. [CrossRef]
60. Miyata, K.; Maejima, K.; Tomoda, K.; Isono, M. Serratia Protease: Part I. Purification and General Properties of the Enzyme. *Agric. Biol. Chem.* **1970**, *34*, 310–318. [CrossRef]
61. Nemiwal, M.; Zhang, T.C.; Kumar, D. Enzyme Immobilized Nanomaterials as Electrochemical Biosensors for Detection of Biomolecules. *Enzym. Microb. Technol.* **2022**, *156*, 110006. [CrossRef]
62. Kumar, S.; Jana, A.K.; Dhamija, I.; Singla, Y.; Maiti, M. Preparation, Characterization and Targeted Delivery of Serratiopeptidase Immobilized on Amino-Functionalized Magnetic Nanoparticles. *Eur. J. Pharm. Biopharm.* **2013**, *85*, 413–426. [CrossRef]
63. Guo, H.; Lei, B.; Yu, J.; Chen, Y.; Qian, J. Immobilization of Lipase by Dialdehyde Cellulose Crosslinked Magnetic Nanoparticles. *Int. J. Biol. Macromol.* **2021**, *185*, 287–296. [CrossRef]
64. Huang, B.; Wang, X.; Fang, H.; Jiang, S.; Hou, H. Mechanically Strong Sulfonated Polybenzimidazole PEMs with Enhanced Proton Conductivity. *Mater. Lett.* **2019**, *234*, 354–356. [CrossRef]
65. Bolivar, J.M.; Woodley, J.M.; Fernandez-Lafuente, R. Is Enzyme Immobilization a Mature Discipline? Some Critical Considerations to Capitalize on the Benefits of Immobilization. *Chem. Soc. Rev.* **2022**, *51*, 6251–6290. [CrossRef] [PubMed]

66. Rodrigues, R.C.; Ortiz, C.; Berenguer-Murcia, Á.; Torres, R.; Fernández-Lafuente, R. Modifying Enzyme Activity and Selectivity by Immobilization. *Chem. Soc. Rev.* **2013**, *42*, 6290–6307. [CrossRef]
67. Wu, D.; Ran, T.; Wang, W.; Xu, D. Structure of a thermostable serralysin from *Serratia* sp. FS14 at 1.1 Å resolution. *Acta Crystallogr. Sect. F Struct. Biol. Commun.* **2016**, *72*, 10–15. [CrossRef] [PubMed]
68. López-Gallego, F.; Guisán, J.M.; Betancor, L. Stabilization of Enzymes by Multipoint Covalent Immobilization on Supports Activated with Glyoxyl Groups. In *Immobilizaion of Enzymes and Cells*; Guisan, J.M., Ed.; Springer: London, UK, 2013; Volume 1051, pp. 59–71. ISBN 9781627035491.
69. Rodriguez-Loya, J.; Lerma, M.; Gardea-Torresdey, J.L. Dynamic Light Scattering and Its Application to Control Nanoparticle Aggregation in Colloidal Systems: A Review. *Micromachines* **2024**, *15*, 24. [CrossRef]
70. Marucco, A.; Prono, M.; Beal, D.; Alasonati, E.; Fisicaro, P.; Bergamaschi, E.; Carriere, M.; Fenoglio, I. Biotransformation of Food-Grade and Nanometric $TiO_2$ in the Oral-Gastro-Intestinal Tract: Driving Forces and Effect on the Toxicity toward Intestinal Epithelial Cells. *Nanomaterials* **2020**, *10*, 2132. [CrossRef]
71. Kamble, S.; Agrawal, S.; Cherumukkil, S.; Sharma, V.; Jasra, R.V.; Munshi, P. Revisiting Zeta Potential, the Key Feature of Interfacial Phenomena, with Applications and Recent Advancements. *ChemistrySelect* **2022**, *7*, e202103084. [CrossRef]
72. Keleştemur, S.; Altunbek, M.; Culha, M. Influence of EDC/NHS Coupling Chemistry on Stability and Cytotoxicity of ZnO Nanoparticles Modified with Proteins. *Appl. Surf. Sci.* **2017**, *403*, 455–463. [CrossRef]
73. Yang, J.Y.; Bae, J.; Jung, A.; Park, S.; Chung, S.; Seok, J.; Roh, H.; Han, Y.; Oh, J.M.; Sohn, S.; et al. Surface Functionalization-Specific Binding of Coagulation Factors by Zinc Oxide Nanoparticles Delays Coagulation Time and Reduces Thrombin Generation Potential in Vitro. *PLoS ONE* **2017**, *12*, e0181634. [CrossRef]
74. Khan, M.F.; Kundu, D.; Hazra, C.; Patra, S. A Strategic Approach of Enzyme Engineering by Attribute Ranking and Enzyme Immobilization on Zinc Oxide Nanoparticles to Attain Thermostability in Mesophilic Bacillus Subtilis Lipase for Detergent Formulation. *Int. J. Biol. Macromol.* **2019**, *136*, 66–82. [CrossRef]
75. Selan, L.; Berlutti, F.; Passariello, C.; Comodi-Ballanti, M.R.; Thaller, M.C. Proteolytic Enzymes: A New Treatment Strategy for Prosthetic Infections? *Antimicrob. Agents Chemother.* **1993**, *37*, 2618–2621. [CrossRef] [PubMed]
76. Klem, H.; Alegre-Requena, J.V.; Paton, R.S. Catalytic Effects of Active Site Conformational Change in the Allosteric Activation of Imidazole Glycerol Phosphate Synthase. *ACS Catal.* **2023**, *13*, 16249–16257. [CrossRef] [PubMed]
77. Solanki, L.A.; Dinesh, S.P.S.; Jain, R.K.; Balasubramaniam, A. Effects of Titanium Oxide Coating on the Antimicrobial Properties, Surface Characteristics, and Cytotoxicity of Orthodontic Brackets–A Systematic Review and Meta Analysis of in-Vitro Studies. *J. Oral Biol. Craniofacial Res.* **2023**, *13*, 553–562. [CrossRef] [PubMed]
78. Gupta, P.V.; Nirwane, A.M.; Belubbi, T.; Nagarsenker, M.S. Pulmonary Delivery of Synergistic Combination of Fluoroquinolone Antibiotic Complemented with Proteolytic Enzyme: A Novel Antimicrobial and Antibiofilm Strategy. *Nanomedicine* **2017**, *13*, 2371–2384. [CrossRef] [PubMed]
79. Rouhani, M.; Valizadeh, V.; Bakhshandeh, H.; Hosseinzadeh, S.A.; Molasalehi, S.; Atyabi, S.M.; Norouzian, D. Improved Anti-Biofilm Activity and Long-Lasting Effects of Novel Serratiopeptidase Immobilized on Cellulose Nanofibers. *Appl. Microbiol. Biotechnol.* **2023**, *107*, 6487–6496. [CrossRef] [PubMed]
80. Mahdiani, H.; Yazdani, F.; Khoramipour, M.; Valizadeh, V.; Bakhshandeh, H.; Dinarvand, R. Preparation and Physicochemical Characterization of Hyaluronic Acid-Lysine Nanogels Containing Serratiopeptidase to Control Biofilm Formation. *Sci. Rep.* **2024**, *14*, 6111. [CrossRef]
81. Filby, B.W.; Weldrick, P.J.; Paunov, V.N. Overcoming Beta-Lactamase-Based Antimicrobial Resistance by Nanocarrier-Loaded Clavulanic Acid and Antibiotic Cotreatments. *ACS Appl. Bio Mater.* **2022**, *5*, 3826–3840. [CrossRef]
82. Papa, R.; Artini, M.; Cellini, A.; Tilotta, M.; Galano, E.; Pucci, P.; Amoresano, A.; Selan, L. A New Anti-Infective Strategy to Reduce the Spreading of Antibiotic Resistance by the Action on Adhesion-Mediated Virulence Factors in Staphylococcus Aureus. *Microb. Pathog.* **2013**, *63*, 44–53. [CrossRef]
83. Mantravadi, H.B. Effectivity of Titanium Oxide Based Nano Particles on E. Coli from Clinical Samples. *J. Clin. Diagn. Res.* **2017**, *11*, DC37–DC40. [CrossRef]
84. Suvarna, V.; Nair, A.; Mallya, R.; Khan, T.; Omri, A. Antimicrobial Nanomaterials for Food Packaging. *Antibiotics* **2022**, *11*, 729. [CrossRef]
85. González-Restrepo, D.; Zuluaga-Vélez, A.; Orozco, L.M.; Sepúlveda-Arias, J.C. Silk Fibroin-Based Dressings with Antibacterial and Anti-Inflammatory Properties. *Eur. J. Pharm. Sci.* **2024**, *195*, 106710. [CrossRef] [PubMed]

Journal of
*Functional Biomaterials*

*Review*

# Unlocking Genome Editing: Advances and Obstacles in CRISPR/Cas Delivery Technologies

**Bibifatima Kaupbayeva [1,*], Andrey Tsoy [1], Yuliya Safarova (Yantsen) [1], Ainetta Nurmagambetova [2], Hironobu Murata [3], Krzysztof Matyjaszewski [3,4] and Sholpan Askarova [1]**

1 Center for Life Sciences, National Laboratory Astana, Nazarbayev University, Astana 010000, Kazakhstan
2 School of Medicine, Nazarbayev University, Astana 020000, Kazakhstan
3 Chemistry Department, Carnegie Mellon University, Pittsburgh, PA 15213, USA
4 Department of Molecular Physics, Faculty of Chemistry, Lodz University of Technology, 90-924 Łódź, Poland
* Correspondence: bibifatima.kaupbayeva@nu.edu.kz; Tel.: +7-7172-705931

**Abstract:** CRISPR/Cas9 (clustered regularly interspaced short palindromic repeats associated with protein 9) was first identified as a component of the bacterial adaptive immune system and subsequently engineered into a genome-editing tool. The key breakthrough in this field came with the realization that CRISPR/Cas9 could be used in mammalian cells to enable transformative genetic editing. This technology has since become a vital tool for various genetic manipulations, including gene knockouts, knock-in point mutations, and gene regulation at both transcriptional and post-transcriptional levels. CRISPR/Cas9 holds great potential in human medicine, particularly for curing genetic disorders. However, despite significant innovation and advancement in genome editing, the technology still possesses critical limitations, such as off-target effects, immunogenicity issues, ethical considerations, regulatory hurdles, and the need for efficient delivery methods. To overcome these obstacles, efforts have focused on creating more accurate and reliable Cas9 nucleases and exploring innovative delivery methods. Recently, functional biomaterials and synthetic carriers have shown great potential as effective delivery vehicles for CRISPR/Cas9 components. In this review, we attempt to provide a comprehensive survey of the existing CRISPR-Cas9 delivery strategies, including viral delivery, biomaterials-based delivery, synthetic carriers, and physical delivery techniques. We underscore the urgent need for effective delivery systems to fully unlock the power of CRISPR/Cas9 technology and realize a seamless transition from benchtop research to clinical applications.

**Keywords:** CRISPR/Cas9; genome editing; functional biomaterials; synthetic polymers; lipid nanoparticles; cell-penetrating peptides; delivery strategies

## 1. Introduction

Clustered regularly interspaced short palindromic repeats associated with protein 9 (CRISPR/Cas9) is a user-friendly gene editing platform. CRISPR/Cas9 was initially found as a prokaryotic defense system against mobile genetic elements such as plasmids or viral genetic material [1]. CRISPR/Cas9 is an essential trait enabling these microorganisms to evade the host's innate immune system [2]. The CRISPR-mediated defense mechanism functions by inserting short DNA fragments of parasite genomes into the CRISPR array of the host to provide sequence-specific protection [3]. The Cas9 protein uses its single guide RNA (sgRNA) to selectively target any DNA site where the protospacer adjacent motif (PAM) is present [4–6]. Cas9 introduces site-specific double-stranded DNA breaks, which are then repaired by endogenous pathways in cells [7]. The sgRNAs can also be engineered to facilitate gene knockouts by delivering insertion or deletion mutations (indels) through nonhomologous end joining (NHEJ) or by promoting the integration of donor sequences via homology-directed repair (HDR) (Figure 1) [8].

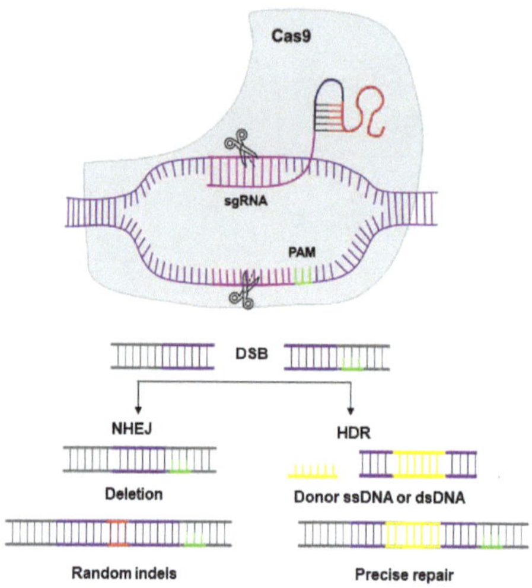


**Figure 1.** Schematic representation of CRISPR/Cas9-mediated gene editing. DSB—double-strand break, NHEJ—nonhomologous end joining, HDR—homology-directed repair, ssDNA—single-stranded DNA, dsDNA—double-stranded DNA.

Cas9 can be introduced into cells in the form of DNA, mRNA (transcribed from a plasmid), or purified protein, each with distinct advantages and disadvantages. Delivering Cas9 via plasmid DNA. which encodes both Cas9 and sgRNA, is a cost-efficient solution that requires only standard laboratory equipment for preparation. This can be advantageous if a longer-term need for Cas9 in the cell is required. However, the plasmid DNA must first be transcribed into RNA and then translated for Cas9 synthesis, which makes it more time-consuming than mRNA or protein methods. In addition, prolonged expression can increase the potential risks of off-target effects and insertional mutagenesis [9,10]. A faster mode of initiating gene editing is the delivery of Cas9 as mRNA, as it does not require transcription. Nevertheless, mRNA is unstable and quickly degraded by RNases. Thus, its expression is transient. Chemical modifications can improve mRNA stability, but transient expression might reduce gene editing efficiency [10,11]. Delivering Cas9 as a purified protein allows for immediate nuclear gene editing and, therefore, has higher efficiency than DNA- or mRNA-based methods. Unfortunately, protein delivery is the shortest-lived and most costly of all three formats, although it carries a lower risk of off-target effects. A fundamental challenge in Cas9 protein delivery is its bacterial origin, as it may carry bacterial endotoxins that trigger severe immune responses, limiting its clinical applications [12,13].

Several strategies for delivering Cas9 are currently being developed and tested. These strategies can be broadly categorized into four groups: viral vectors, biomaterials-based carriers, synthetic carriers, and physical methods.

Gene delivery using viral vectors is well established. While their wild-type versions cause diseases in humans, they have been engineered to be non-pathogenic while retaining the ability to robustly deliver genetic material into host cells without affecting their viability. The most utilized biological transfection vectors are adeno-associated virus (AAV), adenovirus (AdVs), and lentivirus (LV). Biomaterials-based carriers, also called nonviral vector-based delivery or chemical transfection for CRISPR/Cas9 systems, include cell-penetrating peptides, biopolymers, and lipid nanoparticles. In contrast, synthetic carriers are synthetic polymer-based delivery systems. Physical CRISPR delivery methods involve either applying direct physical mechanoporation (micro- and nano-injections, passing constrictions that can facilitate CRISPR delivery) or external forces such as electrical, acoustic, laser/thermal, or magnetic fields. These techniques permeabilize the cell membrane, enhancing the uptake of target molecules.

Each delivery method has its strengths and limitations, making their evaluation crucial when selecting the most appropriate approach for specific applications. Alongside successful delivery and high editing efficiency, safety is one of the most critical concerns in clinical trials. In this regard, our review introduces current CRISPR/Cas9 delivery strategies, with a focus on functional biomaterials and synthetic carriers, and discusses their applications in gene therapy, as well as their limitations and future prospects.

## 2. Viral Vectors for the Delivery of CRISPR Components

### 2.1. Adeno-Associated Virus Vectors

AAVs have been predominantly utilized to deliver the CRISPR/Cas9 system for several reasons. First, they have a good safety profile because their genomes remain episomal after the transduction [14]. Therefore, they have been approved for several human trials in gene augmentation therapies [15]. AAVs also display lower immunogenicity compared to other viral vehicles [16]. Additionally, even high doses of these molecules cause mild toxicity in animal models [17].

However, AAVs offer a limited packaging capacity of 4.7 kb, preventing the use of larger genes. Scientists enhanced the AAV delivery approach by developing a dual AAV system to address this issue. This expanded the capacity to approximately 9 kb [18]. Yang et al. illustrated the use of a dual AAV system to deliver the CRISPR/Cas9 technology, utilizing one vector to introduce SaCas9 and another to provide sgRNA targeting ornithine transcarbamylase (OTC) in mice with partial OTC deficiency, which affects the urea cycle in the liver [19]. Following the injection of two AAVs into newborn mice, the researchers found that the OTC mutation was reverted in 10% of hepatocytes, resulting in improved survival rates among the mice.

While using the dual AAV system addressed the limited carrying capacity found in a single AAV, specific genes still surpass the 9 kb limit imposed by this dual AAV strategy. Koo et al. demonstrated a trans-splicing method with triple AAVs to introduce the human dystrophin muscle dysregulation 1 gene (*DMD*) into dystrophic *mdx* mice [20]. Three separate AAVs were used to carry the *DMD* and the full-length gene was joined together upon inverted terminal repeats (ITR)-mediated trans-splicing. The results demonstrated the expression of human dystrophin in mice. Maddalena et al. showed retinal gene delivery through a triple AAV vector aimed at treating Usher syndrome type 1D and Alstrom syndrome, which are linked to mutations in the CDH23 and ALMS1 genes, respectively [18]. They demonstrated successful transduction of HEK293 cells, achieved 4% transduction of mouse photoreceptors, and 40% transduction of pig retina.

### 2.2. Adenovirus

Compared to AAVs, AdVs have a larger packaging capacity, reaching up to 8 kb [21]. Additionally, AdV is a non-integrating virus with an episomal genome, which minimizes undesired mutations caused by random insertions. Therefore, AdV-mediated delivery of CRISPR/Cas9 has been employed to establish disease models, generate resources for drug discovery, and address current health conditions.

For instance, in 2014, Maddalo et al. used intratracheal administration of AdV-delivered CRISPR/Cas9 to generate a model of non-small cell lung cancer by triggering the formation of an Eml4-Alk fusion gene [22]. Similarly, in 2015, Wang et al. created a mouse model of nonalcoholic steatohepatitis (NASH) by using AdV-delivered SpCas9 to target the Pten gene. The NASH phenotype emerged from the mutation in Pten and the immune reactions against SpCas9 [23]. In drug discovery, Voets et al. utilized AdV to disable the SMAD3 gene in normal human lung fibroblasts and bronchial epithelial cells using a low multiplicity of infection, as low as 20 [24]. In treating established diseases, Ding et al. demonstrated the reduction of plasma cholesterol levels by inducing loss-of-function mutations in the proprotein convertase subtilisin/kexin type 9 (PCSK9) gene in mouse livers [25]. There have been successful attempts to revive muscle function in muscle progenitor cells derived from patients with Duchenne muscular dystrophy in vitro [26] and in *mdx* mice in vivo [27,28]. Additionally, Li et al. engineered HIV-resistant primary CD4+ T cells by introducing the CCR5Δ32 variant into their cell membranes using AdV-delivered CRISPR/Cas9 [29].

However, AdVs pose a significant risk due to their high immunogenicity. Previous research has indicated that they provoke robust immune and inflammatory reactions in animal models, limiting their clinical potential [30]. Therefore, AdV vectors have been subjected to several optimizations. First-generation recombinant AdVs lack the viral gene E1 [14]. These vectors induce both acute and chronic immune responses. The viral capsid initiates the acute response, whereas the chronic response is triggered by viral gene expression. The second-generation vectors have been designed to reduce chronic immune responses by deleting viral genes E2 and E4. These vectors typically have a packaging capacity of approximately 8 kb [15,16]. The latest generation of AdV vectors, helper-dependent or gutless AdV vectors, lacks all viral genes except for inverted terminal repeats (ITRs) and encapsulation sequences. This design enables them to accommodate up to 35 kb of genetic material, making them well-suited for delivering the entire CRISPR/Cas9 system within a single vector [31,32]. Significantly, these vectors do not trigger long-lasting immune reactions. However, the viral capsid can still trigger acute phase immune responses. Additionally, since most individuals have been exposed to adenoviruses from early childhood and have developed neutralizing antibodies against common serotypes, the concentration of genes delivered in gene augmentation therapy typically decreases to about 10% within 24 months as a result of acute immune responses, and the presence of neutralizing antibodies [21,33]. This phenomenon ultimately limits the effectiveness of gene augmentation therapy [34].

### 2.3. Lentiviruses

LV vectors can accommodate genetic material up to approximately 7 kb in size, making them capable of hosting the SpCas9 gene, which is approximately 4.2 kb, along with additional sgRNA molecules. The production of LVs is also less complex than AAVs, and their transduction process is highly efficient across a broad spectrum of cell types [35]. In addition, LV vectors are devoid of all viral genes and do not trigger the immune response [36,37]. These advantages position LV vectors as an optimal choice for delivery in vitro and ex vivo compared to other viral vectors [35].

The lentiviral expression vector containing SpCas9 and sgRNA, utilized to alter targeted genomic sites, introduced a novel approach to assess gene function across the entire genome. For example, Shalem et al. demonstrated that delivering a genome-scale CRISPR/Cas9 knockout (GECKO) library targeting 18,080 genes using 64,751 sgRNAs allowed for positive and negative human cell selection [38]. These screens identified genes essential for cell viability in cancer and pluripotent stem cells. Another CRISPR/Cas9 library screening conducted with lentiviral vectors identified additional tumor-suppressing mutations through a functional search for targets associated with acute leukemia [39]. A new set of lentivirus vectors combined with CRISPR/Cas9 has been developed for lesion therapy in the treatment of HIV-1, HBV, and HSV-1 [40]. Furthermore, vectors have also been employed in correcting hereditary diseases such as cystic fibrosis and various neurodegenerative disorders [40].

However, the potential of LV systems for unpredictable incorporation into the host cell genome poses a challenge. Integration near oncogenes can activate them, potentially leading to tumorigenesis [41]. This limitation prevents LV-mediated delivery of CRISPR/Cas9 for in vivo gene editing in clinical studies [42]. Indeed, tragic incidents in clinical trials have been documented as a result of insertional mutations caused by retroviruses [43–46], underscoring the inherent risks associated with using LVs in patients.

Another common hurdle for using viral vectors is posed by the liver's barrier function. Kupffer cells and liver sinusoidal endothelial cells have been shown to sequester most of the administered dose, thus preventing efficient delivery to the target tissues [47,48]. This results in the need for higher viral doses, which raises safety concerns. For instance, the use of high doses of AAV gene therapy led to the death of two pediatric patients [49]. To overcome this unintended liver capture of viral vectors, Kataoka et al. explored the direct stealth coating of liver sinusoidal wall cells with two-armed poly(ethylyene glycol)-conjugated oligo(l-lysine) (two-arm-PEG-Oligo-Lys) [50]. Preinjection of two-arm-PEG-OligoLys resulted in improved gene transfection efficiency in target tissues.

## 3. Biomaterials-Based Carriers

Biomaterials-based carriers can be broadly categorized into three groups: cell-penetrating peptides (CPPs), lipid nanoparticles (LNPs), and biopolymers (Figure 2). These carriers have become increasingly popular for drug delivery due to their ability to control release, protect therapeutic payloads against degradation, potentially reduce immunogenicity/cellular uptake, etc., as well as add functionality to make active components bioavailable [47]. This has made biomaterials-based vectors a prevalent clinical platform for delivering low-molecular-weight drugs and protein/peptide therapeutics that have shown safety and efficacy in gene therapy through numerous clinical trials.

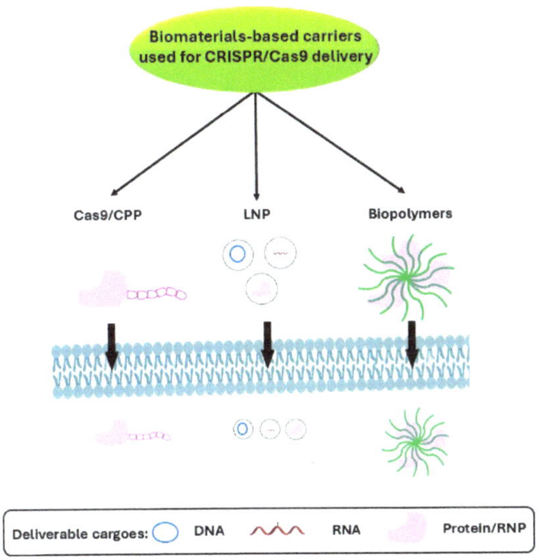


**Figure 2.** Biomaterials-based carriers used for the delivery of CRISPR/Cas9 systems.

The first group of biomaterials used for CRISPR/Cas9 delivery, cell-penetrating peptides (CPPs), have shown great promise for improving the delivery of CRISPR/Cas9 components into target cells. These short, versatile peptides facilitate cellular uptake, allowing for efficient transport of the Cas9 protein and guide RNA. By leveraging the unique properties of CPPs, researchers can enhance the bioavailability and specificity of CRISPR/Cas9, potentially minimizing off-target effects and improving therapeutic effectiveness. The second class of biomaterials gaining considerable attention as CRISPR/Cas9 component carriers in cells are lipid nanoparticles (LNPs). These biomaterials encapsulate the Cas9 and gRNA, increasing their protection from degradation and enhancing cellular uptake. By utilizing LNPs, researchers can achieve targeted delivery and improved stability, potentially leading to more precise and efficient genome editing outcomes. The third group of biomaterials used for CRISPR/Cas9 delivery are biopolymers. These molecules rely on the non-covalent nanoparticle formation of polymers with CRISPR components. Biopolymer-based vectors offer several advantages, such as the ability to deliver multiple gRNAs at a time and the use of targeting ligands for functionalization with specific features that can facilitate CRISPR cargo delivery towards specific tissues and cells, including enough room for loading large payloads. Despite recent research showing some limitations in their ability to deliver CRISPR-Cas9 complexes, biopolymeric vectors may be inherently safe and have a large packaging capacity [51].

### 3.1. CRISPR/Cas9 Delivery by Cell-Penetrating Peptides

Cell-penetrating peptides (CPPs), also known as protein transduction domains, are short peptides capable of penetrating living cells. First discovered in 1988, the transcriptional protein HIV transactivator Tat was the first peptide sequence capable of crossing cellular membranes [52,53]. CPPs act as a delivery platform, carrying their cargo into the cell through perturbation of the cellular membrane lipid bilayer, or endocytosis [54,55]. Notably, CPPs such as HIV-1 Tat, penetratin, and oligoarginine are the best tools for transporting therapeutic biomolecules, generally termed biodrugs, into cells [56]. Researchers also investigated the capability of CPPs to act as penetration enhancers for poorly permeable polymers with low cell/membrane penetrability [57–59]. The precise processes of direct translocation, endosomal uptake, and endosomal escape of CPPs continue to be subjects of active investigation, with ongoing research into their applications in cargo transport [60–67].

A diverse array of CPPs with significant sequence variation exists, prompting extensive research into their chemical and biophysical properties that govern membrane permeation. These peptides are categorized based on their origin, function, sequence, uptake mechanism, and biomedical applications. Physicochemically, CPPs can be categorized into three main groups: amphiphilic CPPs, cationic CPPs, and hydrophobic CPPs [68]. Recent advancements in understanding CPP properties have been integrated into databases and software for predicting the cell entry capabilities of different CPPs [69–72]. General trends guiding these predictions include a preference for higher and lower arginine and lysine contents, as well as predictions of their secondary structures [70].

Over 40% of all CPPs identified are amphiphilic CPPs. Amphiphilic CPPs feature polar and nonpolar amino acid regions, with the nonpolar segment enriched in hydrophobic amino acids like alanine, valine, leucine, and isoleucine [73]. These peptides mainly facilitate intracellular transport and tend to concentrate in the nucleus [74]. Cationic CPPs possess a positive charge, allowing strong affinity with the cytoplasmic membrane under normal physiological pH conditions. Cationic CPPs bind to negatively charged cell membranes via electrostatic interactions and are transported into cells through a receptor-independent mechanism [75]. These CPPs typically possess a highly positive net charge, primarily composed of short basic chains of arginine and lysine, which play crucial roles in facilitating the internalization of various therapeutic cargoes [76]. The third category of CPPs consists of hydrophobic peptides characterized by a significant number of nonpolar amino acid residues. Hydrophobic CPPs are relatively uncommon and typically feature structures with a high proportion of nonpolar residues. These peptides possess hydrophobic amino acids, which are key in membrane translocation. Examples of hydrophobic CPPs are C105Y [77], Bip4 [78], Kaposi fibroblast growth factor (K-FGF) [79], and fibroblast growth factor 12 (FGF-12) [80]. Unlike many amphipathic cationic CPPs, the amino acid sequence of hydrophobic CPPs has been shown to have minimal impact on cellular uptake [78].

There are primarily two methods to conjugate CPPs with cargo. In the first method, the CPP/cargo sequence is expressed in *E. coli*, followed by the purification of the resulting recombinant fusion protein [81,82]. Ramakrishna et al. proposed incorporating a CPP into the SpCas9 protein [83]. However, genetically attaching SpCas9 with a CPP composed of four Gly, nine Arg, and four Leu made purifying the protein in adequate quantities challenging. To address this, a Cys residue was attached to the C-term of SpCas9 with minimal genetic modification. The primary amine (-$NH_2$) group in the CPP attached through maleimide reacted with the free thiol group in the C-term cysteine of SpCas9, forming a CPP-SpCas9 conjugate through a thioether bond.

The second approach involves mixing CRISPR-RNPs with peptide reagents and applying them to cells in ex vivo culture [84,85]. Human cells, such as embryonic stem cells, dermal fibroblasts, HEK 293T cells, HeLa cells, and embryonic carcinoma cells, were exposed to the CPP-SpCas9 conjugate and CPP-sgRNA complex, either in a sequential or simultaneous manner. This CPP-mediated translocation system resulted in gene disruption ranging from 8.7% to 14% with minimized off-target effects, suggesting that CPP-mediated delivery could enhance CRISPR/Cas9 genome editing [84].

Using this method, genes were also knocked out in white blood cells by delivering Cas9 or Cas12a ribonucleoproteins or adenine base editors. Engineered cells demonstrated antitumor efficacy in mice, and the yield of edited primary human lymphocytes was significantly increased. This approach, named peptide-enabled RNP delivery for CRISPR engineering (PERC), enables highly efficient and precise multiplexed T-cell engineering, offering several benefits compared to other delivery technologies. PERC is effective with adenine base editors, Cas9, and Cas12a nucleases, indicating broad compatibility with various CRISPR effectors. It is as straightforward to introduce as viral transduction and allows for precise editing of multiple genes simultaneously. Furthermore, PERC has shown promise in correcting pathogenic mutations associated with inborn immune defects when used with base editing enzymes [85].

Although considered a cost-effective approach, CPPs show low editing efficiency, low specificity, limited stability, immunogenicity, and endosomal trapping. The methods require further optimization to advance the use of CPPs in clinical research. CPPs' efficiencies to cross the cellular membranes vary depending on cell type and delivered cargo. Furthermore, challenges related to translocating the CRISPR/Cas9 complex into the nucleus must be addressed once it enters the cell.

### 3.2. Lipid-Based Delivery Systems

A promising strategy for drug delivery is to use advanced drug carriers known as lipid nanoparticles (LNPs), which encapsulate biological macromolecules, including nucleic acids (DNA or RNA) and proteins (Figure 3). Common approaches include enveloping the following: (1) plasmid DNA (pDNA) that encodes Cas9 and sgRNA, (2) Cas9 mRNA along with sgRNA, either together or individually, and (3) Cas9/sgRNA as a ribonucleoprotein (RNP) complex. Each method features unique benefits and drawbacks, necessitating specific formulation criteria for LNPs to maintain optimal compatibility and functionality [86].

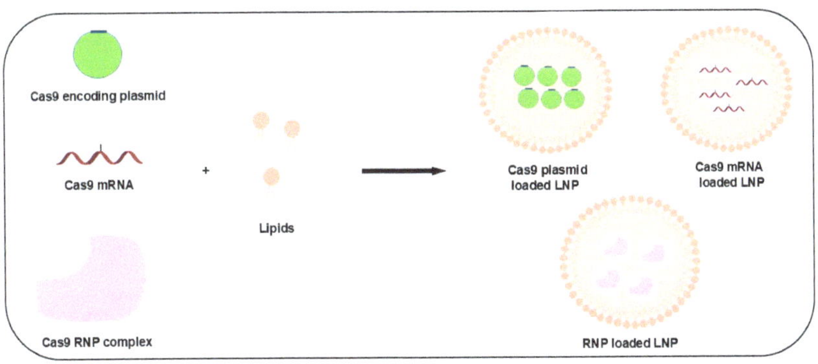


**Figure 3.** Schematic on the synthesis of LNP for CRISPR/Cas9 delivery system.

Kulkarni et al. developed an LNP composition of pDNA encoding Cas9 and gRNA using DLin-MC3-DMA, replacing the saturated helper lipid distearoylphosphatidylcholine (DSPC) with unsaturated phosphatidylcholine (PC) helper lipids. They also assessed the effectiveness of various compositions containing ionizable positively charged lipids combined with unsaturated PC helper lipids. Among these, the most effective composition for primary mesenchymal embryonic cells derived from chicken embryos used DLin-KC2-DMA and 1-stearoyl-2-oleoyl-sn-glycero-3-phosphocholine (SOPC). This composition resulted in a transfection effectiveness of 90% and a cell viability of over 85%, in contrast to 50% transfection efficiency and 33% cell viability observed with lipofectamine [87].

Several challenges in pDNA delivery, such as volume of plasmid for encapsulation, penetration of cell membranes, nonspecific interactions with serum or extracellular proteins, and cytotoxicity, have been addressed by enhancing encapsulation efficiency. This was achieved by compressing the volume of plasmids using chondroitin sulfate and protamine to create a dense core [88]. Their LNP composition included cholesterol, the permanently cationic lipid 1,2-Dioleoyl-3-trimethylammonium propane (DOTAP), and the helper lipid 1,2-dioleoyl-sn-glycero-3-phosphoethanolamine (DOPE). Combining DOTAP and DOPE facilitated increased transfection by fostering electrostatic interactions with cellular membranes. Additional modification with DSPE-PEG decreased toxicity, enhanced stability and solubility, extended half-life, and minimized immune response. The ratio of DOTAP to DOPE was crucial in determining physicochemical parameters. This formulation was tested on cancer cells (A375 melanoma cell line, PC3 prostate cancer cell line, and MCF-7 breast cancer cell line) with overexpressed polo-like kinase 1 (PLK-1). Flow cytometry demonstrated approximately 47% transfection efficiency in A375 cells, and high-throughput sequencing identified 1 to 20 indels in the gene of interest. This composition demonstrated superior genome editing effectiveness in vitro and in vivo compared to lipofectamine [88].

Siegwart et al. have addressed the challenges of co-delivering different-sized Cas9 mRNA (4.5 kb) and sgRNA (0.1 kb) in vivo [89] by developing a selective organ targeting (SORT) strategy that enables tissue-specific gene editing. SORT can be engineered to target-deliver mRNA, Cas9 mRNA in complex with sgRNA, and Cas9 RNP to the lung, spleen, and liver in mice.

Targeting the PLK1 gene via LNP has successfully facilitated gene editing both in vitro and in vivo, even without plasmid condensation agents. Li et al. utilized a reporter gene system to transfect HepG2-Luc cells and mice with HepG2-Luc xenograft tumors using a novel ionizable LNP composition [90]. By adding a step to improve the stability of LNPs, this composition effectively encapsulated CRISPR/Cas9 pDNA targeting PLK1. This method resulted in a 32% reduction in mRNA levels in vitro, decreased tumor growth rate, decreased PLK1 mRNA expression levels, and increased programmed cell death in tumor cells in vivo [90].

There is an increasing emphasis on delivering Cas9 mRNA rather than pDNA for gene editing in both in vitro and in vivo applications. LNPs are being used to encapsulate Cas9 mRNA and gRNA together or separately. Finn et al. explored how modifying the tertiary structure of Cas9 sgRNA can improve editing effectiveness in vivo, explicitly targeting the Ttr gene, which is highly expressed in rare amyloidosis disorders [91]. In another study, Qiu et al. generated an LNP-mediated delivery system for Cas9 mRNA, targeting the liver to disrupt the angiopoietin-like 3 (Angptl3) gene [92]. The group employed bioreducible LNPs to deliver both Cas9 mRNA and sgRNA, demonstrating high in vitro editing efficiency and significant decrease of the Pcsk9 gene in vivo. The system featured a tail-branched bioreducible lipidoid (306-O12B) combined with excipient lipids to co-deliver SpCas9 mRNA and sgRNA targeting Angptl3 in a single administration. The 306-O12B LNP effectively delivered Cas9 mRNA and sgAngptl3 to hepatocytes in wild-type C57BL/6 mice, achieving an editing efficiency of 38.5% and a 65.2% reduction in ANGPTL3 protein levels in serum. Furthermore, Angptl3 knockdown in the liver resulted in substantial reductions in low-density lipoprotein cholesterol (LDL-C) and triglyceride (TG) levels, without any indication of off-target mutations or liver toxicity at the nine most likely predicted sites [92].

LNPs have been effectively used to deliver adenine base editor mRNA and sgRNA for targeting PCSK9 in vivo. An LNP composition similar to ONPATTRO, which encapsulates base editor mRNA and sgRNA targeting PCSK9, demonstrated up to 67% editing efficiency in rodents and s34% in macaques [93]. Notably, the editing was predominantly confined to hepatic tissues, with minimal off-target effects observed in non-hepatic tissues in both species, indicating the formulation's tissue specificity.

Although there was a temporary rise in serum transaminase levels, indicating potential liver cell injury, the animals showed no symptoms, and the elevated levels resolved quickly [93].

Kenjo et al. employed an in vivo lipid screening technique to discover a new ionizable lipid, TCL053, for delivering mRNA via intramuscular injection [94]. Their LNP formulations with TCL053 encapsulated Cas9 mRNA and sgRNA separately. They were tested in a humanized mouse model of Duchenne muscular dystrophy (DMD), which involved a mouse model with Dmd1 exon 44 deletion and the addition of human DMD1 exon 45. This composition achieved approximately 10% exon skipping effectiveness in the tibialis anterior muscle, about five times higher than that observed with MC3-based LNPs. While serum cytokine levels increased 6 to 24 h after administration, these levels returned to normal within 7 days. The formulation's low immunogenicity allowed for the safe readministration of the LNPs once, twice, or three times at monthly intervals, resulting in cumulative DMD1 editing [94].

Wei et al. created a technique for generating and engineering altered lipid nanoparticles that effectively deliver the Cas9/gRNA RNP complex to various tissues [95]. Intravenous administration facilitated tissue-specific, multiplexed modification of six genes in the lungs of mice. The high efficacy of these carriers was leveraged to develop cancer models specific to organs in the livers and lungs of mice through targeted gene deletions. Additionally, the RNPs successfully restored dystrophin expression in dystrophin-deficient mice and sharply reduced PCSK9 levels in the blood serum and livers of C57BL/6 mice with these advanced carriers [95]. The 5A2-DOT-10 LNPs, which encapsulated Cas9/sgDMD RNPs, were administered weekly into the Tibialis Anterior (TA) muscles of mice with a DMD exon 44 deletion, resulting in a 4.2% recovery of dystrophin protein as quantified by Western blot analysis. Furthermore, in the group treated with 5A2-DOT-5 LNPs that encapsulated Cas9/sgPCSK9 RNPs, the T7EI assay demonstrated successful indel formation at the PCSK9 gene loci [95].

Wang et al. modified their LNP composition to include bioreducible lipids that can effectively deliver polyanionic RNPs to green fluorescent protein (GFP)-expressing HEK cells [96]. These bioreducible lipids enhance the endosomal escape of the cargo, achieving more than 50% efficiency in reducing enhanced green fluorescent protein (eGFP) signals. Nuclear localization signals (NLSs) on Cas9 facilitate its efficient transport into the nucleus, followed by genome editing [96]. The study highlights that employing a combinatorial approach to screen distinct LNP formulations, including anionic proteins and the formation of Cas9 with polyanionic sgRNAs, could lead to developing a highly effective gene-editing delivery system [96].

Zuris et al. have developed a technique utilizing standard cationic lipid nucleic acid transfection reagents to effectively introduce polyanionic proteins into human cells, even in the presence of serum [97]. This method effectively introduced several proteins, such as Cre recombinase, TALE- and Cas9-based transcription activators, and Cas9:sgRNA nuclease complexes. Results demonstrated that unmodified Cas9:sgRNA complexes achieved up to 80% genome editing efficiency, demonstrating higher specificity than DNA transfection. Additionally, this technique has proven effective for delivering RNP proteins into the inner ear of mice in vivo, leading to significant recombination and genome editing within hair cells [97].

Although concerns regarding lower transfection efficacy, stability, and the potential to trigger immune responses remain [98], the rapid advancements in research on LNPs and their successful use in delivering mRNA in the Pfizer and Moderna vaccines for SARS-CoV-2 is expected to advance the clinical application of LNP carriers. Beyond the lipids used in COVID-19 vaccines, significant efforts are underway to generate safe and effective ionizable lipids to enhance in vivo delivery. Currently, Intellia Therapeutics is at the forefront of translating LNP-mediated delivery of CRISPR therapeutics using mRNA into clinical settings, and it is expected that the application of new LNP-RNP systems will broaden into various therapeutic domains in the future.

### 3.3. Biopolymers

Recently, biopolymers have been considered promising CRISPR/Cas9 delivery vehicles due to their biocompatibility and low toxicity [99,100]. Proteins (e.g., albumin, collagen), polysaccharides (e.g., chitosan, alginate), and nucleic acids are among the natural polymers being explored for this purpose [100]. Zhang et al. reported one of the first chitosan-mediated delivery systems for gene therapy [101]. Chitosan was pegylated with poly(ethylene glycol) monomethyl ether (mPEG). These copolymer conjugates demonstrated the ability to shield DNA from DNase I degradation and achieved maximum transfection effectiveness. PEGylated chitosan was capable of carrying DNA through the mucus model. This can be important in the realm of lung diseases.

In various studies, the chitosan derivative carboxymethyl chitosan is used due to improved solubility and protonation of its amino groups, making it suitable for pH-dependent release [102]. Furthermore, carboxyl groups could be modified with a ternary polymer to induce the targeting moiety of the gene delivery system [103]. Whereas in most systems, chitosan is not used as a single molecule for Cas9 delivery, the decoration of the polymer construct with chitosan helps endosomal transport through the cell membrane. For instance, in a study by Srivastav et al. [104], chitosan-coated PLGA nanoparticles showed profound efficiency in genome editing, providing 70% improvement compared to the control according to the experimental settings [105].

Alginate, a naturally derived polymer, is widely recognized for its stability and ability to form water hydrogels, making it appealing for biomedical applications. It is mucoadhesive and mucopenetrating, enhancing its effectiveness in drug delivery systems. Additionally, alginate is FDA-approved, further supporting its use in clinical settings. However, its limitations include low encapsulation efficiency and a short lifetime. Despite these challenges, alginate offers significant advantages, including a high affinity to the CD44 receptor and the ability to be easily functionalized. It is also degraded by hyaluronidase, which can be advantageous in controlled degradation and drug release scenarios. These properties collectively make alginate a versatile but sometimes limited choice for certain therapeutic applications. Alallam et al. employed alginate nanoparticles (ALG NPs) as a CRISPR/Cas9 gene editing delivery system. Using an electrospray technique, the researchers successfully encapsulated two CRISPR plasmids within ALG NPs, achieving a mean nanoparticle size of 228 nm and a zeta potential of −4.42 mV. The encapsulation efficiency exceeded 99% while preserving the integrity of the CRISPR plasmids. The CRISPR-loaded ALG NPs demonstrated cytocompatibility and successfully delivered the Cas9 transgene into HepG2 cells, effectively editing the GFP gene by inducing double-strand breaks [106].

Cyclodextrin is a versatile polymer known for its ease of modification, making it highly adaptable for various biomedical applications. It is particularly effective in encapsulating bioactive molecules, thereby improving the stability of these encapsulated cargoes. This enhances the efficacy and shelf life of the therapeutic agents it carries. However, cyclodextrin typically requires additional modification for applications involving DNA condensation, as its natural structure does not inherently support this function. Notably, a supramolecular polymer system using disulfide-bridged biguanidyl adamantine and β-cyclodextrin-conjugated poly(ethylene imine) effectively mediates the controlled intracellular delivery of Cas9 RNP, achieving high genome-editing activity in both 293T cells and colorectal cancer (CRC) cells [107]. Additionally, when decorated with hyaluronic acid (HA), this system successfully targets mutant KRAS, significantly suppressing tumor growth in mouse models and offering a prospective therapeutic strategy for colorectal cancer treatment [107]. Cationic polymers, such as polyethyleneimine-β-cyclodextrin, have

efficiently delivered large plasmids that encode Cas9 and sgRNA, resulting in successful genome editing at specific loci [108]. These polymer-based systems provide advantages over viral vectors, including larger packaging capacity and improved safety profiles [51].

Protamine is another advantageous material for gene delivery studies and therapeutic applications owing to its high DNA condensation potential and inherent pharmacological activity. However, a significant disadvantage of protamine is its aggregating nature in circulation, which reduces efficacy and may cause adverse side effects. Despite this limitation, protamine remains essential in drug delivery due to its unique properties. A novel biomimetic core-shell system mimicking cell membranes was designed for light-controlled and precise gene editing. This system explicitly targets the elevated levels of hypoxia-inducible factor-1 alpha (HIF-1$\alpha$) linked to cancer metastasis and resistance to treatment. This system combines protamine and calcium ions for efficient CRISPR/Cas9 delivery, with a hidden shell modified for tumor targeting and light-triggered gene editing. The system facilitates endosomal escape upon laser activation and releases the CRISPR/Cas9 assembly in the cytoplasm, allowing for precise gene editing. This approach significantly improves the therapeutic effectiveness of chemotherapy medications, reduces cancer spread, and offers an approach to cancer treatment. The system demonstrated enhanced antimetastatic effects in neoplastic H1299 cells and improved the in vivo efficacy of paclitaxel, offering a promising strategy for cancer therapy through precise gene disruption [109]. Another study highlighted an innovative approach to enhancing the delivery effectiveness of protamine-based transporters by incorporating lipids. A PEG phospholipid-altered positively charged lipid nanoparticle was developed, featuring a protamine, plasmid, and chondroitin sulfate core with a cationic lipid capsule. This design effectively shielded DNA and RNA from degradation. It facilitated release from endosomes, achieving a transfection efficiency of 47.4% in A375 cells in vitro and significantly suppressing tumor development in vivo through intertumoral injection [88].

While all the methods discussed above focus on utilizing polymer-based carriers to transport the RNP complex, an alternative and intriguing approach is directly modifying the Cas9 surface with polymers. In 2021, Kang et al. explored this by decorating the Cas9 surface with branched PEI, demonstrating that it could effectively complex with gRNA [21] and a DNA donor template for HDR [110]. The reported HDR efficiency was approximately 31%, with minimal cytotoxicity. This was the first Cas9 surface modification with polymers, which the authors called a "minimal carrier-assisted" delivery technique. This direct modification approach offers several advantages: polymers can continuously shield Cas9 from the immune system, enhancing biocompatibility. Additionally, polymers can stabilize the RNP complex and protect both the gRNA and donor DNA, potentially improving the effectiveness and safety of the gene-editing process.

Thus, polymers provide greater rigidity and stability than lipid nanoparticles (LNPs), and they can be engineered into various nanostructures with customizable sizes, charges, and compositions. The outer shell of polymer nanoparticles can be functionalized with unique ligands or antibodies, enabling precise delivery to particular cell types or tissues, which enhances the precision of CRISPR/Cas9 transport. Additionally, polymers are advantageous due to their low toxicity and minimal immunogenicity. Among polymers, natural biopolymers are often favored over synthetic ones for CRISPR/Cas9 delivery due to their superior biocompatibility and biodegradability, making them safer for in vivo applications.

## 4. Synthetic Polymer-Based Carriers

Recent research shows promising results in using synthetic polymer-based delivery systems for CRISPR/Cas9 gene editing. These benefits include customized design, reduced immunogenicity, direct functionalization, and high-yield fabrication without the difficulties of stoichiometric control between CRISPR components that are inherent to lipid-protein nanoparticles [111,112].

Polyethylenimine (PEI) is extensively utilized due to its strong cationic nature, making it ideal for gene transfection [113]. For instance, branched PEI-25K successfully delivered CRISPR/Cas9 plasmids to Neuro2a cells to target the Sck26a4 locus, mediating targeted gene editing [114]. PEI-functionalized magnetic nanoparticles effectively transfected HEK293 cells, achieving genome editing rates comparable to lipofectamine [115]. Polyethyleneimine-β-cyclodextrin (PC) efficiently delivered large Cas9/sgRNA plasmids, successfully editing two genomic loci: the hemoglobin subunit beta, achieving up to 19.1% editing efficiency, and rhomboid 5 homolog 1, with 7% efficiency [108]. Carbon dots conjugated with PEI1.8k and arginine (CD-PEI1.8k-Arg) outperformed native PEI in delivering CRISPR complex across various cell lines, maintaining efficiency in high serum concentrations and low plasmid doses. This system also effectively knocked out the GFP gene and showed potential for local brain tissue delivery [116]. Moradi et al. designed nanoparticles by combining an arginine-disulfide linker with low-molecular-weight polyethyleneimine (PEI1.8k), creating PEI1.8k-Arg nanoparticles. These nanoparticles enhance plasmid release and membrane permeability and facilitate nuclear distribution, resulting in improved transfection effectiveness compared to unmodified PEI1.8k.

The transporting system was influential not only in conventional cells (HEK 293T) but also in cells that are considered challenging to transfect, such as primary cells (HUVECs), cancer cells (HeLa), and neuronal cells (PC-12), achieving between 5- and 10-fold increases in transfection compared to the standard polymeric transfection agent [117]. These studies highlight the versatility and effectiveness of PEI-based carriers for CRISPR/Cas9 delivery, paving the way for improved gene editing applications. Li et al. proposed a method of precise genome editing that could be imaging-guided and stimuli-triggered, making the process visible and controllable [118]. The complex structure of the polymer construct with the alkyl side chains and fluorinated PEI formed the hydrophobic core that holds Cas9 via electrostatic interactions. Additionally, glucocorticoid dexamethasone was introduced into the polymer backbone to dilate the nuclear pores upon encountering the nuclear glucocorticoid receptors. The construct's elegance is finely tuned through the photothermal transducing property of polymer brush chains that are triggered by laser irradiation. Studies conducted in vitro on HEK-293T cells and HCT 116 cell lines showed that the approach is not cytotoxic, and in vivo data confirmed that the strategy is viable, allowing for genome editing to be carried out under physically visible control [118].

Polylactic-co-glycolic acid (PLGA)-based nanoparticles can also potentially deliver CRISPR/Cas9 components for gene editing. Jo et al. proved that these nanoparticles carry large CRISPR-Cas9 plasmids and release them in primarily bone-derived macrophages within 24 h [119]. PLGA nanoparticles were exploited to efficiently deliver Cas9 protein and sgRNA to hematopoietic stem and progenitor cells, resulting in gene editing and enhanced fetal hemoglobin expression without causing cellular cytotoxicity [120].

Recent studies have used PEG-based transporting platforms for CRISPR/Cas9 gene editing. PEGylated nanoparticles based on α-helical polypeptides resulted in effective cellular uptake and release from endosomes, yielding a 47.3% gene editing efficiency in vitro and 35% knockout in vivo [121]. PEGylated PLANAs, a class of modified peptide/lipid-associated nucleic acids (PLANAs), exhibited reduced toxicity and a transfection efficacy equivalent to commercial reagents for CRISPR/Cas9 ribonucleoprotein delivery [122]. Liver-targeted polymeric micellar nanoparticles containing pCas9 (PEG-polycarbonate and cholesterol-modified PEI) exhibited superior cellular uptake, biocompatibility, in vivo retention within the tumor (via passive targeting), gene editing capability, and antitumor activity following IV administration to mice [123]. Moreover, Kataoka et al. demonstrated the challenging co-delivery of Cas9 mRNA and sgRNA using a poly(ethylene glycol)-shielded polyion complex by co-encapsulating sgRNA with Cas9 mRNA in a single platform [124]. Following intraparenchymal administration, this platform enabled efficient genome editing in mouse brain parenchymal cells.

Poly(beta-amino ester) (PBAE) polymers represent a novel type of nonviral vector for CRISPR/Cas9-based gene editing and other therapeutic nucleic acids. These biodegradable polymers have several advantages, including high transfection efficiency, large packaging capacity, and safety [125]. PBAEs can effectively deliver plasmid DNA encoding Cas9 and sgRNA for gene knockout and deletion [126] and base editors for precise gene editing [127]. Modifications to PBAEs, such as carboxylation and guanidylation, have enhanced their ability to deliver proteins and CRISPR/Cas9 ribonucleoproteins [128,129]. Recent advancements include cyclization-enhanced PBAEs for improved gene editing in disease models [130] and highly branched PBAEs for targeted genomic excision [51]. These developments emphasize the prospects of PBAEs as robust and efficient transporting vehicles for various gene editing applications in vitro and in vivo [131]. In a 2022 study by El-Kharrag et al., RNP complexes targeting the CD33 gene were transported to CD34+ cells utilizing polymer nanoparticles based on PBAEs, resulting in an 85% cell survival rate and a CD33 expression reduction ranging from 13% to 85%. Compared to electroporation, the nanoparticle delivery method showed higher cell survival (85% vs. 72%), more significant CD33 expression reduction (88% vs. 76%), and superior long-term multilineage engraftment potential [132].

Highly branched poly(β-amino ester) polymers have demonstrated potential in delivering CRISPR/Cas9 components, achieving up to 40% targeted genomic deletion in human cells [51]. Rui et al. reported a novel category of carboxylated branched poly(β-amino ester) capable of self-assembling into nanoparticles for effective cellular transport of CRISPR/Cas9 RNPs. In vitro, nanoparticles facilitated swift cellular uptake, effective endosomal release, and the delivery of functional proteins into the cytosol. RNP delivery in vivo triggered increased levels of gene editing at low RNP doses [128]. Authors suggest that encapsulating protein cargo within polymeric nanoparticles can reduce immune reactions by shielding the protein from circulating neutralizing antibodies. This protection may facilitate CRISPR gene editing in patients with an existing immune response. Overall, PBAEs possess key features for gene delivery, such as a reversible positive charge for nucleic acid binding, high buffering capacity, and rapid degradability. Still, their instability in physiological environments can limit transfection efficiency. However, their chemical versatility allows for modifications and blending with other materials to enhance stability and tailor them for specific delivery applications.

Poly [2-dimethylaminoethyl methacrylate] (pDMAEMA)-based polymers can efficiently condense plasmid DNA into nanoparticles, facilitating cellular uptake and transfection [133,134]. These polymers exhibit excellent transfection efficiency while maintaining low levels of cytotoxicity compared to commercial transfection reagents [135,136]. The proton sponge effect of pDMAEMA aids in endosomal release, contributing to its superior transfection capabilities [137]. Recent advancements include the development of hyperbranched and stimuli-responsive polymeric carriers for controlled CRISPR/Cas9 transport [136,138].

In response to the shortcomings of traditional polymer-based delivery systems, researchers have sought new strategies capitalizing on the virtues of both polymers and lipids. An promising alternative strategy involves synthesizing hybrid polymers, where lipids are grafted to a polymeric core-shell. These synthetic polymer-based delivery system advancements have demonstrated efficient transfection and gene editing capabilities, often surpassing commercial liposome-based reagents [135,138,139]. As a model system, the cationic lipid-assisted nanoparticle (CLAN) was optimized for macrophage delivery of Cas9 mRNA (mCas9) and sgRNA targeting NLRP3. This method resulted in the successful knockdown of NLRP3 gene expression that inhibited activation of the NLRP3 inflammasome upon diverse stimuli and uncovered the possibility of utilizing CLAN nano complexes as immune responses and modulatory tools through targeted gene delivery [140]. Zhang et al. used a similar strategy to enclose mCas9/gCD40 genes into PEG-b-PLGA-based CLANs for reprogramming dendritic cells to decrease transplant rejection [108]. Similarly, CLAN systems present inhibited netrin-1 expression in type 2 diabetic symptoms [141].

While most polymer carriers encapsulate RNPs through electrostatic interactions, our current research focuses on covalent modification using a "grafting from" approach

(Figure 4). This method employs atom-transfer radical polymerization (ATRP) to attach polymers to the surface of Cas9, modifying the enzyme with polymer chains. The advantage of this method is that it effectively immunoisolates and stabilizes both Cas9 and the sgRNA within the complex [142]. The "grafting from" technique allows for the growth of cell-permeable polymers to efficiently deliver the CRISPR/Cas9 system into cells [143]. Furthermore, our previous work has demonstrated that incorporating peptide linkers into the polymer sidechains, which can be cleaved by proteases, enables the controlled release of the enzyme core [144]. Similarly, Cas9 can be modified to facilitate its release in the nucleus. Additionally, incorporating nuclear localization signal peptides into the polymer sidechains can improve the complex's ability to cross the nuclear envelope effectively. Overall, with the swift advancement in CRISPR technologies and the progress in nonviral delivery systems, these challenges are anticipated to be addressed shortly, paving the way for widespread integration of CRISPR/Cas9-based genome editing therapies into clinical practice.

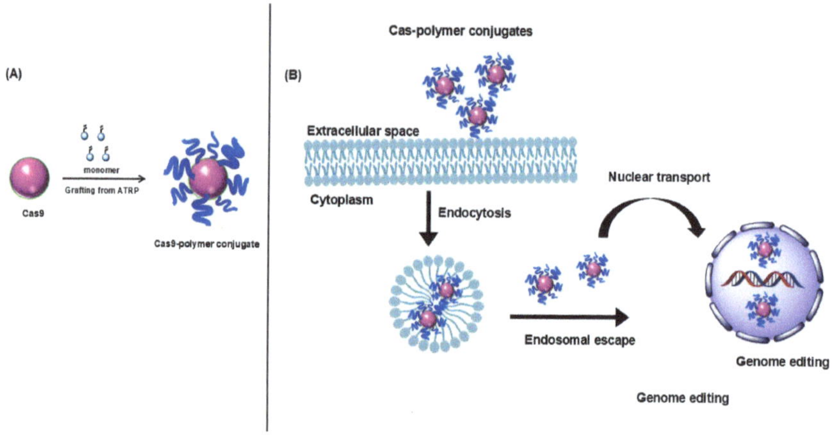


**Figure 4.** "Grafting from" Cas9. (**A**) ATRP-synthesis of Cas9-polymer conjugates. (**B**) Delivery of Cas9-polymer conjugates into cells.

The application of ATRP has emerged as a promising strategy in gene therapy [119,145]. Its robustness allows for precise control over polymer architecture [146,147], size [144], charge [148,149], and hydrophilicity [149], facilitating the synthesis of tailored carriers. Recently, ATRP has been developed to be more biocompatible by reducing the copper catalyst concentration required for the process and using low-energy green light irradiation [150].

Matyjaszewski et al. demonstrated that cationic nanogels containing DMAEMA and a cross-linker with reducible disulfide moieties, synthesized via ATRP, are highly effective for delivering pDNA and short interfering RNA (siRNA) [151]. Additionally, annealing complementary RNA strands with siRNA and conjugating with polymers from both sides can solve problems regarding endonuclease digestion and facilitate cellular uptake [152]. The researchers further showed the synthesis of block polymers with positively charged sulfonium (meth)acrylate and poly(ethylene oxide) using ATRP as a siRNA carrier. Block copolymers successfully formed polyplexes with siRNA and protected the siRNA against nuclease digestion. The efficiency of mRNA knockdown was evident from glyceraldehyde 3-phosphate dehydrogenase (*Gapdh*) decreased expression in murine preosteoblasts [153]. Hollinger et al. demonstrated that ATRP-synthesized cationic nanogel-siRNA polyplexes are efficient in in vivo knockdown of GFP in a mouse model [154].

ATRP also enables the synthesis of star polymers, which are widely used in gene delivery. These are branched polymers with multiple arms attached to one central core. Star polymers, consisting of poly(ethylene glycol) methyl ether methacrylate (PEGMA), peptide (Gly-Arg-Gly-Asp-Ser) modified PEG acrylate (GRGDS-PEG-Acryl), fluorescein o-methacrylate (FMA), and ethylene glycol dimethacrylate (EGDMA) were synthesized via ATRP [155]. These polymers demonstrated 90% cell viability after 24 h incubation with MC3T3-E1.4 cells. Additionally, peptide modification of the polymers resulted in 100% cellular uptake of the star polymers observed by flow cytometry. ATRP-prepared star polymers with PEGMA, DMAEMA, and a disulfide methacrylate cross-linker showed over 80% biocompatibility, even at high concentrations, and successful cellular uptake [156]. Further, star polymers synthesized from DMAEMA and EGDMA were combined with either pDNA or siRNA to form polyplexes [157]. This study demonstrated that low molar ratios of star polymers enabled the intracellular delivery of nucleic acids.

Recently, the synthesis of a new acylation agent that enables the incorporation of ATRP initiator into short synthetic RNA and natural biomass RNA was reported [158]. These RNA-initiator conjugates were subsequently used to grow polymers via photoinduced ATRP, allowing fine tuning of the properties of RNA-polymer hybrids. While creating nucleic acid-polymer conjugates via ATRP offers many applications, the synthesis is limited to grafting the polymers from the terminus of nucleic acids. To overcome this hurdle, Matyjaszewski et al. presented a novel serinol-based α-bromoisobutyryl (SBiB) phosphoramidite, which enables the multiple attachments of polymerization initiator groups at any site on an oligonucleotide [159]. This approach enables the synthesis a wider variety of nucleic acid-polymer hybrids. Moreover, the researchers demonstrated a way to circumvent the intrinsic instability of RNA molecules by adding protecting groups on the 2′-hydroxyl positions [160]. This resulted in the ATRP synthesis of highly stable RNA-polymer hybrids with the potential to expand the field of RNA-based polymeric materials.

Das et al. developed a method of modifying the surface of exosomes with oligonucleotide tethers [161]. They showed that the cellular uptake of the exosomes could be adjusted with tethered aptamer while the targeting specificity could be adjusted with tethered protein. Notably, the developed strategy is independent of the exosome source, making it universally applicable.

The development of a fluorescent nanotag capable of detecting protein targets in confocal microscopy and flow cytometry has been demonstrated by ATRP synthesis of bottlebrush polymers with hundreds of duplex DNA strands [162]. Hundreds of fluorescent dyes were covalently attached to DNA duplexes and tethered to a single antibody probe without risking self-quenching.

Matyjaszewski and Das demonstrated the synthesis of protein-polymer conjugates with noncovalent bonds mediated by DNA [163]. Despite being noncovalent, the DNA-mediated method offers precise pairing and assembly characteristics inherent to DNA. The same group reported the solid-phase synthesis of DNA-polymer hybrids, broadening the scope of advanced polymer-bioconjugate functional materials [164].

In summary, ATRP has proven to be a robust and versatile method for synthesizing polymers with precise control over their properties, making it a valuable tool in gene therapy. Its ability to create customized carriers and facilitate efficient nucleic acid delivery underscores its significant potential in advancing therapeutic applications.

## 5. Physical Transfection Methods for CRISPR/Cas9 System Delivery

### 5.1. Mechanoporation

Mechanoporation uses mechanical or shear forces to generate pores in cellular membranes. Microinjection is a conventional method of mechanical transfection for delivering CRISPR/Cas9 into cells [165–167]. This method injects CRISPR/Cas9 directly into cells using a microneedle under microscopic visualization. Direct transfer via microinjection of the CRISPR/Cas9 complex provides the benefit of transporting the entire CRISPR/Cas9 system, including components of various sizes, such as proteins. This method bypasses the limitations associated with size constraints that may exist with other delivery approaches. For instance, Ma et al. [168] demonstrated that microinjection was effectively used to knock out four genes (ApoE, B2m, Prf1, and Prkdc) in rats in a single step. The microinjection technique achieved this by co-injecting Cas9 mRNA and sgRNAs into zygotes. In a similar study, sgRNA has been effectively introduced alongside Cas9 protein targeting ovine myostatin (MSTN) by microinjecting it into the cytoplasm of ovine zygotes, aiming to disrupt the MSTN genomic sequence across the entire embryo; this approach effectively knocked out MSTN in sheep [166]. However, despite its effectiveness, microinjection presents challenges due to its demanding technical requirements, as it involves manually injecting a single cell [169].

One way to overcome the limitation of single-cell transfection is a microfluidic-based biophysical mechanoporation technique that involves passing several cells at increased velocities through narrow micrometer-scale openings. This process disrupts the plasma membrane, delivering different cargoes directly across the cytosol of various cells. For example, Sharei et al. utilized microfabricated silicon channels to generate temporary openings for introducing materials into cells [104]. Their method involved passing a mixture of delivery materials and cells through a microfluidic channel containing a constriction with a width of approximately 30–80% of the diameter of the cells. This approach facilitated the formation of temporary pores in the cells, enabling efficient delivery of materials. In a similar study, Han et al. developed a series of microfluidic silicon devices featuring a series of narrowing channels with varying dimensions formed by structures of different shapes [170]. The study showed that this method effectively facilitated the delivery of CRISPR components into traditionally challenging cell types like immune and stem cells.

Navigating cells towards nanoscale cell-penetrating structures is another mechanoporation technique that efficiently transfects larger numbers of cells by directly penetrating the cell membrane. In particular, silicon nanoneedles measuring 200 nm in diameter and coated with Cas9-sgRNA have been employed successfully [171]. Furthermore, silicon nanoneedles have been employed to convey plasmid DNA-encoding vascular endothelial growth factor into mouse muscles, thereby enhancing tissue neovascularization [172]. In this study, cells were interfaced with nanoneedles either by seeding them over the nanoneedles or pressing them over a monolayer of cells [172]. These nanoneedles puncture the plasma membrane, enabling the delivery of Cas9 complexes into the cells for targeted gene editing or manipulation. A key advantage of this strategy is that it transfects adherent cells in a monolayer rather than requiring them to be in suspension.

However, all the abovementioned mechanoporation techniques typically introduce materials into the cytoplasm, necessitating following transport of these materials into the nucleus for effective genome editing, which can lead to undesired transcription reactions. While specific research groups have demonstrated the ability to use the microinjection technique to directly deliver CRISPR/Cas9 constructs into the nucleus [173], this approach is low throughput and requires a highly skilled technician. A method called force-controlled fluidic injection (FCFI) into single-cell nuclei for improved CRISPR delivery has been developed to tackle this challenge. FCFI technology combines microfluidics and force microscopy by incorporating microscopic channels into force-sensitive probes. This integration allows for precise handling of liquid volumes at the femtoliter scale and enables force-controlled manipulations of microscopic objects, offering improved control over CRISPR delivery into cell nuclei [174]. However, micro- and nano-injections restrict their use for in vivo transport due to the efficiency of transfection being limited to individual cells.

### 5.2. Electroporation

Electroporation is the second extensively utilized physical transfection method for delivering genetic materials into cells [86,175]. This technique involves the application of a strong electric field across a cell membrane. The electric field surpasses the membrane's capacitance, leading to the transient opening of nanometer-sized pores or swift disruption of the lipid bilayers, thereby facilitating efficient intracellular transport. Since this method does not require microinjection skills, it allows for the simultaneous treatment of a considerably greater amount of cells or embryos. For instance, Hashimoto et al. achieved effective genome editing in mouse embryos by optimizing the electroporation conditions for introducing RNAs of the CRISPR/Cas9 complex into zygotes [176].

Similarly, Alghadban et al. noted enhancements in mutagenesis efficiency for producing ssODN repair templates, along with increased rates of embryo survival and development, when administering CRISPR/Cas9 systems as ribonucleoproteins (RNPs) through zygote electroporation [177]. Wu et al. corrected a cataract-inducing mutation by CRISPR-Cas9-mediated gene modification in stem cells of spermatogonial mouse [178]. Rathbone et al. studied the impacts of electroporating Cas9 RNPs targeting Hpd, the gene encoding hydroxyphenylpyruvate dioxygenase, into primary mouse and human hepatocytes. They reported increased levels of gene editing in both cell types [179].

However, electroporation technology demands specific conditions tailored to different cell types. Applying strong currents can damage cells through excessive heat exposure, ionic imbalances, and pH alterations, rendering this method unfit for cells sensitive to stress. Therefore, meticulous evaluation and identification of suitable conditions are imperative for electroporation to achieve effective transfection while preserving cell integrity.

Xu et al. devised a novel tube-shaped cuvette to address several drawbacks associated with electroporation. This method targeted the knockout of β2-microglobulin (B2M), a crucial component of major histocompatibility complex (MHC) class I molecules, within primary human mesenchymal stem cells. The study demonstrated a remarkable 80.2% reduction in B2M expression by delivering Cas9/gRNA RNP and a single-stranded oligodeoxynucleotide (ssODN), introducing a frameshift mutation. Additionally, the technique significantly decreased the surface expression of the protein in mesenchymal stem cells, dropping from 95.6% to 59.9% [180]. In a separate investigation, nanostructure-mediated electroporation has facilitated the downsizing of physical transfection methods, leading to improved efficiency and precision. Moreover, it ensures uniform treatment of cells with minimal effects on viability, contrasting with the uneven cell permeabilization associated with bulk electroporation [181]. Notably, in gene editing applications in vivo, electroporation has effectively transported genetic materials into the mouse retina [182].

It is worth noting that all of the abovementioned studies were conducted using in vitro and ex vivo approaches. There are only a few reports of successful application of electroporation techniques for delivering Cas9-mediated systems in vivo. For example, Wu et al. utilized electroporation on mouse tail skin to restore C7 function in recessive dystrophic epidermolysis bullosa (RDEB) mice. They noted a rise in epidermal–dermal adhesion from 30% to 60% within 3 to 5 days following a single administration. Nevertheless, FACS analysis of tdTomato+ epidermal cells treated using this strategy showed fluorescence in 2% of the cells. Moreover, the enhanced epidermal–dermal adhesion observed in treated mice was not maintained beyond 5 days, raising concerns about the longevity of these gene edits [183].

While the success of the electroporation technique and its modifications hold promise for CRISPR/Cas9 gene editing for in vivo applications, several significant limitations need to be addressed before it can be considered safe and efficient for human use in clinical settings. These limitations include potential damage to surrounding tissues associated with the procedure and a limited comprehension of off-target effects. To overcome the limitations associated with high-voltage electroporation, researchers are exploring alternative methods of cellular poration, such as thermoporation [184], optoporation [185], and acoustoporation [186], which aim to retain the scalability and ease of use of electroporation while mitigating its drawbacks.

### 5.3. Hydrodynamic Injection

While mechanoporation and electroporation are primarily used with in vitro or ex vivo cultured cells, hydrodynamic injection has been successfully employed for in vivo CRISPR/Cas9 complex delivery. Hydrodynamic injection entails administering a substantial volume of solution containing the CRISPR/Cas9 system into the animal's circulatory system [187]. This sudden rise in hydrodynamic pressure temporarily enhances the permeability of endothelial and parenchymal cells, enabling the CRISPR/Cas9 complex to penetrate cells in various tissues, such as the heart [85,86], liver [87–91], and lungs [188].

As an example, Schuh et al. demonstrated that hydrodynamic injection of a liposomal complex transporting the CRISPR/Cas9 plasmid and a donor vector in newborn Mucopolysaccharidosis type I mice resulted in a remarkable rise in serum alpha-L-iduronidase levels (IDUA) for up to 6 months. After hydrodynamic injection, they observed a marked biodistribution of the complexes in the lungs and heart. This supported the findings of elevated IDUA activity and decreased accumulation of glycosaminoglycans, particularly in these tissues [188]. However, this technically simple method can be rather distressing to the organism, often causing cardiac impairment, liver enlargement, and increased blood pressure [189]. To mitigate the hemodynamic side effects due to the rapid administration of a large volume, it is vital to moderate the conditions to ensure safety. One effective strategy is to bypass the blood vessels of the target organ and directly inject the solution. This approach achieved through catheterization and surgical techniques in large animals has allowed protein expression levels in tissues to resemble closely those achieved in gold-standard models. These potential outcomes in delivering CRISPR constructs have sparked renewed clinical enthusiasm in the gene transfer technique [189].

In summary, while physical transfection methods offer advantages, they have significant limitations for in vivo applications due to their invasive nature, making them primarily suitable for in vitro systems. Nevertheless, recent advancements in microtechnology and nanotechnology have introduced innovative physical transfection methods, presenting potential opportunities to expand the application of these techniques for use in human settings [190,191].

## 6. Conclusions and Future Perspectives

A significant milestone in CRISPR/Cas9 technology was achieved in 2023, when the US FDA approved the first CRISPR/Cas9-edited cell-based gene therapy, Gasgevy™ (Vertex Pharmaceuticals), for treating sickle cell disease and beta-thalassemia in patients aged 12 years and older [192]. Despite the remarkable achievements in gene therapy through the CRISPR/Cas9 system, ensuring the safe and effective application of this technology presents a conundrum. The most pressing challenge of this technology remains its delivery systems. Although several different techniques are currently being employed to deliver CRISPR into cells, each comes with its own strengths and weaknesses (Table 1). Therefore, the need for a universal platform for CRISPR/Cas9 has become more urgent than ever.

**Table 1.** Characteristics of CRISPR/Cas9 delivery systems.

| Delivery Method | Delivery Formats | Advantages | Disadvantages | Application |
|---|---|---|---|---|
| Adeno-associated virus vectors (AAV) | DNA | Low immunogenicity even at high doses | Limited packaging capacity requires more than one vector | Gene therapy for various genetic diseases |
| Adenoviral vectors (AdV) | DNA | Increased packaging capacity within one vector | Triggers acute immune response | Gene therapy for genetic diseases |
| Lentiviral vectors (LV) | DNA | Increased packaging capacity and low immunogenicity | Undesirable off-target effects observed in conjunction with CRISPR-Cas9 | Primarily utilized for the development of screening tools |
| Lipid nanoparticles (LNPs) | DNA, mRNA, RNP | Low off-target effects, easy to produce, low cost, FDA-approved | Endosomal degradation of cargo, requires optimization | In vitro and in vivo genome editing |
| Cell-penetrating peptides (CPPs) | RNP | Low off-target effects | Low efficiency, immunogenicity | Genome editing for cells in vitro |
| Polymer-based delivery | DNA, mRNA, RNP | Low off-target effects, easy to produce, large packaging capacity | Variable efficiency, cytotoxicity | In vitro genome editing |

Generally, the most efficient gene editing outcomes with limited off-target effects are achieved by providing the RNP complex rather than plasmid DNA or mRNA. However, the direct delivery of RNP complexes presents several challenges. First, the hydrophobicity of the nucleic acids means they do not readily dissolve in water and cannot pass through cell membranes efficiently. Second, the negative charge that the phosphate backbone gives nucleic acids can limit their ability to be delivered into cells, as the cell membrane is also negatively charged. Additionally, nucleic acids are easily degraded by enzymes, mainly nucleases from plasma and intracellular nucleases, which limits their in vivo stability and efficacy in reaching target cells [193]. The immune system may further complicate delivery, as nucleic acids and bacterial-origin enzymes are potentially immunogenic, producing antibodies against both the nucleic acids and Cas9. To overcome these challenges, delivering CRISPR/Cas9 RNP complexes via functional biomaterials and synthetic carriers may significantly enhance the efficiency and potency of gene editing applications.

**Author Contributions:** Conceptualization, B.K., K.M. and S.A.; writing—original draft preparation, B.K., A.T., Y.S., A.N. and H.M.; writing—review and editing, B.K., K.M. and S.A.; funding acquisition, B.K. and K.M. All authors have read and agreed to the published version of the manuscript.

**Funding:** This research was funded by the Science Committee Ministry of Science and Higher Education of the Republic of Kazakhstan, grant number AP14871448, and NSF grant DMR 2202747.

**Institutional Review Board Statement:** Not applicable.

**Informed Consent Statement:** Not applicable.

**Data Availability Statement:** Not applicable.

**Conflicts of Interest:** The authors declare no conflicts of interest.

## References

1. Sorek, R.; Lawrence, C.; Wiedenheft, B. CRISPR-mediated adaptive immune systems in bacteria and archaea. *Annu. Rev. Biochem.* **2013**, *82*, 237–266. [CrossRef] [PubMed]
2. Seed, K.D.; Lazinski, D.W.; Calderwood, S.B.; Camilli, A. A bacteriophage encodes its own CRISPR/Cas adaptive response to evade host innate immunity. *Nature* **2013**, *494*, 489–491. [CrossRef] [PubMed]
3. Dimitriu, T.; Szczelkun, M.D.; Westra, E.R. Evolutionary Ecology and Interplay of Prokaryotic Innate and Adaptive Immune Systems. *Curr. Biol.* **2020**, *30*, 1189–1202. [CrossRef] [PubMed]
4. Wang, H.-X.; Li, M.; Lee, C.M.; Chakraborty, S.; Kim, H.-W.; Bao, G.; Leong, K.W. CRISPR/Cas9-Based Genome Editing for Disease Modeling and Therapy: Challenges and Opportunities for Nonviral Delivery. *Chem. Rev.* **2017**, *117*, 9874–9906. [CrossRef] [PubMed]
5. Knott, G.J.; Doudna, J.A. CRISPR-Cas guides the future of genetic engineering. *Science* **2018**, *361*, 866–869. [CrossRef] [PubMed]
6. Zhang, F.; Wen, Y.; Guo, X. CRISPR/Cas9 for genome editing: Progress, implications and challenges. *Hum. Mol. Genet.* **2014**, *23*, R40–R46. [CrossRef]
7. Jiang, F.; Doudna, J.A. CRISPR-Cas9 Structures and Mechanisms. *Annu. Rev. Biophys.* **2017**, *46*, 505–529. [CrossRef]
8. Jiang, W.; Marraffini, L.A. CRISPR-Cas: New Tools for Genetic Manipulations from Bacterial Immunity Systems. *Annu. Rev. Microbiol.* **2015**, *69*, 209–228. [CrossRef]
9. Chen, F.; Alphonse, M.; Liu, Q. Strategies for nonviral nanoparticle-based delivery of CRISPR/Cas9 therapeutics. *Wiley Interdiscip. Rev. Nanomed. Nanobiotechnol.* **2020**, *12*, e1609. [CrossRef]
10. Wu, X.; Kriz, A.J.; Sharp, P.A. Target specificity of the CRISPR-Cas9 system. *Quant. Biol.* **2014**, *2*, 59–70. [CrossRef]
11. Yin, H.; Song, C.-Q.; Suresh, S.; Wu, Q.; Walsh, S.; Rhym, L.H.; Mintzer, E.; Bolukbasi, M.F.; Zhu, L.J.; Kauffman, K.; et al. Structure-guided chemical modification of guide RNA enables potent non-viral in vivo genome editing. *Nat. Biotechnol.* **2017**, *35*, 1179–1187. [CrossRef] [PubMed]
12. Liang, X.; Potter, J.; Kumar, S.; Zou, Y.; Quintanilla, R.; Sridharan, M.; Carte, J.; Chen, W.; Roark, N.; Ranganathan, S.; et al. Rapid and highly efficient mammalian cell engineering via Cas9 protein transfection. *J. Biotechnol.* **2015**, *208*, 44–53. [CrossRef]
13. You, L.; Tong, R.; Li, M.; Liu, Y.; Xue, J.; Lu, Y. Advancements and Obstacles of CRISPR-Cas9 Technology in Translational Research. *Mol. Ther. Methods Clin. Dev.* **2019**, *13*, 359–370. [CrossRef] [PubMed]
14. Wilmott, R.W.; Amin, R.S.; Perez, C.R.; Wert, S.E.; Keller, G.; Boivin, G.P.; Hirsch, R.; De Inocencio, J.; Lu, P.; Reising, S.; et al. Safety of adenovirus-mediated transfer of the human cystic fibrosis transmembrane conductance regulator cDNA to the lungs of nonhuman primates. *Hum. Gene Ther.* **1996**, *3*, 301–3018. [CrossRef] [PubMed]
15. Armentano, D.; Sookdeo, C.C.; Hehir, K.M.; Gregory, R.J.; George, J.A.S.; Prince, G.A.; Wadsworth, S.C.; Smith, A.E. Characterization of an Adenovirus Gene Transfer Vector Containing an E4 Deletion. *Hum. Gene Ther.* **1995**, *6*, 1343–1353. [CrossRef]

16. Engelhardt, J.F.; Ye, X.; Doranz, B.; Wilson, J.M. Ablation of E2A in recombinant adenoviruses improves transgene persistence and decreases inflammatory response in mouse liver. *Proc. Natl. Acad. Sci. USA* **1994**, *91*, 6196–6200. [CrossRef]
17. Lau, C.H.; Suh, Y. In vivo genome editing in animals using AAV-CRISPR system: Applications to translational research of human disease. *F1000Research* **2017**, *20*, 2153. [CrossRef]
18. Maddalena, A.; Tornabene, P.; Tiberi, P.; Minopoli, R.; Manfredi, A.; Mutarelli, M.; Rossi, S.; Simonelli, F.; Naggert, J.K.; Cacchiarelli, D.; et al. Triple Vectors Expand AAV Transfer Capacity in the Retina. *Mol. Ther.* **2018**, *26*, 524–541. [CrossRef]
19. Yang, Y.; Wang, L.; Bell, P.; McMenamin, D.; He, Z.; White, J.; Yu, H.; Xu, C.; Morizono, H.; Musunuru, K.; et al. A dual AAV system enables the Cas9-mediated correction of a metabolic liver disease in newborn mice. *Nat. Biotechnol.* **2016**, *34*, 334–338. [CrossRef]
20. Koo, T.; Popplewell, L.; Athanasopoulos, T.; Dickson, G. Triple trans-splicing adeno-associated virus vectors capable of transferring the coding sequence for full-length dystrophin protein into dystrophic mice. *Hum. Gene. Ther.* **2014**, *25*, 98–108. [CrossRef]
21. Rosewell, A.; Vetrini, F.; Ng, P. Helper-Dependent Adenoviral Vectors. *J. Genet. Syndr. Gene Ther.* **2011**, *5*, 423–450. [CrossRef] [PubMed]
22. Maddalo, D.; Manchado, E.; Concepcion, C.P.; Bonetti, C.; Vidigal, J.A.; Han, Y.-C.; Ogrodowski, P.; Crippa, A.; Rekhtman, N.; de Stanchina, E.; et al. In vivo engineering of oncogenic chromosomal rearrangements with the CRISPR/Cas9 system. *Nature* **2014**, *516*, 423–427. [CrossRef] [PubMed]
23. Wang, D.; Mou, H.; Li, S.; Li, Y.; Hough, S.; Tran, K.; Li, J.; Yin, H.; Anderson, D.G.; Sontheimer, E.J.; et al. Adenovirus-Mediated Somatic Genome Editing of Pten by CRISPR/Cas9 in Mouse Liver in Spite of Cas9-Specific Immune Responses. *Hum. Gene Ther.* **2015**, *26*, 432–442. [CrossRef] [PubMed]
24. Voets, O.; Tielen, F.; Elstak, E.; Benschop, J.; Grimbergen, M.; Stallen, J.; Janssen, R.; van Marle, A.; Essrich, C. Highly efficient gene inactivation by adenoviral CRISPR/Cas9 in human primary cells. *PLoS ONE* **2017**, *12*, e0182974. [CrossRef] [PubMed]
25. Ding, Q.; Strong, A.; Patel, K.M.; Ng, S.-L.; Gosis, B.S.; Regan, S.N.; Cowan, C.A.; Rader, D.J.; Musunuru, K. Permanent Alteration of PCSK9 With In Vivo CRISPR-Cas9 Genome Editing. *Circ. Res.* **2014**, *115*, 488–492. [CrossRef]
26. Maggio, I.; Stefanucci, L.; Janssen, J.M.; Liu, J.; Chen, X.; Mouly, V.; Gonçalves, M.A.F.V. Selection-free gene repair after adenoviral vector transduction of designer nucleases: Rescue of dystrophin synthesis in DMD muscle cell populations. *Nucleic Acids Res.* **2016**, *44*, 1449–1470. [CrossRef]
27. Xu, L.; Park, K.H.; Zhao, L.; Xu, J.; El Refaey, M.; Gao, Y.; Zhu, H.; Ma, J.; Han, R. CRISPR-mediated Genome Editing Restores Dystrophin Expression and Function in mdx Mice. *Mol. Ther.* **2016**, *24*, 564–569. [CrossRef]
28. Maggio, I.; Liu, J.; Janssen, J.M.; Chen, X.; Gonçalves, M.A.F.V. Adenoviral vectors encoding CRISPR/Cas9 multiplexes rescue dystrophin synthesis in unselected populations of DMD muscle cells. *Sci. Rep.* **2016**, *6*, 37051. [CrossRef]
29. Li, C.; Guan, X.; Du, T.; Jin, W.; Wu, B.; Liu, Y.; Wang, P.; Hu, B.; Griffin, G.E.; Shattock, R.J.; et al. Inhibition of HIV-1 infection of primary CD4+ T-cells by gene editing of CCR5 using adenovirus-delivered CRISPR/Cas9. *J. Gen. Virol.* **2015**, *96*, 2381–2393. [CrossRef]
30. Wang, Y.; Shao, W. Innate Immune Response to Viral Vectors in Gene Therapy. *Viruses* **2023**, *15*, 1801. [CrossRef]
31. Parks, R.J.; Chen, L.; Anton, M.; Sankar, U.; Rudnicki, M.A.; Graham, F.L. A helper-dependent adenovirus vector system: Removal of helper virus by Cre-mediated excision of the viral packaging signal. *Proc. Natl. Acad. Sci. USA* **1996**, *93*, 13565–13750. [CrossRef] [PubMed]
32. Palmer, D.; Ng, P. Improved system for helper-dependent adenoviral vector production. *Mol. Ther.* **2003**, *8*, 846–852. [CrossRef] [PubMed]
33. Tatsis, N.; Ertl, H.C.J. Adenoviruses as vaccine vectors. *Mol. Ther.* **2004**, *10*, 616–629. [CrossRef] [PubMed]
34. Brunetti-Pierri, N.; Ng, P. Gene therapy with helper-dependent adenoviral vectors: Lessons from studies in large animal models. *Virus Genes* **2017**, *53*, 684–691. [CrossRef]
35. Kotterman, M.A.; Chalberg, T.W.; Schaffer, D.V. Viral Vectors for Gene Therapy: Translational and Clinical Outlook. *Annu. Rev. Biomed. Eng.* **2015**, *17*, 63–89. [CrossRef]
36. Bennett, J. Immune response following intraocular delivery of recombinant viral vectors. *Gene Ther.* **2003**, *10*, 977–982. [CrossRef]
37. Pauwels, K.; Gijsbers, R.; Toelen, J.; Schambach, A.; Willard-Gallo, K.; Verheust, C.; Debyser, Z.; Herman, P. State-of-the-art lentiviral vectors for research use: Risk assessment and biosafety recommendations. *Curr. Gene Ther.* **2009**, *9*, 459–474. [CrossRef]
38. Shalem, O.; Sanjana, N.E.; Hartenian, E.; Shi, X.; Scott, D.A.; Mikkelson, T.; Heckl, D.; Ebert, B.L.; Root, D.E.; Doench, J.G.; et al. Genome-scale CRISPR-Cas9 knockout screening in human cells. *Science* **2014**, *343*, 84–87. [CrossRef]
39. Heckl, D.; Kowalczyk, M.S.; Yudovich, D.; Belizaire, R.; Puram, R.V.; McConkey, M.E.; Thielke, A.; Aster, J.C.; Regev, A.; Ebert, B.L. Generation of mouse models of myeloid malignancy with combinatorial genetic lesions using CRISPR-Cas9 genome editing. *Nat. Biotechnol.* **2014**, *32*, 941–946. [CrossRef]
40. Choi, J.G.; Dang, Y.; Abraham, S.; Ma, H.; Zhang, J.; Guo, H.; Cai, Y.; Mikkelsen, J.G.; Wu, H.; Shankar, P.; et al. Lentivirus pre-packed with Cas9 protein for safer gene editing. *Gene Ther.* **2016**, *23*, 627–633. [CrossRef]
41. Popescu, N.C.; Zimonjic, D.; DiPaolo, J.A. Viral integration, fragile sites, and proto-oncogenes in human neoplasia. *Hum. Genet.* **1990**, *84*, 383–386. [CrossRef] [PubMed]
42. Rothe, M.; Modlich, U.; Schambach, A. Biosafety Challenges for Use of Lentiviral Vectors in Gene Therapy. *Curr. Gene Ther.* **2013**, *13*, 453–468. [CrossRef] [PubMed]
43. Check, E. Gene therapy put on hold as third child develops cancer. *Nature* **2005**, *433*, 561. [CrossRef] [PubMed]

44. Hacein-Bey-Abina, S.; Garrigue, A.; Wang, G.P.; Soulier, J.; Lim, A.; Morillon, E.; Clappier, E.; Caccavelli, L.; Delabesse, E.; Beldjord, K.; et al. Insertional oncogenesis in 4 patients after retrovirus-mediated gene therapy of SCID-X1. *J. Clin. Investig.* **2008**, *118*, 3132–3142. [CrossRef]
45. Hacein-Bey-Abina, S.; Von Kalle, C.; Schmidt, M.; McCormack, M.P.; Wulffraat, N.; Leboulch, P.; Lim, A.; Osborne, C.S.; Pawliuk, R.; Morillon, E.; et al. LMO2-Associated Clonal T Cell Proliferation in Two Patients after Gene Therapy for SCID-X1. *Science* **2003**, *302*, 415–419. [CrossRef]
46. Check, E. Regulators split on gene therapy as patient shows signs of cancer. *Nature* **2002**, *419*, 545–546. [CrossRef]
47. Jacobs, F.; Wisse, E.; De Geest, B. The role of liver sinusoidal cells in hepatocyte-directed gene transfer. *Am. J. Pathol.* **2010**, *176*, 14–21. [CrossRef]
48. Ganesan, L.P.; Mohanty, S.; Kim, J.; Clark, K.R.; Robinson, J.M.; Anderson, C.L. Rapid and efficient clearance of blood-borne virus by liver sinusoidal endothelium. *PLoS Pathog.* **2011**, *7*, e1002281. [CrossRef]
49. High-dose AAV gene therapy deaths. *Nat. Biotechnol.* **2020**, *38*, 910. [CrossRef]
50. Dirisala, A.; Uchida, S.; Toh, K.; Li, J.; Osawa, S.; Tockary, T.A.; Liu, X.; Abbasi, S.; Hayashi, K.; Mochida, Y.; et al. Transient stealth coating of liver sinusoidal wall by anchoring two-armed PEG for retargeting nanomedicines. *Sci. Adv.* **2020**, *6*, eabb8133. [CrossRef]
51. O'Keeffe Ahern, J.; Lara-Sáez, I.; Zhou, D.; Murillas, R.; Bonafont, J.; Mencía, Á.; García, M.; Manzanares, D.; Lynch, J.; Foley, R.; et al. Non-viral delivery of CRISPR–Cas9 complexes for targeted gene editing via a polymer delivery system. *Gene Ther.* **2022**, *29*, 157–170. [CrossRef] [PubMed]
52. Frankel, A.D.; Pabo, C.O. Cellular uptake of the tat protein from human immunodeficiency virus. *Cell* **1988**, *55*, 1189–1193. [CrossRef] [PubMed]
53. Green, M.; Loewenstein, P.M. Autonomous functional domains of chemically synthesized human immunodeficiency virus tat trans-activator protein. *Cell* **1988**, *55*, 1179–1188. [CrossRef] [PubMed]
54. Trehin, R.; Merkle, H.P. Chances and pitfalls of cell penetrating peptides for cellular drug delivery. *Eur. J. Pharm. Biopharm.* **2004**, *58*, 209–223. [CrossRef] [PubMed]
55. Zorko, M.; Langel, U. Cell-penetrating peptides: Mechanism and kinetics of cargo delivery. *Adv. Drug Deliv. Rev.* **2005**, *57*, 529–545. [CrossRef]
56. Khafagy, E.S.; Morishita, M. Oral biodrug delivery using cell-penetrating peptide. *Adv. Drug Deliv. Rev.* **2012**, *64*, 531–539. [CrossRef]
57. Kamei, N.; Morishita, M.; Eda, Y.; Ida, N.; Nishio, R.; Takayama, K. Usefulness of cell-penetrating peptides to improve intestinal insulin absorption. *J. Control. Release* **2008**, *132*, 21–25. [CrossRef]
58. Kamei, N.; Morishita, M.; Takayama, K. Importance of intermolecular interaction on the improvement of intestinal therapeutic peptide/protein absorption using cell-penetrating peptides. *J. Control. Release* **2009**, *136*, 179–186. [CrossRef]
59. Khafagy, E.S.; Morishita, M.; Kamei, N.; Eda, Y.; Ikeno, Y.; Takayama, K. Efficiency of cell-penetrating peptides on the nasal and intestinal absorption of therapeutic peptides and proteins. *Int. J. Pharm.* **2009**, *381*, 49–55. [CrossRef]
60. Bechara, C.; Sagan, S. Cell-penetrating peptides: 20 years later, where do we stand? *FEBS Lett.* **2013**, *587*, 1693–1702. [CrossRef]
61. Komin, A.; Russell, L.M.; Hristova, K.A.; Searson, P.C. Peptide-based strategies for enhanced cell uptake, transcellular transport, and circulation: Mechanisms and challenges. *Adv. Drug Deliv. Rev.* **2017**, *110–111*, 52–64. [CrossRef] [PubMed]
62. Stanzl, E.G.; Trantow, B.M.; Vargas, J.R.; Wender, P.A. Fifteen years of cell-penetrating, guanidinium-rich molecular transporters: Basic science, research tools, and clinical applications. *Acc. Chem. Res.* **2013**, *46*, 2944–2954. [CrossRef] [PubMed]
63. Ramsey, J.D.; Flynn, N.H. Cell-penetrating peptides transport therapeutics into cells. *Pharmacol. Ther.* **2015**, *154*, 78–86. [CrossRef] [PubMed]
64. Madani, F.; Lindberg, S.; Langel, U.; Futaki, S.; Graslund, A. Mechanisms of cellular uptake of cell-penetrating peptides. *J. Biophys.* **2011**, *2011*, 414729. [CrossRef]
65. Guidotti, G.; Brambilla, L.; Rossi, D. Cell-Penetrating Peptides: From Basic Research to Clinics. *Trends Pharmacol. Sci.* **2017**, *38*, 406–424. [CrossRef]
66. Kauffman, W.B.; Fuselier, T.; He, J.; Wimley, W.C. Mechanism Matters: A Taxonomy of Cell Penetrating Peptides. *Trends Biochem. Sci.* **2015**, *40*, 749–764. [CrossRef]
67. Kalafatovic, D.; Giralt, E. Cell-Penetrating Peptides: Design Strategies beyond Primary Structure and Amphipathicity. *Molecules* **2017**, *22*, 1929. [CrossRef]
68. Pooga, M.; Langel, U. Classes of Cell-Penetrating Peptides. *Methods Mol. Biol.* **2015**, *1324*, 3–28. [CrossRef]
69. Sanders, W.S.; Johnston, C.I.; Bridges, S.M.; Burgess, S.C.; Willeford, K.O. Prediction of cell penetrating peptides by support vector machines. *PLoS Comput. Biol.* **2011**, *7*, e1002101. [CrossRef]
70. Gautam, A.; Singh, H.; Tyagi, A.; Chaudhary, K.; Kumar, R.; Kapoor, P.; Raghava, G.P. CPPsite: A curated database of cell penetrating peptides. *Database* **2012**, *2012*, bas015. [CrossRef]
71. Holton, T.A.; Pollastri, G.; Shields, D.C.; Mooney, C. CPPpred: Prediction of cell penetrating peptides. *Bioinformatics* **2013**, *29*, 3094–3096. [CrossRef] [PubMed]
72. Wei, L.; Xing, P.; Su, R.; Shi, G.; Ma, Z.S.; Zou, Q. CPPred-RF: A Sequence-based Predictor for Identifying Cell-Penetrating Peptides and Their Uptake Efficiency. *J. Proteome Res.* **2017**, *16*, 2044–2053. [CrossRef] [PubMed]

73. Fernandez-Carneado, J.; Kogan, M.J.; Pujals, S.; Giralt, E. Amphipathic peptides and drug delivery. *Biopolymers* **2004**, *76*, 196–203. [CrossRef] [PubMed]
74. Elliott, G.; O'Hare, P. Intercellular trafficking of VP22-GFP fusion proteins. *Gene Ther.* **1999**, *6*, 149–151. [CrossRef] [PubMed]
75. Tünnemann, G.; Ter-Avetisyan, G.; Martin, R.M.; Stöckl, M.; Herrmann, A.; Cardoso, M.C. Live-cell analysis of cell penetration ability and toxicity of oligo-arginines. *J. Pept. Sci.* **2008**, *14*, 469–476. [CrossRef]
76. Green, M.; Ishino, M.; Loewenstein, P.M. Mutational analysis of HIV-1 Tat minimal domain peptides: Identification of trans-dominant mutants that suppress HIV-LTR-driven gene expression. *Cell* **1989**, *58*, 215–223. [CrossRef]
77. Rhee, M.; Davis, P. Mechanism of uptake of C105Y, a novel cell-penetrating peptide. *J. Biol. Chem.* **2006**, *281*, 1233–1240. [CrossRef]
78. Gomez, J.A.; Chen, J.; Ngo, J.; Hajkova, D.; Yeh, I.J.; Gama, V.; Miyagi, M.; Matsuyama, S. Cell-Penetrating Penta-Peptides (CPP5s): Measurement of Cell Entry and Protein-Transduction Activity. *Pharmaceuticals* **2010**, *3*, 3594–3613. [CrossRef]
79. Dokka, S.; Toledo-Velasquez, D.; Shi, X.; Wang, L.; Rojanasakul, Y. Cellular delivery of oligonucleotides by synthetic import peptide carrier. *Pharm. Res.* **1997**, *14*, 1759–1764. [CrossRef]
80. Nakayama, F.; Yasuda, T.; Umeda, S.; Asada, M.; Imamura, T.; Meineke, V.; Akashi, M. Fibroblast growth factor-12 (FGF12) translocation into intestinal epithelial cells is dependent on a novel cell-penetrating peptide domain: Involvement of internalization in the in vivo role of exogenous FGF12. *J. Biol. Chem.* **2011**, *286*, 25823–25834. [CrossRef]
81. Derossi, D.; Joliot, A.H.; Chassaing, G.; Prochiantz, A. The third helix of the Antennapedia homeodomain translocates through biological membranes. *J. Biol. Chem.* **1994**, *269*, 10444–10450. [CrossRef] [PubMed]
82. Derossi, D.; Calvet, S.; Trembleau, A.; Brunissen, A.; Chassaing, G.; Prochiantz, A. Cell internalization of the third helix of the Antennapedia homeodomain is receptor-independent. *J. Biol. Chem.* **1996**, *271*, 18188–18193. [CrossRef] [PubMed]
83. Ramakrishna, S.; Kwaku Dad, A.B.; Beloor, J.; Gopalappa, R.; Lee, S.K.; Kim, H. Gene disruption by cell-penetrating peptide-mediated delivery of Cas9 protein and guide RNA. *Genome Res.* **2014**, *24*, 1020–1027. [CrossRef] [PubMed]
84. Suresh, B.; Ramakrishna, S.; Kim, H. Cell-Penetrating Peptide-Mediated Delivery of Cas9 Protein and Guide RNA for Genome Editing. *Methods Mol. Biol.* **2017**, *1507*, 81–94. [CrossRef] [PubMed]
85. Foss, D.V.; Muldoon, J.J.; Nguyen, D.N.; Carr, D.; Sahu, S.U.; Hunsinger, J.M.; Wyman, S.K.; Krishnappa, N.; Mendonsa, R.; Schanzer, E.V.; et al. Peptide-mediated delivery of CRISPR enzymes for the efficient editing of primary human lymphocytes. *Nat. Biomed. Eng.* **2023**, *7*, 647–660. [CrossRef]
86. Zhang, S.; Shen, J.; Li, D.; Cheng, Y. Strategies in the delivery of Cas9 ribonucleoprotein for CRISPR/Cas9 genome editing. *Theranostics* **2021**, *11*, 614–648. [CrossRef]
87. Kulkarni, J.A.; Myhre, J.L.; Chen, S.; Tam, Y.Y.C.; Danescu, A.; Richman, J.M.; Cullis, P.R. Design of lipid nanoparticles for in vitro and in vivo delivery of plasmid DNA. *Nanomed. Nanotechnol. Biol. Med.* **2017**, *13*, 1377–1387. [CrossRef]
88. Zhang, L.; Wang, P.; Feng, Q.; Wang, N.; Chen, Z.; Huang, Y.; Zheng, W.; Jiang, X. Lipid nanoparticle-mediated efficient delivery of CRISPR/Cas9 for tumor therapy. *NPG Asia Mater.* **2017**, *9*, e441. [CrossRef]
89. Cheng, Q.; Wei, T.; Farbiak, L.; Johnson, L.T.; Dilliard, S.A.; Siegwart, D.J. Selective organ targeting (SORT) nanoparticles for tissue-specific mRNA delivery and CRISPR–Cas gene editing. *Nat. Nanotechnol.* **2020**, *15*, 313–320. [CrossRef]
90. Li, C.; Yang, T.; Weng, Y.; Zhang, M.; Zhao, D.; Guo, S.; Hu, B.; Shao, W.; Wang, X.; Hussain, A.; et al. Ionizable lipid-assisted efficient hepatic delivery of gene editing elements for oncotherapy. *Bioact. Mater.* **2022**, *9*, 590–601. [CrossRef]
91. Finn, J.D.; Smith, A.R.; Patel, M.C.; Shaw, L.; Youniss, M.R.; van Heteren, J.; Dirstine, T.; Ciullo, C.; Lescarbeau, R.; Seitzer, J.; et al. A Single Administration of CRISPR/Cas9 Lipid Nanoparticles Achieves Robust and Persistent In Vivo Genome Editing. *Cell Rep.* **2018**, *22*, 2227–2235. [CrossRef] [PubMed]
92. Qiu, M.; Glass, Z.; Chen, J.; Haas, M.; Jin, X.; Zhao, X.; Rui, X.; Ye, Z.; Li, Y.; Zhang, F.; et al. Lipid nanoparticle-mediated codelivery of Cas9 mRNA and single-guide RNA achieves liver-specific in vivo genome editing of Angptl3. *Proc. Natl. Acad. Sci. USA* **2021**, *118*, e2020401118. [CrossRef] [PubMed]
93. Rothgangl, T.; Dennis, M.K.; Lin, P.J.C.; Oka, R.; Witzigmann, D.; Villiger, L.; Qi, W.; Hruzova, M.; Kissling, L.; Lenggenhager, D.; et al. In vivo adenine base editing of PCSK9 in macaques reduces LDL cholesterol levels. *Nat. Biotechnol.* **2021**, *39*, 949–957. [CrossRef] [PubMed]
94. Kenjo, E.; Hozumi, H.; Makita, Y.; Iwabuchi, K.A.; Fujimoto, N.; Matsumoto, S.; Kimura, M.; Amano, Y.; Ifuku, M.; Naoe, Y.; et al. Low immunogenicity of LNP allows repeated administrations of CRISPR-Cas9 mRNA into skeletal muscle in mice. *Nat. Commun.* **2021**, *12*, 7101. [CrossRef] [PubMed]
95. Wei, T.; Cheng, Q.; Min, Y.-L.; Olson, E.N.; Siegwart, D.J. Systemic nanoparticle delivery of CRISPR-Cas9 ribonucleoproteins for effective tissue specific genome editing. *Nat. Commun.* **2020**, *11*, 3232. [CrossRef]
96. Wang, M.; Zuris, J.A.; Meng, F.; Rees, H.; Sun, S.; Deng, P.; Han, Y.; Gao, X.; Pouli, D.; Wu, Q.; et al. Efficient delivery of genome-editing proteins using bioreducible lipid nanoparticles. *Proc. Natl. Acad. Sci. USA* **2016**, *113*, 2868–2873. [CrossRef]
97. Zuris, J.A.; Thompson, D.B.; Shu, Y.; Guilinger, J.P.; Bessen, J.L.; Hu, J.H.; Maeder, M.L.; Joung, J.K.; Chen, Z.-Y.; Liu, D.R. Cationic lipid-mediated delivery of proteins enables efficient protein-based genome editing in vitro and in vivo. *Nat. Biotechnol.* **2015**, *33*, 73–80. [CrossRef]
98. Whitehead, K.A.; Langer, R.; Anderson, D.G. Knocking down barriers: Advances in siRNA delivery. *Nat. Rev. Drug Discov.* **2009**, *8*, 129–138. [CrossRef]
99. Lin, M.; Wang, X. Natural Biopolymer-Based Delivery of CRISPR/Cas9 for Cancer Treatment. *Pharmaceutics* **2024**, *16*, 62. [CrossRef]

100. Jiang, Z.; Song, Z.; Cao, C.; Yan, M.; Liu, Z.; Cheng, X.; Wang, H.; Wang, Q.; Liu, H.; Chen, S. Multiple Natural Polymers in Drug and Gene Delivery Systems. *Curr. Med. Chem.* **2024**, *31*, 1691–1715. [CrossRef]
101. Zhang, H.; Bahamondez-Canas, T.F.; Zhang, Y.; Leal, J.; Smyth, H.D.C. PEGylated Chitosan for Nonviral Aerosol and Mucosal Delivery of the CRISPR/Cas9 System In Vitro. *Mol. Pharm.* **2018**, *15*, 4814–4826. [CrossRef] [PubMed]
102. Kalliola, S.; Repo, E.; Srivastava, V.; Zhao, F.; Heiskanen, J.P.; Sirviö, J.A.; Liimatainen, H.; Sillanpää, M. Carboxymethyl Chitosan and Its Hydrophobically Modified Derivative as pH-Switchable Emulsifiers. *Langmuir ACS J. Surf. Colloids* **2018**, *34*, 2800–2806. [CrossRef] [PubMed]
103. Park, S.C.; Nam, J.P.; Kim, Y.M.; Kim, J.H.; Nah, J.W.; Jang, M.K. Branched polyethylenimine-grafted-carboxymethyl chitosan copolymer enhances the delivery of pDNA or siRNA in vitro and in vivo. *Int. J. Nanomed.* **2013**, *8*, 3663–3677. [CrossRef]
104. Sharei, A.; Zoldan, J.; Adamo, A.; Sim, W.Y.; Cho, N.; Jackson, E.; Mao, S.; Schneider, S.; Han, M.-J.; Lytton-Jean, A.; et al. A vector-free microfluidic platform for intracellular delivery. *Proc. Natl. Acad. Sci. USA* **2013**, *110*, 2082–2087. [CrossRef] [PubMed]
105. Srivastav, A.; Gupta, K.; Chakraborty, D.; Dandekar, P.; Jain, R. Efficiency of Chitosan-Coated PLGA Nanocarriers for Cellular Delivery of siRNA and CRISPR/Cas9 Complex. *J. Pharm. Innov.* **2022**, *17*, 180–193. [CrossRef]
106. Alallam, B.; Altahhan, S.; Taher, M.; Mohd Nasir, M.H.; Doolaanea, A.A. Electrosprayed Alginate Nanoparticles as CRISPR Plasmid DNA Delivery Carrier: Preparation, Optimization, and Characterization. *Pharmaceuticals* **2020**, *13*, 158. [CrossRef] [PubMed]
107. Wan, T.; Chen, Y.; Pan, Q.; Xu, X.; Kang, Y.; Gao, X.; Huang, F.; Wu, C.; Ping, Y. Genome editing of mutant KRAS through supramolecular polymer-mediated delivery of Cas9 ribonucleoprotein for colorectal cancer therapy. *J. Control. Release Off. J. Control. Release Soc.* **2020**, *322*, 236–247. [CrossRef]
108. Zhang, Z.; Wan, T.; Chen, Y.; Chen, Y.; Sun, H.; Cao, T.; Songyang, Z.; Tang, G.; Wu, C.; Ping, Y.; et al. Cationic Polymer-Mediated CRISPR/Cas9 Plasmid Delivery for Genome Editing. *Macromol. Rapid Commun.* **2019**, *40*, e1800068. [CrossRef]
109. Qiao, L.; Gao, M.; Yi, X.; Peng, H.; Zhang, R.; Yao, W.; Sun, G.; He, X. Biomimetic gene editing system for precise tumor cell reprogramming and augmented tumor therapy. *J. Control. Release Off. J. Control. Release Soc.* **2023**, *356*, 663–677. [CrossRef]
110. Kang, Y.K.; Lee, J.; Im, S.H.; Lee, J.H.; Jeong, J.; Kim, D.K.; Yang, S.Y.; Jung, K.; Kim, S.-G.; Chung, H.J. Cas9 conjugate complex delivering donor DNA for efficient gene editing by homology-directed repair. *J. Ind. Eng. Chem.* **2021**, *102*, 241–250. [CrossRef]
111. Carboni, V.; Maaliki, C.; Alyami, M.; Alsaiari, S.; Khashab, N. Synthetic Vehicles for Encapsulation and Delivery of CRISPR/Cas9 Gene Editing Machinery. *Adv. Ther.* **2019**, *2*, 1800085. [CrossRef]
112. Chen, G.; Abdeen, A.A.; Wang, Y.; Shahi, P.K.; Robertson, S.; Xie, R.; Suzuki, M.; Pattnaik, B.R.; Saha, K.; Gong, S. A biodegradable nanocapsule delivers a Cas9 ribonucleoprotein complex for in vivo genome editing. *Nat. Nanotechnol.* **2019**, *14*, 974–980. [CrossRef]
113. Pandey, A.P.; Sawant, K.K. Polyethylenimine: A versatile, multifunctional non-viral vector for nucleic acid delivery. *Mater. Sci. Eng. C Mater. Biol. Appl.* **2016**, *68*, 904–918. [CrossRef] [PubMed]
114. Ryu, N.; Kim, M.A.; Park, D.; Lee, B.; Kim, Y.R.; Kim, K.H.; Baek, J.I.; Kim, W.J.; Lee, K.Y.; Kim, U.K. Effective PEI-mediated delivery of CRISPR-Cas9 complex for targeted gene therapy. *Nanomed. Nanotechnol. Biol. Med.* **2018**, *14*, 2095–2102. [CrossRef]
115. Rohiwal, S.S.; Dvorakova, N.; Klima, J.; Vaskovicova, M.; Senigl, F.; Slouf, M.; Pavlova, E.; Stepanek, P.; Babuka, D.; Benes, H.; et al. Polyethylenimine based magnetic nanoparticles mediated non-viral CRISPR/Cas9 system for genome editing. *Sci. Rep.* **2020**, *10*, 4619. [CrossRef] [PubMed]
116. Hashemzadeh, I.; Hasanzadeh, A.; Radmanesh, F.; Khodadadi Chegeni, B.; Hosseini, E.S.; Kiani, J.; Shahbazi, A.; Naseri, M.; Fatahi, Y.; Nourizadeh, H.; et al. Polyethylenimine-Functionalized Carbon Dots for Delivery of CRISPR/Cas9 Complexes. *ACS Appl. Bio Mater.* **2021**, *4*, 7979–7992. [CrossRef] [PubMed]
117. Moradi, F.; Hasanzadeh, A.; Radmanesh, F.; Rajai Daryasarei, S.; Hosseini, E.S.; Kiani, J.; Shahbazi, A.; Nourizadeh, H.; Eslami, M.; Dorgalaleh, A.; et al. Smart arginine-equipped polycationic nanoparticles for p/CRISPR delivery into cells. *Nanotechnology* **2021**, *33*, 075104. [CrossRef]
118. Li, L.; Yang, Z.; Zhu, S.; He, L.; Fan, W.; Tang, W.; Zou, J.; Shen, Z.; Zhang, M.; Tang, L.; et al. A Rationally Designed Semiconducting Polymer Brush for NIR-II Imaging-Guided Light-Triggered Remote Control of CRISPR/Cas9 Genome Editing. *Adv. Mater.* **2019**, *31*, e1901187. [CrossRef]
119. Averick, S.; Mehl, R.A.; Das, S.R.; Matyjaszewski, K. Well-defined biohybrids using reversible-deactivation radical polymerization procedures. *J. Control. Release* **2015**, *205*, 45–57. [CrossRef]
120. Cruz, L.J.; van Dijk, T.; Vepris, O.; Li, T.; Schomann, T.; Baldazzi, F.; Kurita, R.; Nakamura, Y.; Grosveld, F.; Philipsen, S.; et al. PLGA-Nanoparticles for Intracellular Delivery of the CRISPR-Complex to Elevate Fetal Globin Expression in Erythroid Cells. *Biomaterials* **2021**, *268*, 120580. [CrossRef]
121. Wang, H.X.; Song, Z.; Lao, Y.H.; Xu, X.; Gong, J.; Cheng, D.; Chakraborty, S.; Park, J.S.; Li, M.; Huang, D.; et al. Nonviral gene editing via CRISPR/Cas9 delivery by membrane-disruptive and endosomolytic helical polypeptide. *Proc. Natl. Acad. Sci. USA* **2018**, *115*, 4903–4908. [CrossRef] [PubMed]
122. Alhazza, A.; Mahdipoor, P.; Hall, R.; Manda, A.; Lohan, S.; Parang, K.; Aliabadi, H.M. Modifying peptide/lipid-associated nucleic acids (PLANAs) for CRISPR/Cas9 ribonucleoprotein delivery. *Eur. J. Pharm. Sci. Off. J. Eur. Fed. Pharm. Sci.* **2024**, *195*, 106708. [CrossRef] [PubMed]
123. Li, Y.; Li, C.; Yan, J.; Liao, Y.; Qin, C.; Wang, L.; Huang, Y.; Yang, C.; Wang, J.; Ding, X.; et al. Polymeric micellar nanoparticles for effective CRISPR/Cas9 genome editing in cancer. *Biomaterials* **2024**, *309*, 122573. [CrossRef] [PubMed]

124. Abbasi, S.; Uchida, S.; Toh, K.; Tockary, T.A.; Dirisala, A.; Hayashi, K.; Fukushima, S.; Kataoka, K. Co-encapsulation of Cas9 mRNA and guide RNA in polyplex micelles enables genome editing in mouse brain. *J. Control. Release* **2021**, *332*, 260–268. [CrossRef] [PubMed]
125. Karlsson, J.; Rhodes, K.R.; Green, J.J.; Tzeng, S.Y. Poly(beta-amino ester)s as gene delivery vehicles: Challenges and opportunities. *Expert. Opin. Drug Deliv.* **2020**, *17*, 1395–1410. [CrossRef]
126. Rui, Y.; Varanasi, M.; Mendes, S.; Yamagata, H.M.; Wilson, D.R.; Green, J.J. Poly(Beta-Amino Ester) Nanoparticles Enable Nonviral Delivery of CRISPR-Cas9 Plasmids for Gene Knockout and Gene Deletion. *Mol. Ther. Nucleic Acids* **2020**, *20*, 661–672. [CrossRef]
127. Chen, Q.; Su, L.; He, X.; Li, J.; Cao, Y.; Wu, Q.; Qin, J.; He, Z.; Huang, X.; Yang, H.; et al. Poly(beta-amino ester)-Based Nanoparticles Enable Nonviral Delivery of Base Editors for Targeted Tumor Gene Editing. *Biomacromolecules* **2022**, *23*, 2116–2125. [CrossRef]
128. Rui, Y.; Wilson, D.R.; Choi, J.; Varanasi, M.; Sanders, K.; Karlsson, J.; Lim, M.; Green, J.J. Carboxylated branched poly(β-amino ester) nanoparticles enable robust cytosolic protein delivery and CRISPR-Cas9 gene editing. *Sci. Adv.* **2019**, *5*, eaay3255. [CrossRef]
129. Wang, X.; Li, Y.; Wang, X.; Sandoval, D.M.; He, Z.; Sáez, I.L.; Wang, W. Guanidyl-Rich Poly(β Amino Ester)s for Universal Functional Cytosolic Protein Delivery and Clustered Regularly Interspaced Short Palindromic Repeats (CRISPR) Cas9 Ribonucleoprotein Based Gene Editing. *ACS Nano* **2023**, *17*, 17799–17810. [CrossRef]
130. Wang, X.; Li, Y.; Sigen, A.; Lyu, J.; Wang, X.; He, Z.; Lara-Sáez, I.; Li, M.; Wang, W. Cyclization-enhanced poly(β-amino ester)s vectors for efficient CRISPR gene editing therapy. *J. Control. Release Off. J. Control. Release Soc.* **2024**, *368*, 444–452. [CrossRef]
131. Sadeqi Nezhad, M. Poly (beta-amino ester) as an in vivo nanocarrier for therapeutic nucleic acids. *Biotechnol. Bioeng.* **2023**, *120*, 95–113. [CrossRef]
132. El-Kharrag, R.; Berckmueller, K.E.; Madhu, R.; Cui, M.; Campoy, G.; Mack, H.M.; Wolf, C.B.; Perez, A.M.; Humbert, O.; Kiem, H.P.; et al. Efficient polymer nanoparticle-mediated delivery of gene editing reagents into human hematopoietic stem and progenitor cells. *Mol. Ther. J. Am. Soc. Gene Ther.* **2022**, *30*, 2186–2198. [CrossRef] [PubMed]
133. Mathew, A.; Cao, H.; Collin, E.; Wang, W.; Pandit, A. Hyperbranched PEGmethacrylate linear pDMAEMA block copolymer as an efficient non-viral gene delivery vector. *Int. J. Pharm.* **2012**, *434*, 99–105. [CrossRef] [PubMed]
134. Jiang, X.; Lok, M.C.; Hennink, W.E. Degradable-brushed pHEMA-pDMAEMA synthesized via ATRP and click chemistry for gene delivery. *Bioconjugate Chem.* **2007**, *18*, 2077–2084. [CrossRef] [PubMed]
135. Timin, A.S.; Muslimov, A.R.; Lepik, K.V.; Epifanovskaya, O.S.; Shakirova, A.I.; Mock, U.; Riecken, K.; Okilova, M.V.; Sergeev, V.S.; Afanasyev, B.V.; et al. Efficient gene editing via non-viral delivery of CRISPR-Cas9 system using polymeric and hybrid microcarriers. *Nanomed. Nanotechnol. Biol. Med.* **2018**, *14*, 97–108. [CrossRef]
136. Xiu, K.; Saunders, L.; Wen, L.; Ruan, J.; Dong, R.; Song, J.; Yang, D.; Zhang, J.; Xu, J.; Chen, Y.E.; et al. Delivery of CRISPR/Cas9 Plasmid DNA by Hyperbranched Polymeric Nanoparticles Enables Efficient Gene Editing. *Cells* **2022**, *12*, 156. [CrossRef]
137. van de Wetering, P.; Moret, E.E.; Schuurmans-Nieuwenbroek, N.M.; van Steenbergen, M.J.; Hennink, W.E. Structure-activity relationships of water-soluble cationic methacrylate/methacrylamide polymers for nonviral gene delivery. *Bioconjugate Chem.* **1999**, *10*, 589–597. [CrossRef]
138. Ma, P.; Wang, Q.; Luo, X.; Mao, L.; Wang, Z.; Ye, E.; Loh, X.J.; Li, Z.; Wu, Y.-L. Recent advances in stimuli-responsive polymeric carriers for controllable CRISPR/Cas9 gene editing system delivery. *Biomater. Sci.* **2023**, *11*, 5078–5094. [CrossRef]
139. Gong, Y.; Tian, S.; Xuan, Y.; Zhang, S. Lipid and polymer mediated CRISPR/Cas9 gene editing. *J. Mater. Chem. B* **2020**, *8*, 4369–4386. [CrossRef]
140. Xu, C.; Lu, Z.; Luo, Y.; Liu, Y.; Cao, Z.; Shen, S.; Li, H.; Liu, J.; Chen, K.; Chen, Z.; et al. Targeting of NLRP3 inflammasome with gene editing for the amelioration of inflammatory diseases. *Nat. Commun.* **2018**, *9*, 4092. [CrossRef]
141. Luo, Y.L.; Xu, C.F.; Li, H.J.; Cao, Z.T.; Liu, J.; Wang, J.L.; Du, X.J.; Yang, X.Z.; Gu, Z.; Wang, J. Macrophage-Specific In Vivo Gene Editing Using Cationic Lipid-Assisted Polymeric Nanoparticles. *ACS Nano* **2018**, *12*, 994–1005. [CrossRef] [PubMed]
142. Kaupbayeva, B.; Murata, H.; Wilson, A.L.; Matyjaszewski, K.; Minden, J.S.; Russell, A.J. Molecular Sieving on the Surface of a Nano-Armored Protein. *Biomacromolecules* **2019**, *20*, 1235–1245. [CrossRef] [PubMed]
143. Murata, H.; Cummings, C.S.; Koepsel, R.R.; Russell, A.J. Polymer-Based Protein Engineering Can Rationally Tune Enzyme Activity, pH-Dependence, and Stability. *Biomacromolecules* **2013**, *14*, 1919–1926. [CrossRef] [PubMed]
144. Kaupbayeva, B.; Murata, H.; Rule, G.S.; Matyjaszewski, K.; Russell, A.J. Rational Control of Protein–Protein Interactions with Protein-ATRP-Generated Protease-Sensitive Polymer Cages. *Biomacromolecules* **2022**, *23*, 3831–3846. [CrossRef] [PubMed]
145. Baker, S.L.; Kaupbayeva, B.; Lathwal, S.; Das, S.R.; Russell, A.J.; Matyjaszewski, K. Atom Transfer Radical Polymerization for Biorelated Hybrid Materials. *Biomacromolecules* **2019**, *20*, 4272–4298. [CrossRef] [PubMed]
146. Kaupbayeva, B.; Boye, S.; Munasinghe, A.; Murata, H.; Matyjaszewski, K.; Lederer, A.; Colina, C.M.; Russell, A.J. Molecular Dynamics-Guided Design of a Functional Protein–ATRP Conjugate That Eliminates Protein–Protein Interactions. *Bioconjugate Chem.* **2021**, *32*, 821–832. [CrossRef]
147. Kapil, K.; Szczepaniak, G.; Martinez, M.R.; Murata, H.; Jazani, A.M.; Jeong, J.; Das, S.R.; Matyjaszewski, K. Visible-Light-Mediated Controlled Radical Branching Polymerization in Water. *Angew. Chem. Int. Ed.* **2023**, *62*, e202217658. [CrossRef]
148. Baker, S.L.; Murata, H.; Kaupbayeva, B.; Tasbolat, A.; Matyjaszewski, K.; Russell, A.J. Charge-Preserving Atom Transfer Radical Polymerization Initiator Rescues the Lost Function of Negatively Charged Protein–Polymer Conjugates. *Biomacromolecules* **2019**, *20*, 2392–2405. [CrossRef]

149. Baker, S.L.; Munasinghe, A.; Murata, H.; Lin, P.; Matyjaszewski, K.; Colina, C.M.; Russell, A.J. Intramolecular Interactions of Conjugated Polymers Mimic Molecular Chaperones to Stabilize Protein–Polymer Conjugates. *Biomacromolecules* **2018**, *19*, 3798–3813. [CrossRef]
150. Szczepaniak, G.; Jeong, J.; Kapil, K.; Dadashi-Silab, S.; Yerneni, S.S.; Ratajczyk, P.; Lathwal, S.; Schild, D.J.; Das, S.R.; Matyjaszewski, K. Open-air green-light-driven ATRP enabled by dual photoredox/copper catalysis. *Chem. Sci.* **2022**, *13*, 11540–11550. [CrossRef]
151. Averick, S.E.; Paredes, E.; Irastorza, A.; Shrivats, A.R.; Srinivasan, A.; Siegwart, D.J.; Magenau, A.J.; Cho, H.Y.; Hsu, E.; Averick, A.A.; et al. Preparation of cationic nanogels for nucleic acid delivery. *Biomacromolecules* **2012**, *13*, 3445–3449. [CrossRef] [PubMed]
152. Averick, S.E.; Paredes, E.; Dey, S.K.; Snyder, K.M.; Tapinos, N.; Matyjaszewski, K.; Das, S.R. Autotransfecting Short Interfering RNA through Facile Covalent Polymer Escorts. *J. Am. Chem. Soc.* **2013**, *135*, 12508–12511. [CrossRef] [PubMed]
153. Mackenzie, M.C.; Shrivats, A.R.; Konkolewicz, D.; Averick, S.E.; McDermott, M.C.; Hollinger, J.O.; Matyjaszewski, K. Synthesis of poly(meth)acrylates with thioether and tertiary sulfonium groups by ARGET ATRP and their use as siRNA delivery agents. *Biomacromolecules* **2015**, *16*, 236–245. [CrossRef] [PubMed]
154. Shrivats, A.R.; Mishina, Y.; Averick, S.; Matyjaszewski, K.; Hollinger, J.O. In Vivo GFP Knockdown by Cationic Nanogel-siRNA Polyplexes. *Bioengineering* **2015**, *2*, 160–175. [CrossRef]
155. Cho, H.Y.; Gao, H.; Srinivasan, A.; Hong, J.; Bencherif, S.A.; Siegwart, D.J.; Paik, H.-j.; Hollinger, J.O.; Matyjaszewski, K. Rapid Cellular Internalization of Multifunctional Star Polymers Prepared by Atom Transfer Radical Polymerization. *Biomacromolecules* **2010**, *11*, 2199–2203. [CrossRef]
156. Cho, H.Y.; Srinivasan, A.; Hong, J.; Hsu, E.; Liu, S.; Shrivats, A.; Kwak, D.; Bohaty, A.K.; Paik, H.J.; Hollinger, J.O.; et al. Synthesis of biocompatible PEG-Based star polymers with cationic and degradable core for siRNA delivery. *Biomacromolecules* **2011**, *12*, 3478–3486. [CrossRef]
157. Cho, H.Y.; Averick, S.E.; Paredes, E.; Wegner, K.; Averick, A.; Jurga, S.; Das, S.R.; Matyjaszewski, K. Star Polymers with a Cationic Core Prepared by ATRP for Cellular Nucleic Acids Delivery. *Biomacromolecules* **2013**, *14*, 1262–1267. [CrossRef]
158. Jeong, J.; Hu, X.; Murata, H.; Szczepaniak, G.; Rachwalak, M.; Kietrys, A.; Das, S.R.; Matyjaszewski, K. RNA-Polymer Hybrids via Direct and Site-Selective Acylation with the ATRP Initiator and Photoinduced Polymerization. *J. Am. Chem. Soc.* **2023**, *145*, 14435–14445. [CrossRef]
159. Jeong, J.; Szczepaniak, G.; Das, S.R.; Matyjaszewski, K. Expanding the architectural horizon of nucleic-acid-polymer biohybrids by site-controlled incorporation of ATRP initiators in DNA and RNA. *Chem* **2023**, *9*, 3319–3334. [CrossRef]
160. Jeong, J.; Szczepaniak, G.; Das, S.R.; Matyjaszewski, K. Synthesis of RNA-Amphiphiles via Atom Transfer Radical Polymerization in the Organic Phase. *Precis. Chem.* **2023**, *1*, 326–331. [CrossRef]
161. Yerneni, S.S.; Lathwal, S.; Shrestha, P.; Shirwan, H.; Matyjaszewski, K.; Weiss, L.; Yolcu, E.S.; Campbell, P.G.; Das, S.R. Rapid On-Demand Extracellular Vesicle Augmentation with Versatile Oligonucleotide Tethers. *ACS Nano* **2019**, *13*, 10555–10565. [CrossRef] [PubMed]
162. Fouz, M.F.; Mukumoto, K.; Averick, S.; Molinar, O.; McCartney, B.M.; Matyjaszewski, K.; Armitage, B.A.; Das, S.R. Bright Fluorescent Nanotags from Bottlebrush Polymers with DNA-Tipped Bristles. *ACS Cent. Sci.* **2015**, *1*, 431–438. [CrossRef] [PubMed]
163. Averick, S.E.; Paredes, E.; Grahacharya, D.; Woodman, B.F.; Miyake-Stoner, S.J.; Mehl, R.A.; Matyjaszewski, K.; Das, S.R. A Protein–Polymer Hybrid Mediated By DNA. *Langmuir* **2012**, *28*, 1954–1958. [CrossRef] [PubMed]
164. Averick, S.E.; Dey, S.K.; Grahacharya, D.; Matyjaszewski, K.; Das, S.R. Solid-Phase Incorporation of an ATRP Initiator for Polymer–DNA Biohybrids. *Angew. Chem. Int. Ed.* **2014**, *53*, 2739–2744. [CrossRef] [PubMed]
165. Martin-Martin, I.; Aryan, A.; Meneses, C.; Adelman, Z.N.; Calvo, E. Optimization of sand fly embryo microinjection for gene editing by CRISPR/Cas9. *PLoS Neglected Trop. Dis.* **2018**, *12*, e0006769. [CrossRef]
166. Crispo, M.; Mulet, A.P.; Tesson, L.; Barrera, N.; Cuadro, F.; dos Santos-Neto, P.C.; Nguyen, T.H.; Crénéguy, A.; Brusselle, L.; Anegón, I.; et al. Efficient Generation of Myostatin Knock-Out Sheep Using CRISPR/Cas9 Technology and Microinjection into Zygotes. *PLoS ONE* **2015**, *10*, e0136690. [CrossRef]
167. Hruscha, A.; Schmid, B. Generation of zebrafish models by CRISPR/Cas9 genome editing. *Methods Mol. Biol.* **2015**, *1254*, 341–350. [CrossRef]
168. Ma, Y.; Shen, B.; Zhang, X.; Lu, Y.; Chen, W.; Ma, J.; Huang, X.; Zhang, L. Heritable Multiplex Genetic Engineering in Rats Using CRISPR/Cas9. *PLoS ONE* **2014**, *9*, e89413. [CrossRef]
169. Sinclair, F.; Begum, A.A.; Dai, C.C.; Toth, I.; Moyle, P.M. Recent advances in the delivery and applications of nonviral CRISPR/Cas9 gene editing. *Drug Deliv. Transl. Res.* **2023**, *13*, 1500–1519. [CrossRef]
170. Han, X.; Liu, Z.; Jo, M.C.; Zhang, K.; Li, Y.; Zeng, Z.; Li, N.; Zu, Y.; Qin, L. CRISPR-Cas9 delivery to hard-to-transfect cells via membrane deformation. *Sci. Adv.* **2015**, *1*, e1500454. [CrossRef]
171. Yamagishi, A.; Matsumoto, D.; Kato, Y.; Honda, Y.; Morikawa, M.; Iwata, F.; Kobayashi, T.; Nakamura, C. Direct Delivery of Cas9-sgRNA Ribonucleoproteins into Cells Using a Nanoneedle Array. *Appl. Sci.* **2019**, *9*, 965. [CrossRef]
172. Chiappini, C.; De Rosa, E.; Martinez, J.O.; Liu, X.; Steele, J.; Stevens, M.M.; Tasciotti, E. Biodegradable silicon nanoneedles delivering nucleic acids intracellularly induce localized in vivo neovascularization. *Nat. Mater.* **2015**, *14*, 532–539. [CrossRef] [PubMed]

173. Chuang, C.K.; Chen, C.H.; Huang, C.L.; Su, Y.H.; Peng, S.H.; Lin, T.Y.; Tai, H.C.; Yang, T.S.; Tu, C.F. Generation of GGTA1 Mutant Pigs by Direct Pronuclear Microinjection of CRISPR/Cas9 Plasmid Vectors. *Anim. Biotechnol.* **2017**, *28*, 174–181. [CrossRef] [PubMed]
174. Guillaume-Gentil, O.; Potthoff, E.; Ossola, D.; Dörig, P.; Zambelli, T.; Vorholt, J.A. Force-Controlled Fluidic Injection into Single Cell Nuclei. *Small* **2013**, *9*, 1904–1907. [CrossRef]
175. Du, Y.; Liu, Y.; Hu, J.; Peng, X.; Liu, Z. CRISPR/Cas9 systems: Delivery technologies and biomedical applications. *Asian J. Pharm. Sci.* **2023**, *18*, 100854. [CrossRef]
176. Hashimoto, M.; Takemoto, T. Electroporation enables the efficient mRNA delivery into the mouse zygotes and facilitates CRISPR/Cas9-based genome editing. *Sci. Rep.* **2015**, *5*, 11315.
177. Alghadban, S.; Bouchareb, A.; Hinch, R.; Hernandez-Pliego, P.; Biggs, D.; Preece, C.; Davies, B. Electroporation and genetic supply of Cas9 increase the generation efficiency of CRISPR/Cas9 knock-in alleles in C57BL/6J mouse zygotes. *Sci. Rep.* **2020**, *10*, 17912. [CrossRef]
178. Wu, Y.; Zhou, H.; Fan, X.; Zhang, Y.; Zhang, M.; Wang, Y.; Xie, Z.; Bai, M.; Yin, Q.; Liang, D.; et al. Correction of a genetic disease by CRISPR-Cas9-mediated gene editing in mouse spermatogonial stem cells. *Cell Res.* **2015**, *25*, 67–79. [CrossRef]
179. Rathbone, T.; Ates, I.; Fernando, L.; Addlestone, E.; Lee, C.M.; Richards, V.P.; Cottle, R.N. Electroporation-Mediated Delivery of Cas9 Ribonucleoproteins Results in High Levels of Gene Editing in Primary Hepatocytes. *CRISPR J.* **2022**, *5*, 397–409. [CrossRef]
180. Xu, X.; Gao, D.; Wang, P.; Chen, J.; Ruan, J.; Xu, J.; Xia, X. Efficient homology-directed gene editing by CRISPR/Cas9 in human stem and primary cells using tube electroporation. *Sci. Rep.* **2018**, *8*, 018–30227. [CrossRef]
181. Shokouhi, A.-R.; Chen, Y.; Yoh, H.Z.; Murayama, T.; Suu, K.; Morikawa, Y.; Brenker, J.; Alan, T.; Voelcker, N.H.; Elnathan, R. Electroactive nanoinjection platform for intracellular delivery and gene silencing. *J. Nanobiotechnology* **2023**, *21*, 273. [CrossRef] [PubMed]
182. Latella, M.C.; Di Salvo, M.T.; Cocchiarella, F.; Benati, D.; Grisendi, G.; Comitato, A.; Marigo, V.; Recchia, A. In vivo Editing of the Human Mutant Rhodopsin Gene by Electroporation of Plasmid-based CRISPR/Cas9 in the Mouse Retina. *Mol. Ther. Nucleic Acids* **2016**, *5*, 92. [CrossRef] [PubMed]
183. Wu, W.; Lu, Z.; Li, F.; Wang, W.; Qian, N.; Duan, J.; Zhang, Y.; Wang, F.; Chen, T. Efficient in vivo gene editing using ribonucleoproteins in skin stem cells of recessive dystrophic epidermolysis bullosa mouse model. *Proc. Natl. Acad. Sci. USA* **2017**, *114*, 1660–1665. [CrossRef] [PubMed]
184. Wang, P.; Zhang, L.; Zheng, W.; Cong, L.; Guo, Z.; Xie, Y.; Wang, L.; Tang, R.; Feng, Q.; Hamada, Y.; et al. Thermo-triggered Release of CRISPR-Cas9 System by Lipid-Encapsulated Gold Nanoparticles for Tumor Therapy. *Angew. Chem. Int. Ed. Engl.* **2018**, *57*, 1491–1496. [CrossRef] [PubMed]
185. Pylaev, T.E.; Avdeeva, E.S.; Khlebtsov, B.N.; Lomova, M.V.; Khlebtsov, N.G. High-throughput cell optoporation system based on Au nanoparticle layers mediated by resonant irradiation for precise and controllable gene delivery. *Sci. Rep.* **2024**, *14*, 3044. [CrossRef]
186. Yoon, S.; Wang, E.P.; Peng, Q.; Wang, Y.; Shung, K. Acoustic-transfection for genomic manipulation of single-cells using high frequency ultrasound. *Sci. Rep.* **2017**, *7*, 5275. [CrossRef]
187. Suda, T.; Yokoo, T.; Kanefuji, T.; Kamimura, K.; Zhang, G.; Liu, D. Hydrodynamic Delivery: Characteristics, Applications, and Technological Advances. *Pharmaceutics* **2023**, *15*, 1111. [CrossRef]
188. Schuh, R.S.; Poletto, É.; Pasqualim, G.; Tavares, A.M.V.; Meyer, F.S.; Gonzalez, E.A.; Giugliani, R.; Matte, U.; Teixeira, H.F.; Baldo, G. In vivo genome editing of mucopolysaccharidosis I mice using the CRISPR/Cas9 system. *J. Control. Release* **2018**, *288*, 23–33. [CrossRef]
189. Sendra, L.; Herrero, M.J.; Aliño, S.F. Translational Advances of Hydrofection by Hydrodynamic Injection. *Genes* **2018**, *9*, 136. [CrossRef]
190. Yan, L.; Zhang, J.; Lee, C.-S.; Chen, X. Micro- and Nanotechnologies for Intracellular Delivery. *Small* **2014**, *10*, 4487–4504. [CrossRef]
191. Sun, M.; Duan, X. Recent advances in micro/nanoscale intracellular delivery. *Nanotechnol. Precis. Eng.* **2020**, *3*, 18–31. [CrossRef]
192. Hoy, S.M. Exagamglogene Autotemcel: First Approval. *Mol. Diagn. Ther.* **2024**, *28*, 133–139. [CrossRef] [PubMed]
193. Dirisala, A.; Uchida, S.; Tockary, T.A.; Yoshinaga, N.; Li, J.; Osawa, S.; Gorantla, L.; Fukushima, S.; Osada, K.; Kataoka, K. Precise tuning of disulphide crosslinking in mRNA polyplex micelles for optimising extracellular and intracellular nuclease tolerability. *J. Drug Target.* **2019**, *27*, 670–680. [CrossRef] [PubMed]

Journal of
*Functional Biomaterials*

MDPI

*Article*

# Sonification of Deproteinized Bovine Bone Functionalized with Genistein Enhances Bone Repair in Peri-Implant Bone Defects in Ovariectomized Rats

**Nathália Dantas Duarte [1], Gabriel Mulinari-Santos [1,2,*], Fábio Roberto de Souza Batista [1], Marcelly Braga Gomes [2], Naara Gabriela Monteiro [1], Ana Cláudia Ervolino da Silva [1], Reinhard Gruber [3], Paulo Noronha Lisboa-Filho [4], Pedro Henrique Silva Gomes-Ferreira [5] and Roberta Okamoto [2,*]**

1 Department of Diagnosis and Surgery, Araçatuba School of Dentistry, São Paulo State University "Júlio de Mesquita Filho", Araçatuba 16015-050, São Paulo, Brazil; nd.duarte@unesp.br (N.D.D.); fabio.rs.batista@unesp.br (F.R.d.S.B.); naara.monteiro@unesp.br (N.G.M.); ana.ervolino@unesp.br (A.C.E.d.S.)
2 Department of Basic Sciences, Araçatuba School of Dentistry, São Paulo State University "Júlio de Mesquita Filho", Araçatuba 16018-805, São Paulo, Brazil; marcelly.braga@unesp.br
3 Department of Oral Biology, University Clinic of Dentistry, Medical University of Vienna, 1090 Wien, Austria; reinhard.gruber@meduniwien.ac.at
4 Department of Physics, Bauru School of Sciences, São Paulo State University "Júlio de Mesquita Filho", Bauru 17033-360, São Paulo, Brazil; paulo.lisboa@unesp.br
5 Department of Dentistry, Ourinhos University Center, Ourinhos 19909-100, São Paulo, Brazil; pedro.gomes@unifio.edu.br
* Correspondence: gabriel.mulinari@unesp.br (G.M.-S.); roberta.okamoto@unesp.br (R.O.)

**Abstract:** Estrogen deficiency is one of several contributing factors to catabolic changes in bone surrounding dental implants, impairing bone repair in defects requiring bone regeneration. Functionalizing bone substitutes is an alternative approach among various strategies to address this challenge. In this study, the aim was to evaluate the effect of functionalizing deproteinized bovine bone (Bio-Oss®, BO) with genistein via sonication on peri-implant bone defects in ovariectomized rats. The animals were randomly distributed according to the treatment into the following four groups (n = 10): BO sonicated with genistein (BOS + GEN), BO sonicated alone (BOS), untreated BO (BO), and blood clot only (CLOT). After twenty-eight days, implant removal torque was determined, and the peri-implant bone parameters were calculated based on computed microtomography. Additionally, the gene expression of bone turnover markers was evaluated. As a main result, the functionalization with genistein increased implant removal torque and the peri-implant bone volume in the BOS + GEN group compared to both BOS and BO groups (both $p < 0.05$). These findings suggest that the sonification of deproteinized bovine bone functionalized with genistein improves bone repair in peri-implant bone defects in ovariectomized rats.

**Keywords:** biocompatibility; bone regeneration; dental implants; genistein; osseointegration; osteoporosis; rat; tibia

## 1. Introduction

Estrogen deficiency is one of the various contributing factors to catabolic bone metabolism, leading to increased bone resorption in postmenopausal women [1,2]. Osteopenia is characterized by reduced bone density, particularly affecting the trabecular bone, which becomes thinner and loses its structural integrity [3]. This condition can progress to osteoporosis with its clinical hallmarks being fragility fractures [4]. Estrogen plays a crucial role in controlling bone remodeling and consequently maintaining bone mass [5]. Osteoporosis is not a contraindication to dental implant treatment; however, it increases marginal peri-implant bone loss [6]. Therefore, since estrogen deficiency is a contributing factor capable of causing catabolic changes in the peri-implant bone [2–5], it is necessary to ensure the peri-implant bone quality and consequent dental implant survival.

Dental implants are frequently placed in areas of alveolar ridge defects, dehiscence, or fenestrations, and bone grafts may be required to fill these peri-implant bone defects [7]. Likewise, bone substitutes are crucial for alveolar ridge preservation, proper implant stability, and bone formation for osseointegration [8]. However, the challenges of bone repair increase with estrogen deficiency [7]. This condition can reduce the differentiation of mesenchymal cells, impair angiogenesis [9], and increase osteoclast activity [10]. Estrogen deficiency may compromise an adequate peri-implant bone repair [11,12]. Also, estrogen deficiency can impair bone regeneration by lowering differentiation and maturation of osteoblasts and the formation of bone matrix [13,14]. Hence, it might be helpful to support the consolidation of bone substitutes in bone defects around dental implants under osteoporotic conditions.

Bio-Oss® is an established bone substitute prepared from deproteinized bovine cancellous bone with the expected osteoconductive properties [15–17]. Despite Bio-Oss® being widely used clinically, stimulating the local bone regeneration is advantageous for its consolidation with the implant and the local bone, particularly in situations of estrogen deficiency [18]. A promising alternative approach among various strategies involves the functionalization of Bio-Oss® with biomolecules to enhance bone regeneration [19]. Biomolecules to enhance bone regeneration using bone substitutes are being verified in estrogen deficiency conditions [20]. Ideally, these biomolecules should overcome the catabolic circumstances of estrogen deficiency.

Genistein ($C_{15}H_{10}O_5$) is a 7-hydroxy isoflavone categorized as an abundant isoflavone from soy [21,22]. This phytoestrogen has a molecular similarity to estrogen [23] and enhances osteoblast differentiation through estrogen receptors [24,25]. Its protective effect on bone is indicated by increasing the expression of osteocalcin [26], in addition to inhibiting osteoclastogenesis by changing the ratio of osteoprotegerin and receptor activator of nuclear factor kappa-B ligand [26,27]. Even though the ability of genistein to support bone regeneration under osteoporotic conditions was not confirmed [27], genistein is an effective treatment for overcoming experimental osteoporosis [25,28]. Our strategy is to distribute genistein within Bio-Oss® equal particles in functionalization by sonification.

Sonification is a novel tool for developing nanoscale biomaterials [7,29]. It uses ultrasound to homogenize and distribute biomolecules, thereby amplifying their physical–chemical properties [30]. Consequently, nanoparticles can improve the cellular interaction in bone, enhancing osteoblast differentiation [29,31]. Sonification is also effective for incorporating biomolecules into bone substitutes [32]. Therefore, in this study, it was investigated how genistein incorporated into Bio-Oss® by sonification affects bone repair in peri-implant defects using ovariectomized rats as a model for estrogen deficiency.

## 2. Materials and Methods

### 2.1. Ethics and Sample Size Calculation

The Ethics Committee approved this research on the use of animals from Araçatuba School of Dentistry, São Paulo State University (FOA/UNESP) under number 0499-2022. Additionally, this research was performed according to the ARRIVE Guidelines [33]. All evaluations were performed under calibration and blinding examination. The sample size of this study was calculated using the power test (OpenEpi, Version 3, Open-Source Calculator), based on results already published with a similar methodology using the values of the removal torque [7]. The means used for the calculation were 4.4 and 6.0 Ncm, with standard deviations of 1.51 and 2.6, with a significance level of 5% and power of 95% in a one-tailed hypothesis test. Therefore, the number of animals enrolled per group in this study was 10. Accordingly, a total of forty female six-month-old animals (*Rattus norvegicus albinus*, Wistar) weighing approximately 300 g were maintained at the Central Bioterium of Araçatuba School of Dentistry from UNESP in temperature-controlled conditions and exposed to a 12 h light–dark cycle. All the animals were kept in cages with water ad libitum and regular feed (Nuvilab, Curitiba, Brazil).

### 2.2. Estrous Cycle

The determination of the estrous cycle was executed before ovariectomy. The ovariectomy was performed on day 0. The peri-implant bone defects and implant placement were performed 30 days after ovariectomy, and the animals were euthanized 28 days after implant surgery. The animals were placed in individual cages for the estrous cycle evaluation, which was conducted daily [34]. To this, one or two drops of saline were introduced into the vagina, which was then aspirated and placed on a histological slide for immediate microscopic analysis to recognize the four phases of the estrous cycle, which are described as proestrus, estrus, metestrus, and diestrus [35]. After three regular cycles, the animals were applied for ovariectomy surgery.

### 2.3. Ovariectomy

Animals were kept on a six-hour preoperative fast. Then, the animals were subjected to sedation and anesthesia through intramuscular administration of ketamine hydrochloride (70 mg/kg; Francotar®, Virbac, São Paulo, Brazil) combined with xylazine hydrochloride (6 mg/kg; Xilazin®, Syntec, Barueri, Brazil). Trichotomy was performed in the abdominal region, followed by antisepsis with a povidone-iodine solution (10%; Rioquímica, São José do Rio Preto, Brazil). An incision was made with a No. 15 blade (Feather Industries, Tokyo, Japan) mounted on a n° 3 scalpel handle (Hu-Friedy, Frankfurt, Germany) in the middle part of the abdomen. After accessing the peritoneal cavity, the adipose tissue was retracted to identify the uterine tube and ovary, which were then collected. The surgical wound was sutured with polyglactin 910 4.0 thread (Ethicon Inc., São José dos Campos, Brazil). Intramuscular antibiotic therapy post-surgery was administered to all animals with benzathine penicillin G (0.2 mL; Pentabiótico® Veterinário Pequeno Porte, Fort Dodge Saúde Animal Ltda., Campinas, Brazil). Analgesia was provided intramuscularly for three days with sodium dipyrone (50–600 IU/kg; D-500®, Zoetis, Parsippany-Troy Hills, NJ, USA) and Tramadol (5 IU/kg; Nulli®, Ourofino Saúde Animal, Cravinhos, Brazil). One week before implant surgery, the estrous cycle was checked to evaluate the success of the ovariectomy, which remained in the diestrus phase. This same surgical technique followed a previous study [36].

### 2.4. Experimental Groups

After ovariectomy, the animals were randomized through a computer-generated list created in Stata 9.0 (StataCorp, College Station, TX, USA) and divided accordingly into the following four experimental groups (n = 10): CLOT control group, peri-implant defect filled with spontaneous blood clot formation; BO group, peri-implant defect filled with BO (Bio-Oss® Small 0.25–1 mm; Geistlich Pharma AG, Wolhusen, Switzerland); BOS group, peri-implant defect filled with BO sonicated alone; BOS + GEN group, peri-implant defect filled with BO and genistein (Sigma-Aldrich, San Luis, CA, USA) sonicated.

### 2.5. Sonification and Functionalization with Genistein

The sonification was performed at the Advanced Materials and Nanotechnology Laboratory, School of Sciences from UNESP. First, the calculation to determine the volume of biomaterial in the bone defect was performed by the physics P.N.L-H. The peri-implant defect created measured 3 mm in diameter and 3.5 mm in depth with a volume of 12.56 $mm^3$. It was subtracted by the implant volume of 5.25 $mm^3$, measuring 1.5 mm in diameter $\times$ 3.5 mm in height. The total volume of the peri-implant bone defect measured 7.31 $mm^3$. The underlying formula was volume = $\pi.r^2.a$. Thus, the result of the total volume of BO for the peri-implant bone defect was 25 mg. BO untreated was used in the BO group, while BO sonicated alone was utilized in the BOS group, and BO sonicated together with 3 mg of synthetic genistein ($\geq$98% purity; Sigma-Aldrich, San Luis, CA, USA) was used in the BOS + GEN group. The samples of BO were weighed as 25 mg on a precision scale (LW303iH, BEL Engineering®, Monza, Italy). Sonification was performed with a Sonics® VCX-750 (Sonics & Materials, Newtown, CT, USA) at 750 W and 20 kHz for 15 min. A variable amplitude of up to 40% with ultrapure water Milli-Q® (Millipore, Burlington, MA, USA) was used for the cavitation bubbles with high solute vapor. The time protocol was three cycles of three minutes each. Later, the bone substitutes were dried at 70 °C (TE-394/2 Model, Tecnal Scientific Equipment, Piracicaba, Brazil). The sonification followed a method as previously described [37]. Samples were sterilized using ultraviolet light for 20 min before the implant surgery.

*2.6. Peri-Implant Bone Defects and Implant Placement*

First, a peri-implant bone defect was created using larger drills in the upper cortical and medullary bones. Next, the bone defect was filled according to each experimental group. Lastly, the implant was placed into the bone defect with anchorage in the lower cortical bone, following a previously successful rat tibia model [7].

For that, animals were fasted for six hours before the surgery and anesthetized by a combination of ketamine hydrochloride (70 mg/kg; Francotar®, Virbac, São Paulo, Brazil) and xylazine hydrochloride (6 mg/kg; Xilazin®, Syntec, Barueri, Brazil). After anesthesia, a trichotomy was performed on the medial area of the right tibia. The antisepsis of the region was performed with a povidone-iodine solution (10%; Rioquímica, São José do Rio Preto, Brazil). A 1.5 cm incision was executed, and the tibial metaphysis was exposed through divulsion. In both tibias, a 1.3 mm bicortical drill was followed by a 3.0 mm drill in the upper cortical and medullary bone, thus maintaining the lower cortical to anchor the implant. Drilling was controlled by an electric motor (BLM 600 Model, Driller, Carapicuíba, Brazil) at a speed of 1000 rpm and contra-angle with 20:1 reduction (Angle Piece 3624N 1:4, Head 67RIC 1:4, KaVo, Biberach, Germany) under irrigation with sodium chloride solution (0.9%; Biosynthetic Ltda., Ribeirão Preto, Brazil).

The defects were filled with the respective biomaterials estimated in each group, except in the CLOT group which was left untreated. Finally, the implants were inserted in the middle of the bone defect. The implants were grade-four titanium (diameter of 1.5 mm and height of 3.5 mm; Titaniumfix®, São José dos Campos, Brazil) with a surface treated by a double acid attack using nitric, hydrofluoric, and sulfuric acid. Wound closure was performed with absorbable thread (Vycril 4.0, Ethicon; Johnson Products, São José dos Campos, Brazil) and monofilament thread (Nylon 5.0, Ethicon; Johnson, São José dos Campos, Brazil). In the immediate postoperative period, each animal received an intramuscular dose of 0.2 mL of penicillin G-benzathine (Fort Dodge Health Animal Ltda., Campinas, Brazil).

*2.7. Euthanasia*

After 28 days following implant surgery, euthanasia was performed according to a previous study [38]. Euthanasia was performed with an intraperitoneal overdose of sodium thiopental (2.5%; 150 mg/kg; Fort Dodge Saúde Animal Ltda., Campinas, Brazil) and lidocaine (2%; 10 mg/kg; Anesthetic; Laboratório Bravet Ltda., Rio de Janeiro, Brazil). The tibias of five animals per group were dissected for removal torque analysis. Next, the peri-implant tissue was collected for reverse transcription polymerase chain reaction (RT-PCR). The tibias of the other five animals per group were collected and stocked in 70% alcohol for micro-computed tomography (micro-CT). All implants were clinically without any signal of inflammation or infection, thereby no group presented any exclusion.

*2.8. Biomechanical Test (Removal Torque)*

The removal torque was executed in five animals per group; thus, a counterclockwise movement was used to analyze the removal torque of implants from the bone using a digital torque wrench (TQ-680 Model; Instrutherm, São Paulo, Brazil) coupled with a critical implant (Conexão Sistemas de Próteses, São Paulo, Brazil). The maximum value of removal torque was recorded in Newton per centimeter (Ncm) until the implant rotated inside the bone, as in the previous study [36].

### 2.9. Micro-CT

The other five animals per group were used for micro-CT. The tibias were scanned using a SkyScan Microtomography (SkyScan 1272; Bruker, Aatselaar, Belgium) from the Multi-User Laboratory of Araçatuba School of Dentistry from UNESP. The images were captured on a camera with a pixel size of 12.45 mm, 2672 × 4000, using 8 µm-thick cuts with a 90 kV X-ray beam, a 111 µA current, a 0.5 mm Al filter, and a 0.4° rotation step. Afterward, the images were reconstructed using NRecon Software (SkyScan v1.6.9.8) with smoothing of 1, ring trace correction of 3, beam strength correction of 5%, and image correction variation of 0. 0 to 0.11. The images were appropriate in a new set of data, positioning all samples standardized in the transverse, longitudinal, and sagittal planes using Data Viewer Software (SkyScan 1.4.4; Leuven, Belgium). The analyses were established using CTAnalyzer Software (SkyScan CTAn, v1.12.4.0; Leuven, Belgium). A region of interest (ROI) between the third and fifth medullary implant threats was used to evaluate 100 slices from its most central portion. Images were converted to gray scale values between 25 and 90 shades representing the new bone formed, excluding the titanium implant and the biomaterials. The parameters evaluated were the percentage of bone volume per tissue volume (BV/TV; %) and the surface of intersection (IS; $mm^3$), following the guideline [39]. The micro-CT analysis was used to characterize the tridimensional bone around the implants using CTvox Software (SkyScan 2.7; Leuven, Belgium). The micro-CT analysis was performed as recently reported [7].

### 2.10. Molecular Analysis (RT-PCR)

The same five tibias of removal-torque were immediately collected, ensuring at least 0.5 cm on each peri-implant side to preserve the bone in contact with the implant. RT-PCR evaluated the gene expression of proteins associated with bone repair. Each sample was washed in phosphate buffer solution and frozen in liquid nitrogen for total RNA extraction using Trizol reagent (Life Technologies Invitrogen, Carlsbad, CA, USA) and stored in a freezer at −80 °C. Following the RNA integrity, purity, and concentration assessment, cDNA was synthesized using 1 µg of RNA through reverse transcriptase reaction (M-MLV RT; Promega Corporation, Madison, AL, USA). The cDNAs from the samples were pipetted for the detection of genes with TaqMan Fast Advanced Mastermix (Applied Biosystems, Waltham, MA, USA) into a PCR plate (96 Well Fast Thermal Cycling; Thermo Fisher Scientific, Waltham, MA, USA). The RT-PCR was performed to assess the expression of osteoprotegerin (OPG; Tnfrsf11b; Rn00563499_m1), receptor activator of nuclear factor kappa B ligand (RANKL; Tnfrsf1; Rn00589289_m1), osteocalcin (OCN; BGGLAP; Rn00566386_g1), and bone sialoprotein (IBSP; IBSP; Rn00561414_m1). The genes and their primer sequences are shown in Table 1. RT-PCR was performed using a Step One Plus detection system from Taqman (Applied Biosystems, Waltham, MA, USA) under the following conditions: 50 °C (2 min), 95 °C (10 min), and 40 cycles of 95 °C (15 s), 60 °C (1 min), followed by the standard denaturation curve. The expression was calculated relative to the expression of mitochondrial ribosomal protein following the ΔΔCT method with ß-actin (Actb Rn00667869_m1) as an endogenous control. The assay was performed in quadruplicate [7].

**Table 1.** Primer sequences used for RT-PCR analysis.

| Gene | Gene Reference | Forward Primer, $5' \rightarrow 3'$ | Reverse Primer, $5' \rightarrow 3'$ |
|---|---|---|---|
| *OPG* | NM_057149.2 | GCACTCCTGGTGTTCTTGGA | TTTGGTCCCAGGCAAACTGT |
| *RANKL* | NM_057149.1 | CGAGCGCAGATGGATCCTAA | GAGCCACGAACCTTCCATCA |
| *IBSP* | NM_012587.2 | GTACCGGCCACGCTACTTTC | ATCTCCAGCCTTCTTGGGTAGC |
| *OCN* | NM_013414.1 | CTCTGAGTCTGACAAAGCCTTCAT | GTAGCGCCGGAGTCTATTCA |
| *ß-actin* | NM_031144.3 | CCACCATGTACCCAGGCATT | CCTAGAAGCATTTGCGGTGC |

### 2.11. Statistical Analysis

Statistical analysis was performed using SigmaPlot 12.5 Software (Systat Software Inc., San Jose, CA, USA). After obtaining all the data, the homoscedasticity test (Shapiro–Wilk) was performed first. A significance level of $p < 0.05$ was considered to confirm the normality distribution of the data. Thus, a one-way ANOVA test was applied for the removal torque, microtomographic, and molecular data, followed by the Tukey post-hoc test for multiple comparisons. Also, a confidence level of $p < 0.05$ was considered significant.

## 3. Results

### 3.1. Removal Torque Values

The implants were successfully installed and stability verified through a removal test. Figure 1 shows that the BOS + GEN had the highest removal torque with 5.4 Ncm, compared to the BOS ($p = 0.006$), BO ($p = 0.001$), and CLOT ($p = 0.0003$) with 3.0 Ncm, 2.3 Ncm, and 2.1 Ncm, respectively.

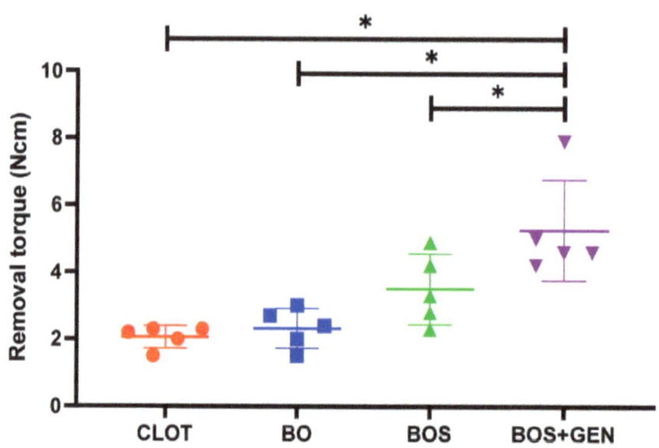


**Figure 1.** Biomechanical test of removal torque. Twenty-eight days after implant placement, each experimental group's removal torque was tested. The removal torque was increased until the implant rotated into the bone, and the highest torque in Newton centimeters was recorded. The statistically significant difference in comparison to the BOS + GEN group ($p < 0.05$) is indicated by *, determined using one-way ANOVA followed by Tukey's *t*-test.

### 3.2. Micro-CT

Consistent with the biomechanical outcomes, BV/TV was highest in the BOS + GEN group with 11.67% compared to CLOT ($p = 0.104$), BOS ($p = 0.017$), and BO ($p = 0.0002$) with 8.12%, 6.47%, and 2.32%, respectively Figure 2A. The IS parameter denoted bone-to-implant contact, and there was no statistical difference between the groups ($p > 0.05$); Tukey; Figure 2B. The representative three-dimensional image of bone repair around the implants installed can be observed in Figure 3.

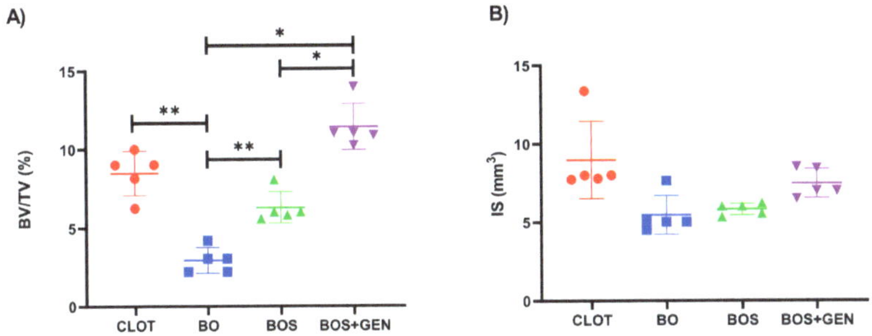


**Figure 2.** Micro-computerized tomography of peri-implant bone. Morphological parameters were estimated as follows: (**A**) percentage of bone volume per tissue volume (BV/TV, %); (**B**) intersection surface (IS; $mm^3$). The statistically significant difference is indicated by * in comparison to the BOS + GEN group. ** denotes a statistically significant difference in comparison to the BO group. The $p < 0.05$ was determined using one-way ANOVA followed by Tukey's $t$-test.

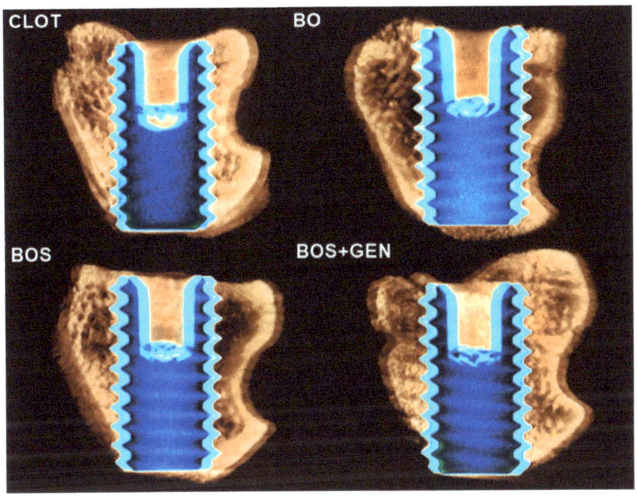


**Figure 3.** The 3D μCT reconstruction of the peri-implant bone area. The μCT images are representative of all four groups, CLOT, BO, BOS, and BOS + GEN, respectively. The microtomography images evidenced that genistein enhanced the peri-implant bone into the medullary implant threats in the BOS + GEN group. The microtomography was executed by applying the CTvox software (SkyScan, Version 2.7).

### 3.3. Molecular Analysis

The relative gene expression of OPG, RANKL, OCN, and IBSP showed higher expression in the BOS and BOS + GEN groups, as shown in Figure 4A–D. Next are the CLOT and BO groups. Then, the statistical differences between the groups were BOS vs. CLOT ($p < 0.0001$; Tukey), BOS vs. BO ($p < 0.0001$; Tukey), BOS vs. BOS + GEN ($p < 0.0001$; Tukey), BOS + GEN vs. CLOT ($p < 0.0001$; Tukey), and BOS vs. BOS + GEN ($p < 0.0001$; Tukey). Besides the exact differences, the relative gene expression of IBSP included the statistical difference between CLOT vs. BO ($p < 0.004$; Tukey).

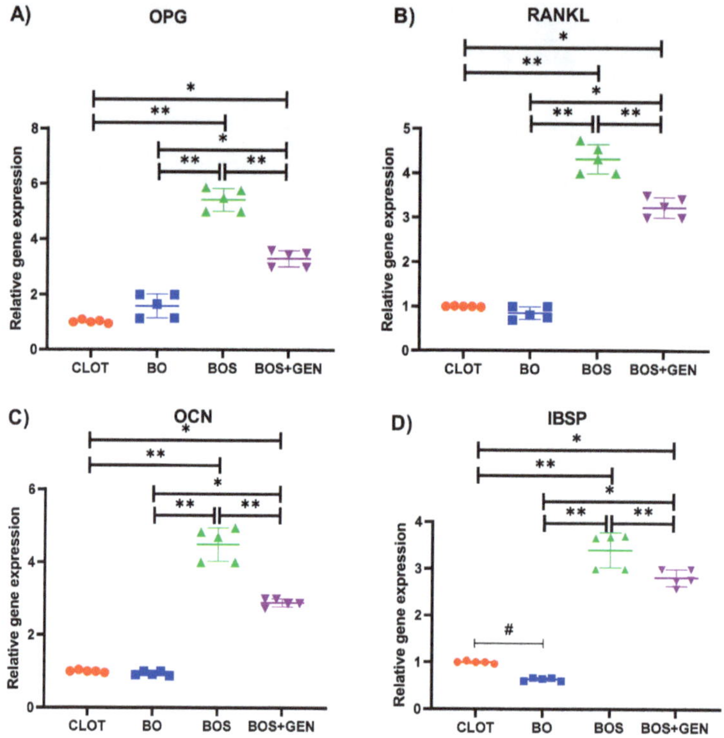


**Figure 4.** Molecular data from RT-PCR analysis of all groups. (**A**) OPG: osteoprotegerin; (**B**) RANKL: receptor activator of nuclear factor kappa-B ligand; (**C**) OCN: osteocalcin; (**D**) IBSP: bone sialoprotein. The * denotes a statistically significant difference in comparison to the BOS*GEN group. The ** denotes a statistically significant difference in comparison to the BOS group. The # denotes a statistically significant difference in comparison to the BO group. The statistically significant difference ($p < 0.05$) was determined using one-way ANOVA followed by Tukey's $t$-test.

## 4. Discussion

Given the increasing life expectancy, dental implants for oral rehabilitation are increasingly necessary [40]. There is a growing population of postmenopausal women necessitating dental implants [40]. Low estrogen levels can compromise bone repair around implants [11,12], in addition to impairing bone regeneration [13]. There is consequently an interest in local therapies to enhance bone repair in peri-implant defects under estrogen deficiency [41]. To this end, we show here that the functionalization of BO by sonification with genistein, compared to all other experimental groups, increased the removal torque of implants in rat tibia. Consistently, μCT revealed a higher BV/TV with BOS + GEN compared to BO or BOS. The improved bone microarchitecture can justify the higher removal torque. In addition, RT-PCR analysis indicates increased bone turnover when sonification with genistein or sonification alone was tested. The RANKL–OPG ratio indicates bone activity [42], thus the constant ratio suggests that genistein has a low impact on osteoclastogenesis. On the other hand, higher levels of OCN and IBSP indicate enhanced osteoblast activity [43,44]. These findings suggest that incorporating genistein improves the consolidation of bone substitutes, leading to enhanced implant stability.

Previous studies have confirmed the positive effects of genistein on osteoblastogenesis [45,46]. Genistein-coated implants resulted in greater bone-to-implant contact in osteoporotic rats [45]. In this study, genistein was identified as a catalyst for enhancing osteogenesis and bone quality with a cohesive network of osteocytes around the implants [45].

Similarly, an in vitro study demonstrated that genistein stimulates osteoblast differentiation by upregulating the expression estrogen receptor-α gene and Runt-related transcription factor 2 [46]. In line with our findings, sonification of other bone substitutes also favored osteogenic differentiation [7,32]. Bioactive glass sonicated with teriparatide enhanced peri-implant bone repair in osteoporotic male rats [7]. Under physiological conditions, bioactive glass sonicated alone also increased peri-implant bone formation by upregulating WNT signaling [32]. Prior studies reinforced an increased cellular reactivity of sonicated nanomaterials mainly by their amplified physical and chemical effects [47,48]. Moreover, nanomaterials can raise the expression of bone proteins as enzyme alkaline phosphatase, Runt-related transcription factor 2 [49]. It can be speculated that genistein loaded by sonification can be an anabolic strategy for bone regeneration, effectively stimulating osteogenesis.

The present results are crucial to fully understanding the experiment. The CLOT group exhibited enhanced bone volume attributed to endogenous bone formed by the blood clot. The higher BV/TV in the CLOT group compared to the BO group can be explained by the void created by the absence of biomaterial within the defect. Furthermore, the quality of bone formation in the absence of bone substitutes remains uncertain, particularly with compromised estrogen levels [50]. Thus, although the CLOT group presented greater BV/TV than the BO and BOS groups, it showed the lowest torque value. Likewise, despite the higher torques observed in the BOS + GEN group, the IS parameter did not indicate a variance in bone-to-implant ratio in the groups. Notably, the biomaterial serves as a scaffold for osteoprogenitor cells, augmenting implant stability [4]. This outcome validates the biomechanical reinforcement of the peri-implant bone by the genistein and solicitation, as evidenced by the higher torque in the BOS + GEN and BOS group. However, there is no difference between the CLOT and the BO group when comparing the torque. Consequently, it is suggested that genistein or sonification alone increases the biomechanical results by augmenting the osteoconductive properties of the bone substitute.

The findings here should be considered within the limitations of this study. The major limitation is that we cannot conclude about the effects of genistein on bone quality. The absence of undecalcified histology is not stipulated in the present study, which could provide valuable perceptions of the bone cells present in each group. A further limitation of this study was that genistein was tested only in deproteinized bovine cancellous bone. The unique time of sonification is also a restriction; however, the sonification time of 15 min demonstrated the best results in our prior study [32]. Additionally, the long bones of rats do not apply for the alveolar bone repair. Moreover, examining at just a one-time point does not provide comprehension of the effects of genistein on bone remodeling. Finally, genistein is considered dose-dependent, where excessive systemic doses have been demonstrated to hinder bone formation [51]. The unique concentration tested provided beneficial results in our study. Thus, future investigations should consider using other bone substitutes and different sonification protocols and drug concentrations before moving to clinical studies.

This study has significant clinical relevance. The main clinical implication is that genistein can be applicable in different scenarios of bone regeneration to overcome estrogen deficiency. Genistein incorporated into deproteinized bovine bone offers a local therapy different from the systemic use of estrogen in postmenopausal women. Estrogen therapy is known to have potential complications in the treatment of postmenopausal women, including cancer and cardiovascular events [52]. Additionally, genistein avoids the side effects of antiresorptive drugs for osteoporosis, such as medication-related osteonecrosis of the jaw [53,54]. Importantly, the use of genistein did not demonstrate systemic or tissue toxicity as in previous in vivo studies [55,56]. Conversely, genistein positively stimulated bone cell proliferation [55]. Genistein also had an antibacterial activity, affecting its acid synthesis and cytoplasmic membrane [55]. From a clinical perspective, genistein could also be beneficial against the presence of microorganisms in bone defects. Thus, it could be interesting in the context of peri-implant diseases. However, the results of this research should be viewed within the circumstances of a pre-clinical animal study. Future studies with an in vitro focus should evaluate the effect of genistein on the biological behavior of osteoblastic cells underlying the formation of the mineralized bone.

## 5. Conclusions

In conclusion, the evidence presented here implies that sonification of deproteinized bovine bone functionalized with genistein improves bone repair in peri-implant bone defects in ovariectomized rats, enhancing implant stability. Thus, these preclinical data demonstrate that genistein, an anti-catabolic drug, can help enhance bone regeneration under osteoporotic conditions in a rat model.

**Author Contributions:** Conceptualization, N.D.D. and R.O.; methodology, F.R.d.S.B., A.C.E.d.S., N.G.M. and M.B.G.; software, P.H.S.G.-F.; validation, N.D.D. and R.O.; formal analysis, N.D.D., N.G.M. and A.C.E.d.S.; investigation, N.D.D. and G.M.-S.; resources, R.O.; data curation, N.D.D., G.M.-S. and R.G.; writing—original draft preparation, N.D.D., G.M.-S. and R.G.; writing—review and editing, N.D.D., G.M.-S. and R.G.; visualization, R.O.; supervision, R.O., P.H.S.G.-F. and P.N.L.-F.; project administration, N.D.D. and R.O. All authors have read and agreed to the published version of the manuscript.

**Funding:** This research was funded by the São Paulo State Research Foundation (FAPESP), grant number 2022/07158-8 and 2023/05814-8. Also, Roberta Okamoto is affiliated with the Research Productivity Scholarship (process: 308408/2023-3).

**Institutional Review Board Statement:** The animal study protocol was approved by the Ethics Committee of Araçatuba School of Dentistry (protocol code 0499-2022 and date of approval 29 July 2022).

**Informed Consent Statement:** Not applicable.

**Data Availability Statement:** The authors will make the raw data supporting this article's conclusions available upon request.

**Acknowledgments:** The authors would like to thank the São Paulo State Research Foundation (FAPESP) for supporting this study (process number 2022/07158-8; 2023/05814-8). Titaniumfix® for supplying the implants. Multi-User Laboratory the Faculty of Dentistry of Araçatuba—UNESP and FINEP (FINEP/CT-INFRA-FINEP Agreement: 01.12.0530.00—PROINFRA 01/2011). In addition, the Laboratory of Advanced Materials and Nanotechnology at the Bauru Faculty of Sciences (FC/UNESP) and Professor Paulo Noronha Lisboa-Filho for assisting the sonification technique. This study was also supported by CNPq—National Council for Scientific and Technological Development—INCT Saúde Oral e Odontologia—Grants n. 406840/2022-9.

**Conflicts of Interest:** The authors declare no conflicts of interest.

## References

1. Huidrom, S.; Beg, M.A.; Masood, T. Post-menopausal Osteoporosis and Probiotics. *Curr. Drug Targets* **2021**, *22*, 816–822. [CrossRef] [PubMed]
2. Lu, L.; Tian, L. Postmenopausal osteoporosis coexisting with sarcopenia: The role and mechanisms of estrogen. *J. Endocrinol.* **2023**, *259*, e230116. [CrossRef]
3. Armas, L.A.G.; Recker, R.R. Pathophysiology of osteoporosis: New mechanistic insights. *Endocrinol. Metab. Clin. N. Am.* **2012**, *41*, 475–486. [CrossRef] [PubMed]
4. Zhang, X.; Wang, Z.; Zhang, D.; Ye, D.; Zhou, Y.; Qin, J.; Zhang, Y. The prevalence and treatment rate trends of osteoporosis in postmenopausal women. *PLoS ONE* **2023**, *18*, e0290289. [CrossRef]
5. Chen, F.; Zhang, Y.; Peng, P.; Huang, X.T.; Qiu, Z.H.; Liu, B.C.; Yang, B.C.; Yang, T.L.; Yang, B.; Guo, Y. Isolation and culture of human primary osteoblasts: Comparing the effects of differences in method details on osteoblast characteristics. *Genes Dis.* **2023**, *11*, 546–549. [CrossRef]
6. Lemos, C.A.A.; Oliveira, A.S.; Faé, D.S.; Oliveira, H.F.F.E.; Rosa, C.D.D.R.D.; Bento, V.A.A.; Verri, F.R.; Pellizzer, E.P. Do dental implants placed in patients with osteoporosis have higher risks of failure and marginal bone loss compared to those in healthy patients? A systematic review with meta-analysis. *Clin. Oral Investig.* **2023**, *27*, 2483–2493. [CrossRef]
7. Gomes-Ferreira, P.H.S.; Micheletti, C.; Frigério, P.B.; Batista, F.R.S.; Monteiro, N.G.; Júnior-Bim, O.; Lisboa-Filho, P.N.; Grandfield, K.; Okamoto, R. PTH 1-34-functionalized bioactive glass improves peri-implant bone repair in orchiectomized rats: Microscale and ultrastructural evaluation. *Biomater. Adv.* **2022**, *134*, 112688. [CrossRef] [PubMed]

8. Agarwal, R.; García, A.J. Biomaterial strategies for engineering implants for enhanced osseointegration and bone repair. *Adv. Drug Deliv. Rev.* **2015**, *94*, 53–62. [CrossRef]
9. Beil, F.T.; Barvencik, F.; Gebauer, M.; Seitz, S.; Rueger, J.M.; Ignatius, A.; Pogoda, P.; Schinke, T.; Amling, M. Effects of estrogen on fracture healing in mice. *J. Trauma.* **2010**, *69*, 1259–1265. [CrossRef]
10. Cheung, W.H.; Miclau, T.; Chow, S.K.; Yang, F.F.; Alt, V. Fracture healing in osteoporotic bone. *Injury* **2016**, *47*, S21–S26. [CrossRef]
11. Du, Z.; Xiao, Y.; Hashimi, S.; Hamlet, S.M.; Ivanovski, S. The effects of implant topography on osseointegration under estrogen deficiency induced osteoporotic conditions: Histomorphometric, transcriptional and ultrastructural analysis. *Acta Biomater.* **2016**, *42*, 351–363. [CrossRef] [PubMed]
12. Glösel, B.; Kuchler, U.; Watzek, G.; Gruber, R. Review of dental implant rat research models simulating osteoporosis or diabetes. *Int. J. Oral Maxillofac. Implant.* **2010**, *25*, 516–524.
13. Mardas, N.; Busetti, J.; de Figueiredo, J.A.; Mezzomo, L.A.; Scarparo, R.K.; Donos, N. Guided bone regeneration in osteoporotic conditions following treatment with zoledronic acid. *Clin. Oral Implant. Res.* **2017**, *28*, 362–371. [CrossRef]
14. Mulinari-Santos, G.; Dos Santos, J.S.; Kitagawa, I.L.; de Souza Batista, F.R.; Botacin, P.R.; Antoniali, C.; Lisboa-Filho, P.N.; Okamoto, R. Estrogen Deficiency Impairs Osseointegration in Hypertensive Rats Even Treated with Alendronate Coated on the Implant Surface. *J. Funct. Biomater.* **2023**, *14*, 471. [CrossRef]
15. Zhuang, G.; Mao, J.; Yang, G.; Wang, H. Influence of different incision designs on bone increment of guided bone regeneration (Bio-Gide® collagen membrane + Bio-Oss® bone powder) during the same period of maxillary anterior tooth implantation. *Bioengineered* **2021**, *12*, 2155–2163. [CrossRef]
16. Van Houdt, C.I.A.; Ulrich, D.J.O.; Jansen, J.A.; Van Den Beucken, J.J.J.P. The performance of CPC/PLGA and Bio-Oss® for bone regeneration in healthy and osteoporotic rats. *J. Biomed. Mater. Res. B Appl. Biomater.* **2018**, *106*, 131–142. [CrossRef]
17. Keil, C.; Gollmer, B.; Zeidler-Rentzsch, I.; Gredes, T.; Heinemann, F. Histological evaluation of extraction sites grafted with Bio-Oss® Collagen: Randomized controlled trial. *Ann. Anat.* **2021**, *237*, 151722. [CrossRef] [PubMed]
18. Wagner, F.; Schuder, K.; Hof, M.; Heuberer, S.; Seemann, R.; Dvorak, G. Does osteoporosis influence the marginal peri-implant bone level in female patients? A cross-sectional study in a matched collective. *Clin. Implant. Dent. Relat. Res.* **2017**, *19*, 616–623. [CrossRef] [PubMed]
19. Spicer, C.D.; Pashuck, E.T.; Stevens, M.M. Achieving Controlled Biomolecule-Biomaterial Conjugation. *Chem. Rev.* **2018**, *118*, 7702–7743. [CrossRef]
20. Zhang, X.; Cui, J.; Cheng, L.; Lin, K. Enhancement of osteoporotic bone regeneration by strontium-substituted 45S5 bioglass via time-dependent modulation of autophagy and the Akt/mTOR signaling pathway. *J. Mater. Chem. B* **2021**, *9*, 3489–3501. [CrossRef]
21. Yu, L.; Rios, E.; Castro, L.; Liu, J.; Yan, Y.; Dixon, D. Genistein: Dual role in women's health. *Nutrients* **2021**, *13*, 3048. [CrossRef] [PubMed]
22. Garbiec, E.; Cielecka-Piontek, J.; Kowalówka, M.; Holubiec, M.; Zalewski, P. Genistein–Opportunities related to an exciting molecule of natural origin. *Molecules* **2022**, *27*, 815. [CrossRef] [PubMed]
23. Mas-Bargues, C.; Borrás, C.; Viña, J. The multimodal action of genistein in Alzheimer's and other age-related diseases. *Free Radic. Biol. Med.* **2022**, *183*, 127–137. [CrossRef]
24. Kuiper, G.G.; Lemmen, J.G.; Carlsson, B.; Corton, J.C.; Safe, S.H.; van der Saag, P.T.; van der Burg, B.; Gustafsson, J.A. Interaction of estrogenic chemicals and phytoestrogens with estrogen receptor beta. *Endocrinology* **1998**, *139*, 4252–4263. [CrossRef]
25. Wu, G.J.; Cherng, Y.G.; Chen, J.T.; Chang, C.C.; Liu, S.H.; Chen, R.M. Genistein triggers translocation of estrogen receptor-alpha in mitochondria to induce expressions of ATP synthesis-associated genes and improves energy production and osteoblast maturation. *Am. J. Chin. Med.* **2021**, *42*, 901–923. [CrossRef]
26. Kauffmann, P.; Rau, A.; Seidlová-Wuttke, D.; Jarry, H.; Schminke, B.; Matthes, S.; Wiese, K.G. Effect of dihydrotestosterone, 17-β-estrogen, genistein and equol on remodeling and morphology of bone in osteoporotic male rats during bone healing. *Bone Rep.* **2020**, *13*, 100300. [CrossRef]
27. Kolios, L.; Sehmisch, S.; Daub, F.; Rack, T.; Tezval, M.; Stuermer, K.M.; Stuermer, E.K. Equol but not genistein improves early metaphyseal fracture healing in osteoporotic rats. *Planta Med.* **2009**, *75*, 459–465. [CrossRef] [PubMed]
28. Inpan, R.; Takuathung, M.N.; Sakuludomkan, W.; Dukaew, N.; Teekachunhatean, S.; Koonrungsesomboon, N. Isoflavone intervention and its impact on bone mineral density in postmenopausal women: A systematic review and meta-analysis of randomized controlled trials. *Osteoporos. Int.* **2024**, *35*, 413–430. [CrossRef]
29. Zou, Z.; Lin, K.; Chen, L.; Chang, J. Ultrafast synthesis and characterization of carbonated hydroxyapatite nanopowders via sonochemistry-assisted microwave process. *Ultrason. Sonochem* **2012**, *19*, 1174–1179. [CrossRef]
30. Arruda, L.B.; Orlandi, M.O.; Lisboa-Filho, P.N. Morphological modifications and surface amorphization in ZnO sonochemically treated nanoparticles. *Ultrason. Sonochem* **2013**, *20*, 799–804. [CrossRef]
31. McMahon, R.E.; Wang, L.; Skoracki, R.; Mathur, A.B. Development of nanomaterials for bone repair and regeneration. *J. Biomed. Mater. Res. B* **2013**, *10*, 387–397. [CrossRef] [PubMed]
32. Gomes-Ferreira, P.H.S.; Lisboa-Filho, P.N.; Silva, A.C.; Bim-Júnior, O.; Batista, F.R.S.; Ervolino-Silva, A.C.; Garcia-Junior, I.R.; Okamoto, R. Sonochemical time standardization for bioactive materials used in peri-implant defects filling. *Ultrason. Sonochem.* **2019**, *56*, 437–446. [CrossRef] [PubMed]

33. Percie du Sert, N.; Hurst, V.; Ahluwalia, A.; Alam, S.; Avey, M.T.; Baker, M.; Browne, W.J.; Clark, A.; Cuthill, I.C.; Dirnagl, U.; et al. The ARRIVE guidelines 2.0: Updated guidelines for reporting animal research. *PLoS Biol.* **2020**, *18*, e3000410.
34. Long, J.A.; Evans, H.M. *The Oestrus Cycle in the Rat and Its Related Phenomena*, 1st ed.; University of California Press: Berkeley, CA, USA, 1922.
35. Maeng, L.Y.; Cover, K.K.; Landau, A.J.; Milad, M.R.; Lebron-Milad, K. Protocol for studying extinction of conditioned fear in naturally cycling female rats. *J. Vis. Exp.* **2015**, *96*, 52202.
36. Mulinari-Santos, G.; de Souza Batista, F.R.; Kirchweger, F.; Tangl, S.; Gruber, R.; Okamoto, R. Losartan reverses impaired osseointegration in spontaneously hypertensive rats. *Clin. Oral Implant. Res.* **2018**, *29*, 1126–1134. [CrossRef]
37. Lisboa-Filho, P.N.; Gomes-Ferreira, P.H.S.; Batista, F.R.S.; Momesso, G.A.C.; Faverani, L.P.; Okamoto, R. Bone repair with raloxifene and bioglass nanoceramic composite in animal experiment. *Connect. Tissue Res.* **2018**, *58*, 97–100. [CrossRef]
38. Inoue, B.K.N.; Paludetto, L.V.; Monteiro, N.G.; Batista, F.R.S.; Kitagawa, I.L.; da Silva, R.S.; Antoniali, C.; Lisboa Filho, P.N.; Okamoto, R. Synergic Action of Systemic Risedronate and Local Rutherpy in Peri-implantar Repair of Ovariectomized Rats: Biomechanical and Molecular Analysis. *Int. J. Mol. Sci.* **2023**, *24*, 16153. [CrossRef]
39. Bouxsein, M.L.; Boyd, S.K.; Christiansen, B.A.; Guldberg, R.E.; Jepsen, K.J.; Müller, R. Guidelines for assessment of bone microstructure in rodents using micro-computed tomography. *J. Bone Miner. Res.* **2010**, *27*, 1468–1486. [CrossRef]
40. Dhayanithi, J.; Rajasekar, A. Comparison of Alveolar Bone Level around Osseointegrated Dental Implants among Premenopausal and Postmenopausal Women: A 2-Year Study. *J. Long. Term. Eff. Med. Implant.* **2024**, *34*, 89–92. [CrossRef]
41. Murphy, E. Estrogen signaling and cardiovascular disease. *Circ. Res.* **2011**, *109*, 687–696. [CrossRef]
42. Yasuda, H. Discovery of the RANKL/RANK/OPG system. *J. Bone Miner. Metab.* **2021**, *39*, 2–11. [CrossRef] [PubMed]
43. Komori, T. Functions of osteocalcin in bone, pancreas, testis, and muscle. *Int. J. Mol. Sci.* **2020**, *21*, 7513. [CrossRef] [PubMed]
44. Chavez, M.B.; Tan, M.H.; Kolli, T.N.; Zachariadou, C.; Farah, F.; Mohamed, F.F.; Chu, E.Y.; Foster, B.L. Bone sialoprotein is critical for alveolar bone healing in mice. *J. Dent. Res.* **2023**, *102*, 187–196. [CrossRef] [PubMed]
45. Micheletti, C.; DiCecco, L.A.; Deering, J.; Chen, W.; Ervolino da Silva, A.C.; Shah, F.A.; Palmquist, A.; Okamoto, R.; Grandfield, K. Mesoscale characterization of osseointegration around an additively manufactured genistein-coated implant. *Sci. Rep.* **2024**, *14*, 15339. [CrossRef]
46. Cepeda, S.B.; Sandoval, M.J.; Crescitelli, M.C.; Rauschemberger, M.B.; Massheimer, V.L. The isoflavone genistein enhances osteo-blastogenesis: Signaling pathways involved. *J. Physiol. Biochem.* **2020**, *76*, 99–110. [CrossRef]
47. Kumar, R.; Kumar, V.B.; Gedanken, A. Sonochemical synthesis of carbon dots, mechanism, effect of parameters, and catalytic, energy, biomedical and tissue engineering applications. *Ultrason. Sonochem.* **2020**, *64*, 105009. [CrossRef]
48. Low, S.S.; Yew, M.; Lim, C.N.; Chai, W.S.; Low, L.E.; Manickam, S.; Tey, B.T.; Show, P.L. Sonoproduction of nanobiomaterials—A critical review. *Ultrason. Sonochem.* **2022**, *82*, 105887. [CrossRef]
49. Bharadwaz, A.; Jayasuriya, A.C. Recent trends in the application of widely used natural and synthetic polymer nanocomposites in bone tissue regeneration. *Mater. Sci. Eng. C Mater. Biol. Appl.* **2020**, *110*, 110698. [CrossRef]
50. Bhatnagar, A.; Kekatpure, A.L. Postmenopausal Osteoporosis: A Literature Review. *Cureus* **2022**, *14*, e29367. [CrossRef]
51. Li, Y.Q.; Xing, X.H.; Wang, H.; Weng, X.L.; Yu, S.B.; Dong, G.Y. Dose-dependent effects of genistein on bone homeostasis in rats' mandibular subchondral bone. *Acta Pharmacol. Sin.* **2012**, *33*, 66–74. [CrossRef]
52. Hilakivi-Clarke, L.; Assis, S.; Warri, A. Exposures to synthetic estrogens at different times during life, and their effect on breast cancer risk. *J. Mammary Gland. Biol. Neoplasia* **2013**, *18*, 25–42. [CrossRef] [PubMed]
53. Martiniakova, M.; Babikova, M.; Omelka, R. Pharmacological agents and natural compounds: Available treatments for osteoporosis. *J. Physiol. Pharmacol.* **2020**, *71*, 1–14.
54. Ruggiero, S.L.; Dodson, T.B.; Aghaloo, T.; Carlson, E.R.; Ward, B.B.; Kademani, D. American Association of Oral and Maxillofacial Surgeons' Position Paper on Medication-Related Osteonecrosis of the Jaws-2022 Update. *J. Oral Maxillofac. Surg.* **2022**, *80*, 920–943. [CrossRef] [PubMed]
55. Mei, S.; Wang, F.; Hu, X.; Yang, K.; Xie, D.; Yang, L.; Wu, Z.; Wei, J. Construction of a hierarchical micro & nanoporous surface for loading genistein on the composite of polyetheretherketone/tantalum pentoxide possessing antibacterial activity and accelerated osteointegration. *Biomater. Sci.* **2021**, *9*, 167–185.
56. Sarasquete, C.; Úbeda-Manzanaro, M.; Ortiz-Delgado, J.B. Toxicity and non-harmful effects of the soya isoflavones, genistein and daidzein, in embryos of the zebrafish, Danio rerio. *Comp. Biochem. Physiology. Toxicol. Pharmacol. CBP* **2018**, *211*, 57–67. [CrossRef]

Journal of
*Functional Biomaterials*

MDPI

*Article*

# Development of Nanocomposite Microspheres for Nasal Administration of Deferiprone in Neurodegenerative Disorders

**Radka Boyuklieva [1,2], Plamen Katsarov [1,2], Plamen Zagorchev [2,3], Silviya Abarova [4], Asya Hristozova [1,5] and Bissera Pilicheva [1,2,*]**

1 Department of Pharmaceutical Sciences, Faculty of Pharmacy, Medical University of Plovdiv, 4002 Plovdiv, Bulgaria; radka.boyuklieva@mu-plovdiv.bg (R.B.); plamen.katsarov@mu-plovdiv.bg (P.K.); asya.hristozova@mu-plovdiv.bg (A.H.)
2 Research Institute, Medical University of Plovdiv, 4002 Plovdiv, Bulgaria; plamen.zagorchev@mu-plovdiv.bg
3 Department of Medical Physics and Biophysics, Faculty of Pharmacy, Medical University of Plovdiv, 4002 Plovdiv, Bulgaria
4 Department of Medical Physics and Biophysics, Faculty of Medicine, Medical University of Sofia, 1000 Sofia, Bulgaria; silviya.m.abarova@gmail.com
5 Department of Analytical Chemistry and Computational Chemistry, Faculty of Chemistry, University of Plovdiv "Paisii Hilendarski", 4000 Plovdiv, Bulgaria
* Correspondence: bisera.pilicheva@mu-plovdiv.bg

**Abstract:** Elevated brain iron levels are characteristic of many neurodegenerative diseases. As an iron chelator with short biological half-life, deferiprone leads to agranulocytosis and neutropenia with a prolonged therapeutic course. Its inclusion in sustained-release dosage forms may reduce the frequency of administration. On the other hand, when administered by an alternative route of administration, such as the nasal route, systemic exposure to deferiprone will be reduced, thereby reducing the occurrence of adverse effects. Direct nose-to-brain delivery has been raised as a non-invasive strategy to deliver drugs to the brain, bypassing the blood–brain barrier. The aim of the study was to develop and characterize nanocomposite microspheres suitable for intranasal administration by combining nano- and microparticle-based approaches. Nanoparticles with an average particle size of 213 ± 56 nm based on the biodegradable polymer poly-ε-caprolactone were developed using the solvent evaporation method. To ensure the deposition of the particles in the nasal cavity and avoid exhalation or deposition into the small airways, the nanoparticles were incorporated into composite structures of sodium alginate obtained by spray drying. Deferiprone demonstrated sustained release from the nanocomposite microspheres and high iron-chelating activity.

**Keywords:** deferiprone; nanocomposite microspheres; nasal administration; nose-to-brain delivery; neurodegenerative disorders

## 1. Introduction

Diseases of the central nervous system (CNS) are still a major challenge to the medical community. Most of the therapeutic agents administered orally or parenterally cannot reach the brain tissue due to the presence of the blood–brain and blood–cerebrospinal barriers. The latter, in combination with the presystemic metabolism, reduces the efficacy of the therapy, requires high doses of medicinal substances, and often causes adverse side effects [1–3].

Metals such as iron (Fe) and copper (Cu) are known to catalyze redox processes in the body. Longer lifespans lead to the accumulation of iron in various parts of the brain, although this is not always associated with toxicity. Iron plays a key role in the physiological functions of the brain, being involved in mitochondrial respiration and myelin and neurotransmitter synthesis. The distribution of iron in the brain is heterogeneous, with the highest concentrations found in the substantia nigra pars compacta and the basal ganglia, where it reaches levels comparable to those in the liver [4]. Various inflammatory processes increase the permeability of the blood–brain barrier and lead to Fe accumulation in the CNS. It is not fully understood why iron accumulation in specific brain regions becomes highly toxic in neurodegenerative diseases. Recent studies of activated microglia have shown that these cells exhibit a propensity to accumulate Fe, which can subsequently lead to cell death [5–7]. This type of cell death mediated by Fe-dependent lipid peroxidation is known as ferroptosis [8]. As cells age, their ability to maintain redox balance declines, leading to the accumulation of free reactive oxygen species (ROS), mitochondrial dysfunction, and neuronal damage.

Deferiprone (DFP) is an iron chelator and is indicated for the treatment of iron overaccumulation in patients with thalassemia major [9]. It belongs to the family of alpha-keto hydroxy pyridines, which are a relatively new class of chelating agents (Figure 1A). DFP binds iron in a molar ratio of 3:1 (Figure 1B). It is one of the few chelators that can cross cellular and subcellular membranes and enter cell organelles, where it binds to accumulated iron reserves and transports the complex-bound iron to plasma transferrin [10]. DFP can bind and eliminate accumulated iron from various parts of the body, including the liver, brain, and heart. DFP exhibits selectivity for iron and almost no affinity for other metals such as zinc, aluminum, and copper. After oral administration, DFP is rapidly and completely absorbed from the upper compartments of the gastrointestinal tract. Peak plasma concentrations of DFP taken in the fasting state are reached approximately 1 h after oral administration. Its elimination occurs mainly by metabolism in the liver, and the major metabolite is a 3-O-glucuronide conjugate that is excreted by the kidney. This metabolite has no iron-binding capacity due to the inactivation of the 3-hydroxy group of DFP. It has a biological half-life of 2–3 h, necessitating the maintenance of effective plasma drug concentrations by administering individual doses at short intervals several times daily [11]. This can be a cause of non-adherence, especially in elderly patients, and compromise treatment success. The development of sustained-release dosage forms of DFP may reduce dosing frequency and improve patients' compliance.

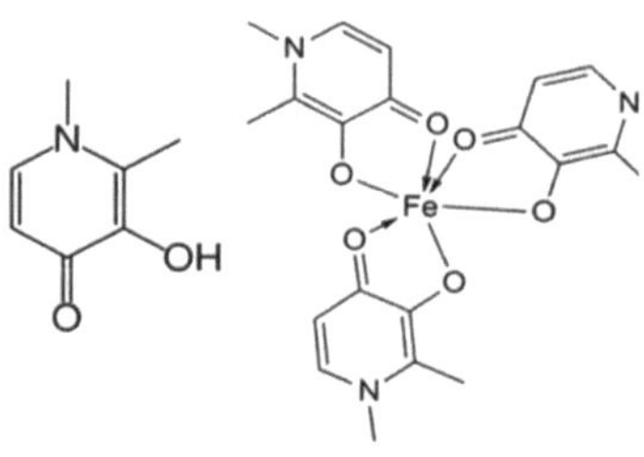

(A) (B)

**Figure 1.** Chemical structure of DFP (**A**) and iron ion binding sites (**B**).

In view of the drawbacks of the oral route, researchers turned to alternative routes of administration. Intranasal administration of drugs eliminates the problems associated with their low absorption, reduced stability, or rapid biotransformation. The olfactory region, located in the hard-to-reach upper part of the nasal cavity, allows substances to bypass the blood–brain barrier and enter the brain directly. This occurs due to the olfactory neurons being in contact with the nasal cavities and the central nervous system simultaneously [12]. Direct nasal administration of some drugs without the use of carriers can provoke serious adverse clinical manifestations. To reach the brain intact, therapeutic agents must be incorporated into appropriate drug delivery systems. Nanosized carriers can carry drugs from the nasal cavity to the brain while protecting them from enzymatic and/or chemical degradation and improving their passage across membrane barriers [13]. Despite the listed advantages, the nanosized structures, due to their small size, follow the respiratory tract and exit the nasal cavity after nasal administration, while microparticles of about

10 μm size after inhalation can deposit in the olfactory region of the nasal cavity [14]. For smaller particles, the site of deposition depends on the velocity at which the particles are inhaled and the turbulence in the airflow [15]. There is some evidence that microparticles improve the delivery of active molecules to the CNS by prolonging the contact time with the nasal mucosa, but due to their larger size, they cannot reach the brain and release the active molecules there [16,17]. Optimizing the size of drug-loaded particles will help their preferential deposition in the olfactory region, and the contact time between the particles and the mucosa will be crucial for the release and absorption of drugs [18,19].

Researchers are expanding the scope of synthesis from basic structures, such as micro- and nanoparticles, to more complex carriers. Nanocomposite microparticles are a new class of drug delivery systems that consist of nanosized particles dispersed into a polymer matrix. By designing the composite structure, carriers with specific physicochemical and mechanical characteristics can be obtained [20]. These structures are a combination of the best properties of their components, exhibiting additional interesting characteristics that the individual ingredients often do not possess.

The aim of the present study is to develop nanocomposite microspheres with optimal bioadhesive and biopharmaceutical properties for the nasal administration of DFP in the therapy of neurodegenerative diseases.

## 2. Materials and Methods

### 2.1. Materials

Deferiprone (DFP, Mw 139.15 g/mol), poly-ε-caprolactone (PCL, Mw 14,000, 80,000 g/mol), sodium alginate (from brown algae, medium viscosity ≥ 2000 cP, 2% (25 °C)), polysorbate 20 (Mw 1220 g/mol), Span 85 (Mw 957.49 g/mol), and human serum albumin (≥96%) were purchased from Sigma-Aldrich (St. Louis, MO, USA). All other reagents and solvents were of analytical grade and used as provided.

### 2.2. Methods

#### 2.2.1. Nanoparticles (NP) Preparation

For the nanoencapsulation of water-soluble substances (such as DFP) by a solvent evaporation technique, the preparation of a W/O emulsion is appropriate. Due to the difficulty in isolating the particles from the oil phase of the emulsion and with a view to their subsequent incorporation into composite structures in the form of aqueous dispersions, the double emulsion technique and the preparation of a W/O/W emulsion type were chosen. The preparation of PCL nanoparticles by double emulsion technique with subsequent evaporation of the solvent was carried out in two steps (Figure 2). In the first step, for the formation of the primary emulsion (W1/O), the internal aqueous phase (W1) without active substance (placebo) or with DFP was emulsified in the oil phase containing the polymer (PCL) dissolved in dichloromethane (DCM) and the emulsifying agent (Span 85) under high-speed homogenization at 17,500 rpm (Miccra MiniBatch D-9, MICCRA GmbH, Heitersheim, Germany) for 3 min. In the second step, the primary emulsion (W1/O) was dispersed into 50 mL of the external aqueous phase (W2) containing purified water and polysorbate 20 as an emulsifying agent. Emulsification was performed under high-speed homogenization at 22,500 rpm for 5 min to form the double emulsion (W1/O/W2). Subsequently, the formed nanoemulsion was stirred with an HS-100D mechanical stirrer (Witeg Labortechnik GmbH, Wertheim, Germany) at a speed of 800 rpm until complete evaporation of dichloromethane, resulting in solidification of the PCL polymer droplets. The obtained NPs were separated by centrifugation in Amicon® ultracentrifuge tubes (Merck KGaA, Darmstadt, Germany) at 3800× $g$ for 20 min at (20 ± 1) °C (Figure 2), washed with petroleum ether to remove residual water, and dried at room temperature for 24 h. The samples were stored in tightly closed containers in a dark place at 20 ± 2 °C for further use.

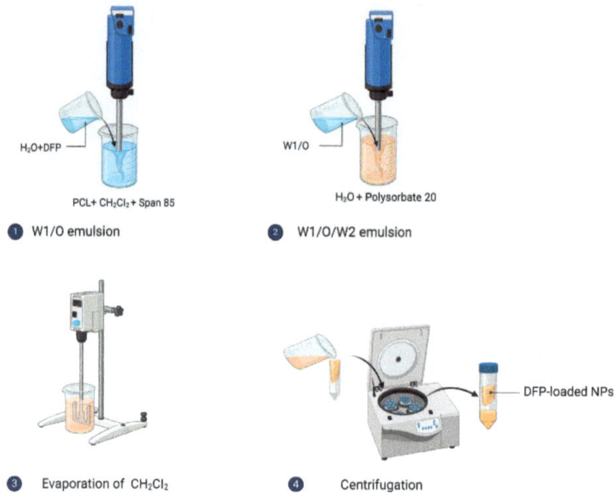


**Figure 2.** Schematic illustration of nanoparticle preparation by double emulsion technique (figure created with BioRender.com).

2.2.2. Preparation of Nanocomposite Microspheres

Alginate microspheres loaded with the formulated PCL nanoparticles were prepared by spray drying using Büchi Mini Spray Dryer B-290 (Büchi Labortechnik AG, Flawil, Switzerland). Briefly, sodium alginate was dissolved in purified water (0.5% or 1% *w*/*v*), and the drug-loaded nanoparticles at an amount corresponding to 200 mg drug content were dispersed into the polymer solution (100 mL). The dispersions were continuously stirred on a magnetic stirrer at 300 rpm and were spray–dried through a 0.7 mm nozzle using pressurized nitrogen (5 bar) and aspiration of 35 $m^3$/h. To achieve a high production yield and mean particle diameter above 5 μm (suitable for nasal administration) [21], the process parameters were varied as follows: drying temperature from 120 °C to 160 °C, feed rate 5 ÷ 7.5 mL/min, and gas flow rate from 400 to 600 L/h. Placebo nanocomposite microparticles without drug substance were also prepared using the described methodology.

*2.3. Characterization Techniques*

2.3.1. Particle Size Analysis, Size Distribution, and Zeta Potential

The size, size distribution, and ζ-potential of the obtained nanoparticles were determined by a Nanotrac particle size analyzer (Microtrac, York, PA, USA) provided with a 3 mW He/Ne laser at 780 nm wavelength. Noninvasive backscattering technology allows for analyzing the size in the range of 0.8 nm to 6.5 μm. The samples from the nanoparticle suspension were directly measured. All the measurements were performed at 25.0 °C at 20 s intervals and were repeated three times.

The size of the nanocomposite microparticles and their size distribution were determined by laser diffraction with an LS 13 320 particle size analyzer (Beckman Coulter, Brea, CA, USA) equipped with a Tornado Dry Powder System. One hundred milligrams of particles were used for each measurement ($n$ = 3).

2.3.2. Scanning Electron Microscopy (SEM)

The formulated nano- and micro-sized particles were analyzed in terms of shape and surface morphology using a scanning electron microscope (Prisma E SEM, Thermo Scientific, Waltham, MA, USA). The dry samples were coated with gold using a sputter coater (Q150T ES Plus, Quorum technologies, West Sussex, UK) and then micrographic images at appropriate magnification were recorded at 15 kV acceleration voltage.

#### 2.3.3. Transmission Electron Microscopy (TEM)

The obtained nanoparticles were also observed using a transmission electron microscope Talos F200C G2 (Talos 1.15.3, Thermo Fisher Scientific, Waltham, MA, USA). The analyzed sample (a suspension of the nanoparticles) was dried for 24 h on a formvar-coated copper grid (200 mesh). The images were taken at 200 kV and recorded with Velox Imaging Software (Velox 2.15.0.45, Waltham, MA, USA).

#### 2.3.4. Fourier-Transform Infrared Spectroscopy (FTIR)

FTIR analysis using a Nicolet iS 10 FTIR spectrometer (Thermo Fisher Scientific, Pittsburgh, PA, USA) was performed in order to evaluate drug–polymer interactions. An ATR accessory (diamond attenuated total reflection) was used to record the spectra of the samples within the range of 600–4000 $cm^{-1}$. OMNIC® software package (Version 7.3, Thermo Electron Corporation, Madison, WI, USA) was utilized for image editing.

#### 2.3.5. Differential Scanning Calorimetry (DSC)

Thermal analysis of the particles was performed using a DSC 204F1 Phoenix (Netzsch Gerätebau GmbH, Selb, Germany). An indium standard (Tm = 156.6 °C, ΔHm = 28.5 J/g) was used to calibrate the temperature and heat flux. The measurements were performed in an argon atmosphere at a heating rate of 10 °C/min.

#### 2.3.6. Production Yield

The production yield of nano- and microparticles was calculated based on the weight of particles obtained (W1) and the total weight of the polymer/polymers (PCL/PCL and sodium alginate) and the drug (W2) by the following equation:

$$Yield\ (\%) = \frac{W1}{W2} \times 100$$

#### 2.3.7. Estimation of Drug Loading (DL) and Entrapment Efficiency (EE)

The amount of DFP included in the nanoparticles and nanocomposite microspheres was determined by high-performance liquid chromatography (HPLC). To separate drug-loaded nanoparticles from the free DFP, the nanoparticle suspension was centrifuged (Sigma Centrifuge 3-18 KS, Osterode am Harz, Germany) in Amicon®Ultra-15 tubes (100 K MWCO) (Merck KGaA, Darmstadt, Germany) for 20 min at 3800× *g* at 20 ± 1 °C. Dichloromethane, methanol, and purified water were added to the nanoparticles from each batch. The samples were placed in a sonication bath (Sonorex Bandelin electronic, Berlin, Germany) to extract DFP. After filtration (PTFE, 0.45 µm), the amount of DFP was determined by HPLC (UltiMate 3000, Thermo Scientific, Waltham, MA, USA) using an Inertsil® ODS-3HPLC column (150 × 4.6 mm, 5 µm, GL Sciences, Tokyo, Japan) under the following conditions: wavelength 280 nm, injection volume 50 µL, flow rate 1 mL/min, column oven temperature 22 °C, and mobile phase PBS pH 2.5 (o-$H_3PO_4$) and acetonitrile in a ratio 67:33 (*v:v*). DFP retention time was 4.86 min; assay duration was 15 min.

To evaluate the DEE of composite structures, dichloromethane, methanol, and water were added to the microparticles. They were placed in a sonication bath to extract DFP. After filtration (PTFE, 0.45 µm), the concentration of DFP was determined according to the described HPLC method.

The drug loading (DL) of the particles was calculated according to the equation:

$$DL(\%) = \frac{\text{Amount of drug in the formulation (mg)}}{\text{Total amount of particles (mg)}} \times 100$$

The drug entrapment efficiency (DEE) was calculated according to the following equation:

$$DEE(\%) = \frac{\text{Actual drug content (mg)}}{\text{Theoretical drug content (mg)}} \times 100$$

#### 2.3.8. In Vitro Drug Release Studies and Release Kinetics

The drug release behavior was studied in vitro using the dialysis bag diffusion technique. Dialysis tubing cellulose membrane (MWCO 12 kDa, Sigma-Aldrich Chemie GmbH, Taufkirchen, Germany) was used. One day before the study, the dialysis membrane was cut into pieces 6 × 2.5 $cm^2$ and hydrated in purified water. In the dialysis bag, 1 mL dispersion of nanoparticles (a certain amount, equivalent to 1.15 mg DFP) in phosphate-buffered saline (PBS, pH 7.4) was placed and the bag was closed with plastic clamps. The dialysis bag was placed in a glass beaker containing an 18 mL acceptor medium (PBS buffer, pH 7.4) and kept on an electromagnetic stirrer at 100 rpm and 37 °C. At predetermined time points, 1 mL from the release medium was withdrawn and replaced with an equal volume of fresh medium. All samples were filtered (0.45 µm PTFE syringe filters, Isolab Laborgeräte Gmb, Eschau, Germany) and analyzed according to the described HPLC methods (Section 2.3.7).

#### 2.3.9. In Vitro Determination of Fe-Chelating Activity of Deferiprone Included in Nanocomposite Microparticles

The ability of DFP to bind free iron ions was determined against the iron indicator ferrozine by the method suggested by Dinis et al. [22]. Ferrozine (3-(2-pyridyl)-5,6-diphenyl-1,2,4-triazine p,p′-disulfonic acid) forms a stable complex with free iron ions (Fe(II)) with a characteristic red color and an absorption maximum at 562 nm. Compounds that bind Fe(II) reduce the amount of free Fe(II) in the solution and lower the concentration of the ferrozine-Fe(II) complex, which also leads to a decrease in the absorbance at 562 nm.

For the test, DFP solution in purified water with a concentration of 1 mg/mL, 0.1 mM $FeSO_4$ solution, and 0.25 mM ferrozine solution were prepared. Placebo (38 mg) and drug-loaded (amount equivalent to 2 mg DFP) nanocomposite microspheres were dispersed in 2 mL purified water. Two milliliters of $FeSO_4$ aqueous solution (0.1 mM) were added, the mixture was shaken, and the reaction was initiated by adding 2 mL of 0.25 mM ferrozine solution. A mixture of 0.1 mM $FeSO_4$ and 0.25 mM ferrozine (1:1) was used as a control. The resulting reaction mixtures were left at room temperature for 10 min then filtered (cellulose acetate, 0.45 µm), and their absorbance was read spectrophotometrically at a wavelength of 562 nm against a blank to exclude interference from the excipients. Fe-chelating activity (Ferrous ions chelating, FIC) was calculated by the following formula:

$$\%\mathbf{FIC} = \frac{A_0 - A_1}{A_0} \times \mathbf{100}$$

where $A_0$ is the absorbance of the control and $A_1$ is the absorbance of the test substances.

#### 2.3.10. Determination of the Ability of DFP-Loaded Nanoparticles to Bind Human Serum Albumin (HSA)

The binding ability of the nanoparticles to human serum albumin was investigated by fluorescence spectroscopy (FS). It is a sensitive method for studying the interaction between drug molecules and HSA, based on the characteristic fluorescent properties of HSA due to three amino acid residues in its structure: tryptophan, tyrosine, and phenylalanine. Upon excitation in the range from 280 nm to 295 nm, albumin emits intensely with a major emission peak at about 340 nm [23]. To investigate the potential interaction between HSA and the model nanoparticles, the fluorescence spectra of albumin were recorded in the absence and presence of increasing amounts of the nanocomposite microspheres. In the case of interaction, the fluorescence intensity of HSA gradually decreases with increasing amounts of nanoparticles [24].

The experiment was carried out at a temperature of 37 °C. Six samples were prepared for the analysis. The nanocomposite microspheres were dispersed in 1.1 mL saline. HSA solution with a concentration of 2.7 mg/mL was prepared. To each sample containing 1 mL of HSA solution, 20, 40, 60, 80, and 100 µL of the nanosuspension were added, respectively, and the samples were diluted with saline to a final volume of 1.1 mL. The samples were incubated for 1 h at 25 °C or 37 °C, after which the fluorescence analysis was performed. The spectra were recorded in the range of 310 ÷ 500 nm.

2.3.11. Mucoadhesive Ability of the Nanocomposite Microspheres

The mucoadhesive ability of the nanocomposite microspheres was investigated by determining the maximum adhesive force applied to a unit area of freshly isolated sheep nasal mucosa (Figure 3) [25–27]. Within one hour after the death of the animal, the nasal mucosa was excised and fixed immobile on a paraffin disc. PBS buffer (pH 7.4) was used as a solution for storing and moistening the mucosa. A cylinder, obtained by compressing microspheres using a hydraulic press, was fixed on a microscopic coverslip. The sample was brought into contact with the mucosal surface tempered at 30 °C ± 0.5 °C for different time intervals (1, 3, 5, 10, 15, and 25 min). The maximum adhesive force applied per unit area was estimated by an interface system, composed of an Isometric force transducer TRI201 (LSI LETICA Scientific Instruments, Panlab S.L., Barcelona, Spain), an amplifier with very high gain, and a filtering system. The voltage obtained at the output of the amplifier was converted to digital form by a microcontroller-operated 13-bit analog-to-digital converter.

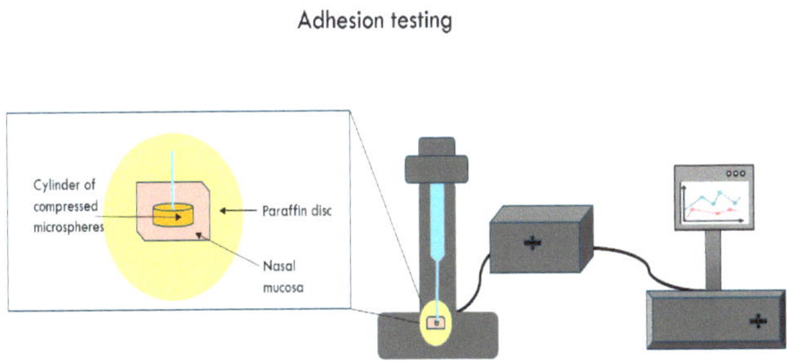


**Figure 3.** Schematic illustration of the experimental set-up for the study of mucoadhesive ability.

Statistical Analysis and Processing of Experimental Data from the Mucoadhesive Test and Fe-Chelating Activity

Statistical analysis was performed using GraphPad Prism v6.01 (GraphPad, Soft, Boston, MA, USA). To determine the statistically significant difference between the average values in the groups, a significance level of $p < 0.05$ was adopted. The data analyzed included results with statistically insignificant standard deviations from the mean, as demonstrated by Friedman's one-factor test, Friedman ANOVA.

## 3. Results and Discussion

### *3.1. Preparation of Poly-ε-Caprolactone Nanoparticles by Double Emulsion/Solvent Evaporation Technique*

The common emulsion solvent evaporation technique by forming an O/W emulsion type was not considered suitable for the inclusion of the water-soluble compound DFP due to its rapid distribution in the external aqueous phase. Therefore, based on the high-water solubility of DFP, a double emulsion technique was used to obtain nanoparticles, and a W/O/W emulsion type was chosen. DCM was used as the oil phase. The conditions of the applied technique (stirring speed, concentration of emulsifying agents, volume of internal and external aqueous phases) were established in preliminary experimental work, in which PCL 14 kDa at a concentration of 0.5% was used (Table 1). At a higher concentration of the polymer, particles with a size outside the desired range were obtained.

**Table 1.** Data from preliminary experimental work. "**Bold**" values indicate changed parameters.

| Conditions | Primary Emulsion's Parameters (W1/O) | | | Double Emulsion's Parameters W1/O/W2 | | | Average Particle Size (nm) ± SD |
|---|---|---|---|---|---|---|---|
| | Inner Phase, W1 (mL) | Stirring Speed (rpm) | Span 85 (%) | Polysorbate 20(%) | Outer Phase, W2 (mL) | Stirring Speed (rpm) | |
| Stirring speed for W1/O | 1.0 | **11,000** | 1.0 | 1.0 | 50.0 | 25,000 | 356 ± 65 |
| | 1.0 | **16,000** | 1.0 | 1.0 | 50.0 | 25,000 | 310 ± 25 |
| | 1.0 | **21,000** | 1.0 | 1.0 | 50.0 | 25,000 | 270 ± 21 |
| Stirring speed for W1/O/W2 | 1.0 | 21,000 | 1.0 | 1.0 | 50.0 | **16,000** | 865 ± 18 |
| | 1.0 | 21,000 | 1.0 | 1.0 | 50.0 | **21,000** | 350 ± 32 |
| | 1.0 | 21,000 | 1.0 | 1.0 | 50.0 | **25,000** | 274 ±12 |
| Concentration of Span 85 | 1.0 | 21,000 | - | 1.0 | 50.0 | 25,000 | unstable W1/O |
| | 1.0 | 21,000 | **0.5** | 1.0 | 50.0 | 25,000 | 480 ± 29 |
| | 1.0 | 21,000 | **1.0** | 1.0 | 50.0 | 25,000 | 290 ± 16 |
| Concentration of Polysorbate 20 | 1.0 | 21,000 | 1.0 | **0.5** | 50.0 | 25,000 | 310 ± 27 |
| | 1.0 | 21,000 | 1.0 | **1.0** | 50.0 | 25,000 | 278 ± 10 |
| | 1.0 | 21,000 | 1.0 | **1.5** | 50.0 | 25 000 | 254 ± 8 |
| Volume of W1 | **1.0** | 21,000 | 1.0 | 1.0 | 50.0 | 25,000 | 285 ± 11 |
| | **1.5** | 21,000 | 1.0 | 1.0 | 50.0 | 25,000 | 310 ± 7 |
| | **2.0** | 21,000 | 1.0 | 1.0 | 50.0 | 25,000 | 369 ± 13 |
| Volume of W2 | 1.0 | 21,000 | 1.0 | 1.0 | **20.0** | 25,000 | 420 ± 21 |
| | 1.0 | 21,000 | 1.0 | 1.0 | **30.0** | 25,000 | 390 ± 19 |
| | 1.0 | 21,000 | 1.0 | 1.0 | **50.0** | 25,000 | 266 ± 8 |

In the preliminary experimental work of our team, it was found that increasing the stirring speed from 11,000 rpm to 16,000 rpm during the first step of emulsification did not significantly affect the final particle size. The size decreased when the stirring speed was further increased to 21,000 rpm, at which speed particles of about 270 nm were obtained. During the second emulsification stage, increasing the stirring speed resulted in a proportional decrease in particle size from 865 nm to 274 nm. This shows that the stirring speed during the second step has a key effect on the particles' size. This hypothesis was also confirmed by Yang et al., who found that in the double emulsion technique, the stirring speed during the second step is a determining factor for the particles' size [28]. However, the stirring speed should not be too high, because instead of multiple, simple emulsion can be obtained [29]. The type and concentration of the emulsifier are important for the stability of the double emulsion. In preliminary tests, the inclusion of a lipophilic and a hydrophilic emulsifier, respectively, in the oil and outer water phases (W2) prevented droplet coalescence during the emulsification stages. One of the samples was prepared without an emulsifier in the oil phase, resulting in a rapid phase separation and inability to form a stable emulsion. Excessive amounts of lipophilic emulsifier may result in the formation of a simple W/O emulsion. A low concentration of the emulsifier in W2 led to an increase in the size of the resulting particles, probably due to the coalescence of the polymer droplets. Conversely, an excessive amount of hydrophilic emulsifier can solubilize the lipophilic phase and accelerate the movement of molecules from the internal to the external aqueous phase. Therefore, the concentration of the hydrophilic emulsifier should be as low as possible [30].

Varying the volume of the internal aqueous phase (W1) did not affect the final size of the particles formed after evaporation of the organic phase, while an increase in the volume of the external aqueous phase (W2) reduced the size of the particles. Larger particles were obtained at a W2 volume of up to 20 mL, and as the volume increased to 50 mL, the particle size decreased. This may be due to a decrease in the viscosity of the emulsion because of the larger volume of the external aqueous phase.

Based on the results of the preliminary experimental work, optimal conditions for obtaining PCL nanoparticles using the double emulsion technique were established (Table 2). Blank nanoparticles from PCL 80 kDa were also obtained under the indicated optimal conditions. Increasing the molecular weight of the polymer expectedly led to some increase in the average particle size, but it remained within the desired range for nose-to-brain delivery.

**Table 2.** Optimal conditions for the preparation of nanoparticles by the double emulsion technique.

| Primary Emulsion's Parameters W1/O | | | | Double Emulsion's Parameters W1/O/W2 | | |
|---|---|---|---|---|---|---|
| Inner Phase, W1 (mL) | Stirring Speed (rpm) | *PCL* (%) | Span 85 (%) | Polysorbate 20 (%) | Outer Phase, W2 (mL) | Stirring Speed (rpm) |
| 1.0 | 21,000 | 0.5 | 1.0 | 1.0 | 50.0 | 25,000 |

## 3.2. *Preparation and Characterization of Deferiprone-Loaded Poly-ε-Caprolactone Nanoparticles*

Two batches of DFP-loaded PCL nanoparticles were developed. The molecular weight of the polymer was varied to determine its influence on drug entrapment efficiency. Low (14,000 g/mol) and high (80,000 g/mol) molecular weight PCLs were used. The nanoparticles' composition is presented in Table 3.

**Table 3.** Composition and characteristics of deferiprone-loaded nanoparticles (means ± SD, $n$ = 3; "-" not included).

| Sample Code | DFP (mg) | PCL (14 kDa) (mg) | PCL (80 kDa) (mg) | DFP: PCL | Mean Diameter (nm) | PDI | ζ-Potential (mV) |
|---|---|---|---|---|---|---|---|
| NP1-DFP | 12.5 | 25.0 | - | 1:2 | 213 ± 56 | 0.820 | −12.70 ± 0.5 |
| NP2-DFP | 12.5 | - | 25.0 | 1:2 | 241 ± 91 | 0.535 | −18.22 ± 0.1 |

The nanoparticles from both batches had a monomodal size distribution (Figure 4) and relatively high ζ-potential values. This implies the presence of electrostatic repulsion between the particles, which prevents their aggregation and stabilizes the dispersion. The average particle size ranged from 213 ± 56 nm to 241 ± 91 nm (Table 3).

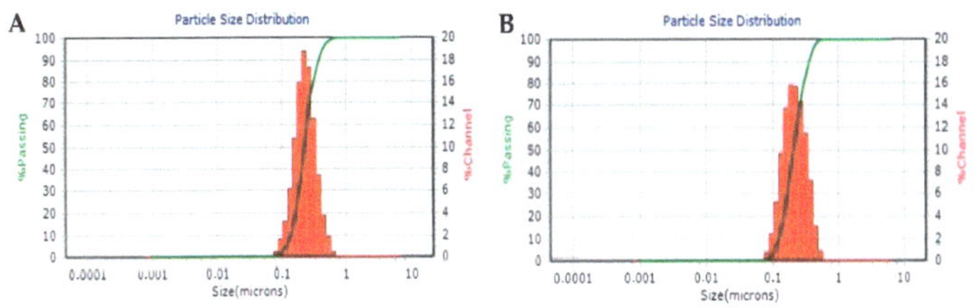


**Figure 4.** DLS histograms of nanoparticles from batches NP1-DFP (**A**) and NP2-DFP (**B**).

### 3.2.1. Drug Loading and Entrapment Efficiency

The water solubility of DFP is strongly affected by pH. It is easily dissolved in polar solutions with acidic pH, but the solubility decreases sharply in a neutral medium. In our preliminary studies, low values for DL and DEE were estimated when purified water with a pH of about 6.0 was used for the preparation of the double emulsion (Table 4). The main disadvantage of the double emulsion technique is the diffusion of the hydrophilic active molecules into the dispersion medium during emulsification. When the goal is to develop a drug-delivery system based on particle design, high drug entrapment is a priority. Hence, the main task was to establish optimal conditions favoring the preferential distribution of the drug in the internal phase of the emulsion. Due to the pH-dependent solubility of DFP, a change in the pH of W1 and W2 was made to increase the amount of substance incorporated into nanoparticles. PBS (pH 2.6) was used for W1, in which DFP has high solubility, and PBS (pH 7.4) was used for W2, in which DFP is less soluble. Changing the pH resulted in an increase in DEE for both batches, as with the batch NP2-DFP prepared with a high molecular weight polymer, DEE was lower (17.15 ± 0.80%), while in the batch NP1-DFP obtained with PCL 14 kDa, DEE was 22.00 ± 2.16%. The lower affinity of hydrophilic molecules such as DFP to the hydrophobic PCL may be the reason for the low encapsulation efficiency. Alex et al. also reported a low encapsulation efficiency of the hydrophilic drug carboplatin in PCL nanoparticles in their work, prepared by double emulsion technique (DEE 27.95 ± 4.21%) [31].

**Table 4.** Effect of pH of W1 (internal aqueous phase) and W2 (external aqueous phase) on entrapment efficiency (DEE), drug loading (DL) (mean values ± SD. $n = 3$).

| Sample Code | pH W1 | pH W2 | DEE (%) | DL (%) |
|---|---|---|---|---|
| NP1-DFP | 6.0 | 6.0 | 3.31 ± 0.97 | 1.62 ± 0.42 |
| NP2-DFP | 6.0 | 6.0 | 2.72 ± 0.12 | 1.34 ± 0.06 |
| NP1-DFP | 2.6 | 7.4 | 22.00 ± 2.16 | 9.08 ± 0.95 |
| NP2-DFP | 2.6 | 7.4 | 17.15 ± 0.80 | 7.40 ± 0.50 |

### 3.2.2. Nanoparticles Shape and Surface Morphology

Figures 5 and 6 show SEM and TEM micrographs of the DFP-loaded NPs. Nanoparticles were spherical in shape with a smooth surface and uniform size distribution. SEM analysis confirms the DLS average diameter of the formulated nanoparticles.

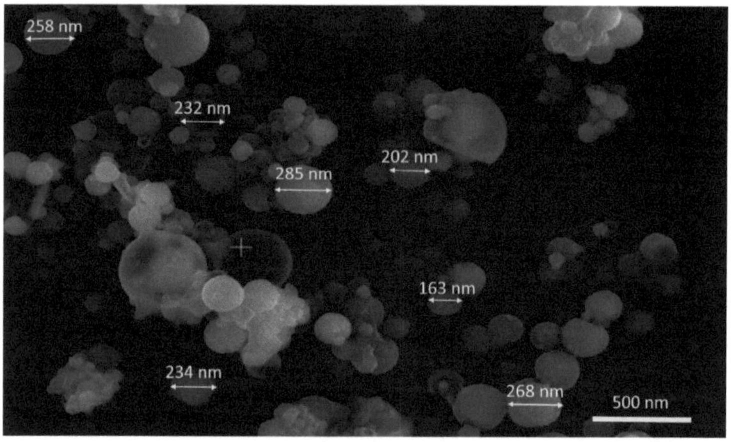


**Figure 5.** SEM micrograph of DFP-loaded nanoparticles from model NP1-DFP (20,000×).

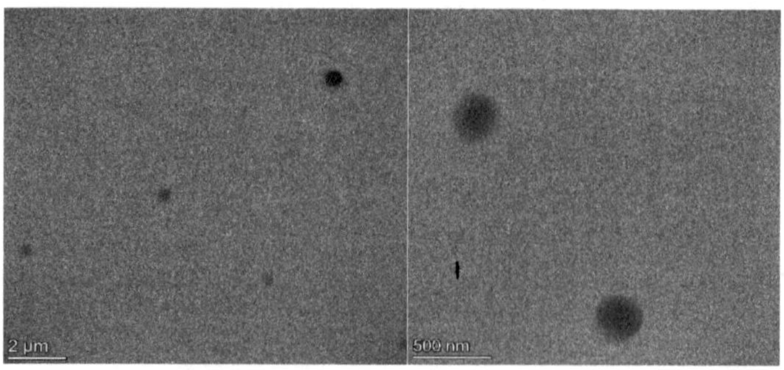


**Figure 6.** TEM micrographs of nanoparticles loaded with DFP from model NP1-DFP (28,000×).

3.2.3. In Vitro Drug Release

The dissolution profiles of DFP from the two PCL-nanoparticle batches are shown in Figure 7. PCL has gained considerable attention as a drug delivery polymer due to its biocompatibility and slow degradation [32,33]. The release retarding effect of the hydrophobic PCL is due to the low penetration of water into the polymer matrix [34]. This effect has been used to control the fast drug release from different particulate dosage forms [35]. It was found that during the first 3 h of the study, about 30% of the drug was released. A reason for this could be the accumulation of the drug at the periphery of the nanoparticles during the intense evaporation of the organic phase [36]. After 3 h, there was a delay in the release, and by the 9th hour, only an additional 10% of the drug was released. Probably, a highly concentrated core of the NPs was formed, which is responsible for the incomplete release [37]. This was due to the relatively slow penetration of water in the PCL matrix. At the end of the 24 h study, about 60% from batch NP1-DFP and about 80% from batch NP2-DFP were released. The release profiles of DFP from the two batches are similar with minor differences attributed to the small variations in drug loading.

To date, only one DFP controlled-release oral dosage form has been developed. Binary matrix tablets containing DFP and thermoplastic polymers (Carbopol 974P and 971P) were prepared by an ultrasound-assisted tableting press. Prolonged release from hydrophilic matrices was successfully achieved, with 50% of the active substance released in 6 h [38]. The inclusion of DFP in PCL NPs leads to a delay in its release without observing a burst effect, which suggests that the drug remains unreleased at the site of administration (nasal cavity) and can be transported to the target site (brain tissue). However, further studies are required to prove this hypothesis.

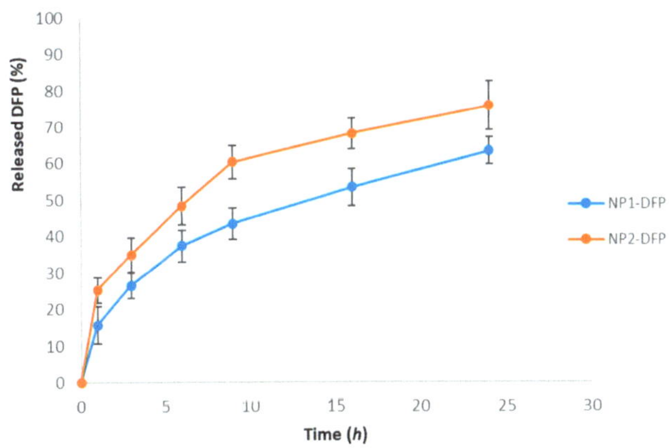


**Figure 7.** DFP release profiles from batches NP1-DFP and NP2-DFP.

### *3.3. Preparation and Characterization of Deferiprone-Loaded Nanocomposite Microspheres*

3.3.1. Optimization of the Microspheres' Preparation

Sodium alginate was selected as the polymer carrier for microencapsulation of the nanoparticles. This natural polysaccharide has good mucoadhesive properties, making alginate microparticles suitable for application on mucous membranes such as the nasal mucosa [39]. Additionally, its biodegradability and hydrophilicity ensure its rapid dissolution in nasal secretions after application, which is essential for the transport of the drug-loaded nanostructures incorporated in the composite systems [13,40].

Spray drying was used to formulate the alginate composites. The technological parameters that influence the characteristics of the obtained microparticles are: the concentration of the starting material for spraying (polymer and drug substance); the rate at which the peristaltic pump feeds the atomizing nozzle; the amount of compressed gas required to disperse the sample in the form of droplets; the temperature of the hot gas used for the drying process; the rate at which the drying air is aspirated [41]. Although spray drying of sodium alginate solutions has been widely applied and proven as an effective microencapsulating method [42], the inclusion of nanoparticles, composed of a water-insoluble polymer such as PCL, can greatly modify the properties of the drying material and may require precise adjusting of the process conditions. Challenges in the technique used were to achieve a high production yield of microparticles, since the method is generally characterized by a great loss of material during pulverization [43]. Considering the nasal route of administration, it was crucial to avoid obtaining particles of very small sizes that could be inhaled into the lungs [21]. To achieve optimal production yield and particle size, spray drying parameters were adjusted within the limits outlined in the literature.

It was estimated that a drying temperature of 140 °C or lower was not effective enough to evaporate the aqueous phase and dry out the droplets sprayed through the nozzle. Consequently, the moist particles adhere to the equipment and cannot be collected as a final powder product. This led to a low yield of microparticles. An inlet temperature of 160 °C was evaluated as optimal for the particle yield. As expected, raising the inlet temperature resulted in a drier product with a higher yield of microparticles. Additionally, at the higher temperature, the obtained particles were larger in size. Although the contact with the hot air during the spray drying process was short, high temperatures are generally not recommended due to the risk to the stability of the drug and the polymers used [43]. In order to ensure the stability of the DFP and the encapsulating polymers, the cyclone of the spray dryer was jacketed with a cooling agent and insulated to maintain a lower temperature on the inner walls, where the dried powder was collected, thus maintaining the outlet temperature below 60 °C.

Another factor that has a strong impact on the yield and the size of microparticles is the gas flow rate. When more gas is passed through, smaller droplets are sprayed through the nozzle, resulting in smaller final dry particles [41,44]. At a rate of 400 L/h, the larger droplets may not dry efficiently, leading to a lower yield. On the other hand, at a rate of 600 L/h, the average particle size became too small. The optimal flow rate was found to be 500 L/h, as it resulted in satisfactory particle size and the highest yield. Producing very small particles can reduce the yield, as some of them are expelled during the process with the aspiration flow.

Two feed rates of the peristaltic pump were studied: 5 mL/min and 10 mL/min. A higher feed rate generally results in larger droplets/particles due to the larger amount of material sprayed. The pump speed should be restricted when the particles are not dry enough [45]. This was confirmed by the results obtained. At a rate of 10 mL/min, the larger droplets formed did not dry sufficiently and an unsatisfactory yield was estimated. This required the speed to be reduced to 5 mL/min, which did not greatly affect the average size of the obtained microparticles.

The microparticles were initially prepared using a 0.5% $w/v$ sodium alginate solution. However, due to small particle size and unsatisfactory yield, the polymer concentration was increased to 1%. The higher polymer concentration led to a larger particle size and a higher yield because there was less liquid to evaporate and a more solid phase to form the powder. However, very high polymer concentrations can lead to challenges in atomization due to the high viscosity and can also reduce drug loading in the particles due to changes in the drug substance and polymer carrier ratio [46].

Based on the study of spray drying parameters, the following conditions were derived for obtaining nanocomposite microparticles from alginate: drying temperature 160 °C, gas flow rate 500 L/h, feed rate 5 mL/min, polymer concentration 1% $v/w$.

#### 3.3.2. Characterization of Nanocomposite Microspheres

The average diameter of the nanocomposite microspheres was 6.05 ± 1.78 µm (Table 5). The morphology of particles was observed via SEM analysis. Spray-dried composite structures were spherical in shape and had a smooth surface (Figure 8). Similar observations were also reported by Bagheri et al. [47]. For intranasally administered powders, optimization of particle size and morphology is necessary to minimize the risk of irritation of the nasal mucosa and to improve powder flowability and nasal deposition [48–50]. The spherical shape is expected to facilitate the delivery of the preparation by nasal devices [45]. High yields of about 86.93% ± 3.04% were obtained, which are considered optimal, taking into account the large losses typical of the production method at a laboratory scale [43,51].

**Table 5.** Characteristics of DFP-loaded nanocomposite microspheres (means ± SD, *n* = 3); drug entrapment efficiency (DEE), drug loading (DL).

| Mean Diameter (μm) | DEE (%) | DL (%) | Yield (%) |
|---|---|---|---|
| 6.05 ± 1.78 | 36.28 ± 0.32 | 5.18 ± 0.06 | 86.93 ± 3.04 |

The particle size distribution of the composite microparticles is presented in Figure 9. A monomodal distribution was observed with a predominance of a fraction of particles with sizes between 2 and 20 μm. A fraction of smaller particle sizes (0.1–1.0 μm) was also observed, which was expected since spray drying is a method that produces microparticles in a relatively wide size range. The size range of the nanocomposite microspheres corresponds to that of nasal powders produced by spray drying [52–54].

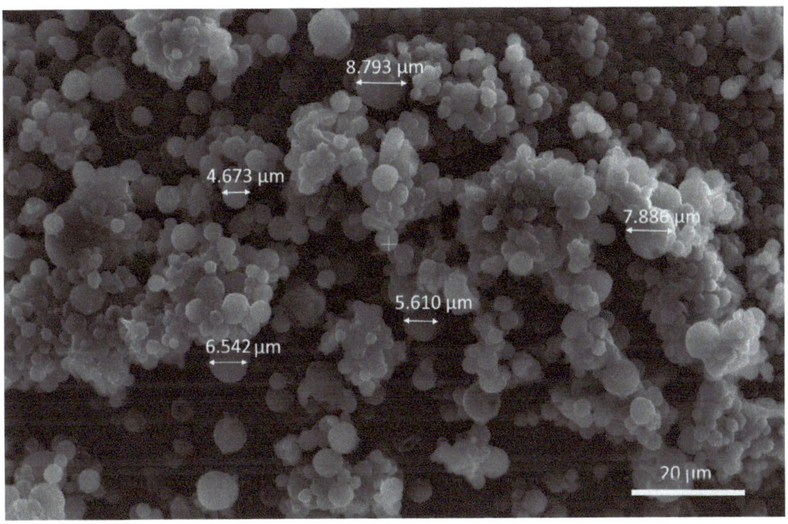


**Figure 8.** SEM micrograph of nanocomposite microspheres from batch M-NP1-DFP (3500×).

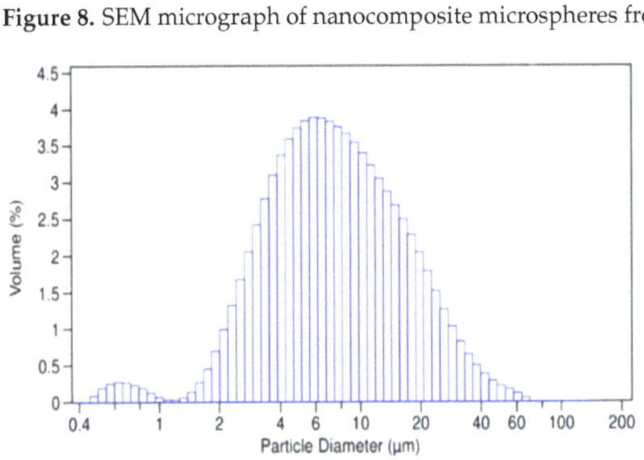


**Figure 9.** Particle size distribution of batch M-NP1-DFP.

3.3.3. In Vitro Drug Release

The release of DFP from nanoparticles was prolonged with only 60% of the drug released in 24 h (Figure 7). The inclusion of nanoparticles in the composite structure led to even further delays in the release of DFP (Figure 10). During the first 3 h, around 10% were released from the composite structure, while at the same time, twice the amount of drug was released from nanoparticles. A plausible explanation is the dissolution of sodium alginate in the release medium, which increases the viscosity and slows down the dissolution and diffusion of DFP. Similar conclusions were reported by other authors, using sodium alginate as a mucoadhesive carrier in nasal gels [55], buccal patches [56], and rectal suppositories [57]. The type of dosage form also influences the drug release rate; for example, alginate was used as a carrier for salbutamol sulfate in sublingual films [58] and tablets [59]. The drug release was found to be prolonged for the films [58] and rapid for the tablets [59].

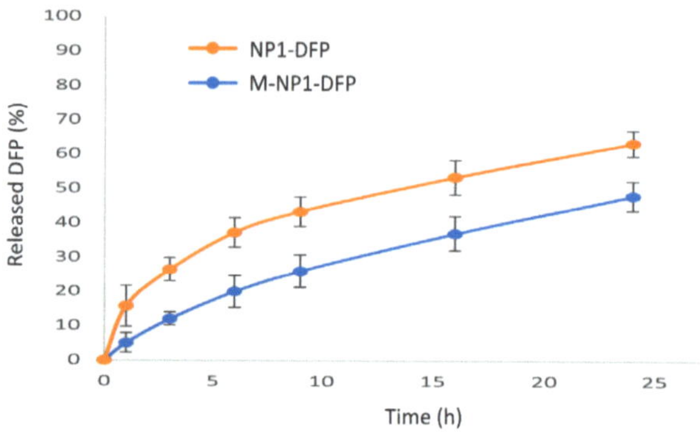


**Figure 10.** Release profiles of DFP from nanoparticles (NP1-DFP) and composite microspheres (M-NP1-DFP).

3.3.4. FTIR Spectroscopy

The infrared spectra of DFP, PCL, sodium alginate, and DFP-loaded nanocomposite microspheres (M-NP1-DFP) are shown in Figure 11. A peak is registered in the spectrum of DFP at 1629 cm$^{-1}$ characteristic of C=O group. A band is observed at 1380 cm$^{-1}$, which together with the band at 1463 cm$^{-1}$ is due to -CH3 groups in the molecule. The characteristic peak of C=C bonds is 1513 cm$^{-1}$, and the presence of C–N bonds in the molecule is confirmed by the peak at 1030 cm$^{-1}$ [60]. In the spectra of PCL, a doublet at 2946 cm$^{-1}$ and 2867 cm$^{-1}$ is observed due to symmetric and asymmetric vibrations of the aliphatic C–H bonds as well as a characteristic band for C=O at 1721 cm$^{-1}$. The valence vibrations of C-C and C-O bonds in the PCL molecule appear at 1293 cm$^{-1}$ [61]. A broad characteristic peak at 3500 cm$^{-1}$ is observed in the spectrum of sodium alginate, which is due to the vibration of the large number of -OH groups in the molecule. Two characteristic peaks at 1603 cm$^{-1}$ and 1411 cm$^{-1}$ are distinguished due to symmetric and asymmetric vibrations of the -COO groups [62]. In the infrared spectrum of batch M-NP1-DFP, the peak at 3253 cm$^{-1}$ confirms the presence of -OH groups. The peaks at 1724 cm$^{-1}$, 1293 cm$^{-1}$, and 1241 cm$^{-1}$ correspond to the indicated characteristic peaks for PCL. The peak at 1629 cm$^{-1}$ corresponding to the C=O group in the DFP molecule is shifted at 1609 cm$^{-1}$, which may be due to overlap with the -COOH groups of alginates. In the ATR spectrum of the composite structure, the remaining characteristic peaks of DFP are also present without significant changes. No new peaks are observed in the ATR spectra of the model system, which shows that during their preparation, no new chemical bonds are formed because of the interaction between the active substances and the polymers.

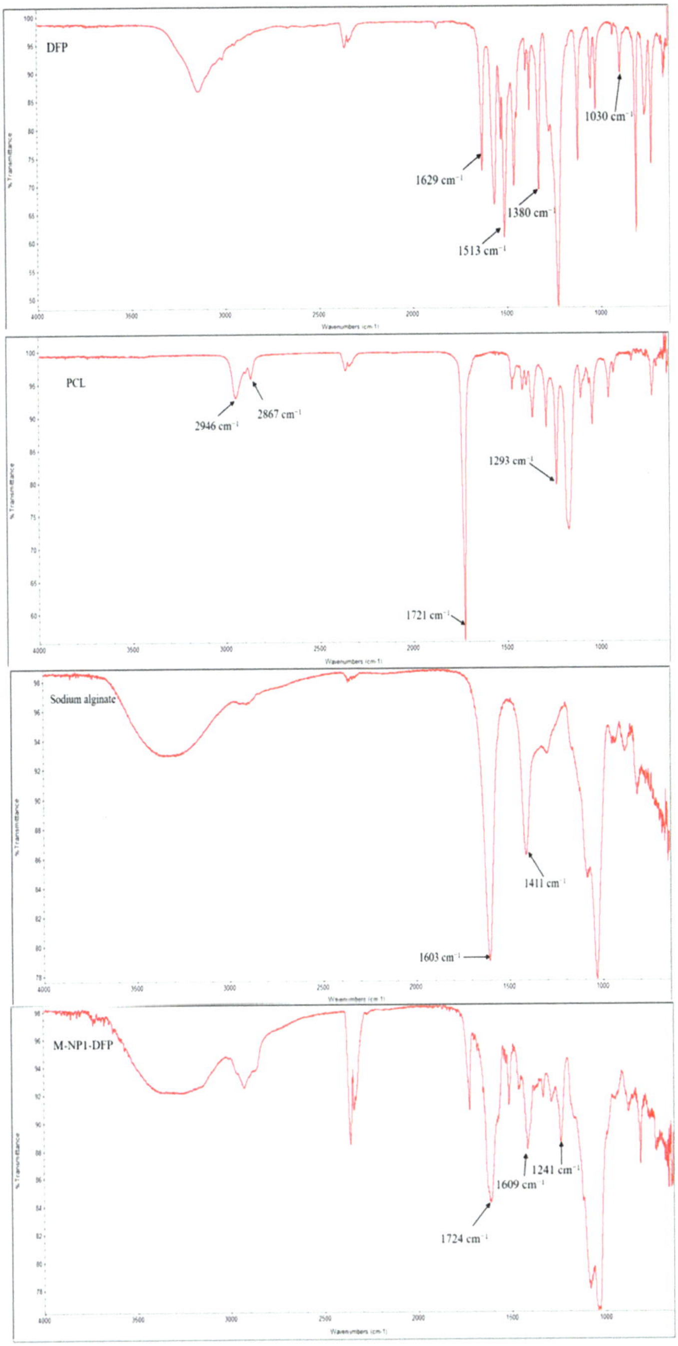


**Figure 11.** FTIR spectra of DFP, PCL, sodium alginate, and nanocomposite microparticles of model M-NP1-DFP.

### 3.3.5. Differential Scanning Calorimetry (DSC)

The physical state of DFP incorporated into nanocomposite microspheres was analyzed using differential scanning calorimetry (DSC). The resulting thermograms are presented in Figure 12 and Table 6. The DSC thermogram of sodium alginate shows an endothermic peak at 111 °C and an exothermic peak at 243 °C. The first peak corresponds to the evaporation of the included water molecules, while the exothermic indicates the oxidative degradation of the polymer (Figure 12A). The thermogram of PCL demonstrated a broad endothermic peak at about 76 °C, which corresponds to the melting temperature of the polymer (Figure 12B). Similar endothermic peaks corresponding to the melting point were also observed in the DFP (284 °C) thermograms (Figure 12C). The thermogram of the microstructures of model M-NP1-DFP contains two endothermic peaks: one at 60 °C, which corresponds to the melting point of PCL and confirms the incorporation of the polymer nanoparticles into the composite, and a second endothermic peak at 165 °C, which is due to the Span 85 used in the preparation of the multiple emulsion (Figure 12D). The exothermic peak at 252 °C is due to the DFP included in the nanoparticles. In the DSC thermogram of the placebo nanocomposite microspheres (M-NP-placebo), one endothermic peak was registered at 60 °C, which is due to the PCL placebo nanoparticles included in the composite structure. The second peak, which is exothermic and recorded at 248 °C, corresponds to the thermal decomposition of the structure-forming polymer, sodium alginate (Figure 12E).

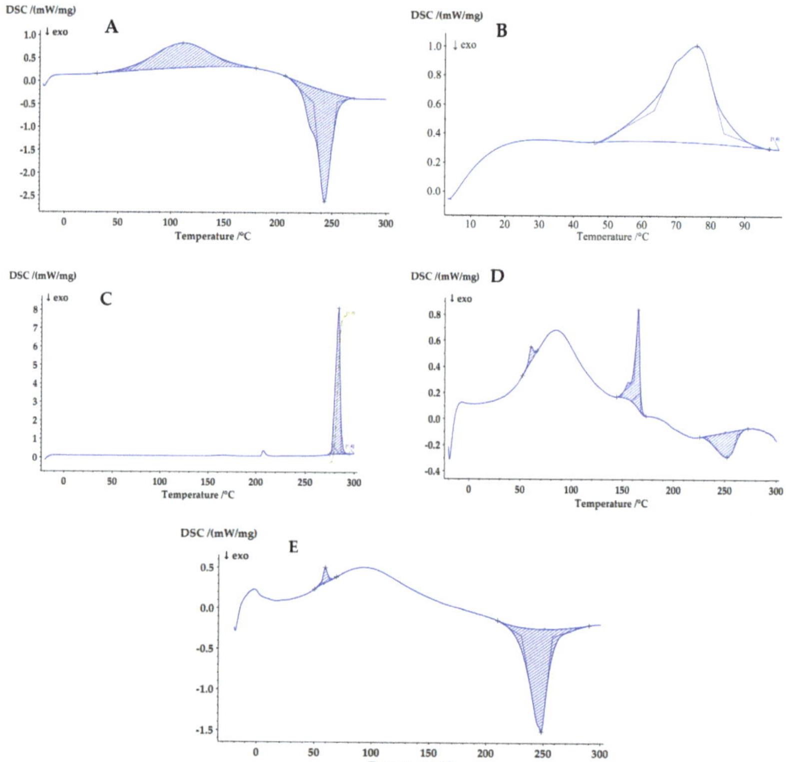


**Figure 12.** DSC thermograms of sodium alginate (**A**), PCL (**B**), DFP (**C**), and particles from batches M-NP1-DFP (**D**) and M-NP-Placebo (**E**).

**Table 6.** DSC thermographic peaks of sodium alginate, PCL, DFP, and particles from batches M-NP1-DFP and M-NP-Placebo.

| Sample | Area (J/g) | Peak (°C) | Onset (°C) | End (°C) | Width (°C) | Height (mW/mg) |
|---|---|---|---|---|---|---|
| Sodium alginate | 200.0<br>−257.2 | 111.0<br>243.0 | 61.6<br>232.9 | 150.2<br>254.5 | 69.3<br>21.6 | 0.543<br>2.414 |
| poly-ε-caprolactone (PCL) | 71.19 | 75.8 | 63.5 | 83.7 | 20.5 | 0.6681 |
| Deferiprone (DFP) | 262.4 | 283.7 | 277.2 | 286.5 | 6.4 | 7.881 |
| Microcomposite particles (M-NP1-DFP) | 3.1<br>29.93<br>−24.39 | 60.2<br>165.2<br>252.4 | 56.8<br>161.2<br>232.4 | 63.7<br>168.0<br>262.2 | 5.3<br>6.2<br>24.7 | 0.1078<br>0.757<br>0.1912 |
| M-NP-Placebo | 5.41<br>−147.8 | 59.3<br>248.3 | 56.4<br>231.1 | 62.9<br>258.0 | 5.0<br>20.8 | 0.185<br>1.264 |

#### 3.3.6. Mucoadhesive Ability

When developing a carrier for nasal administration, its mucoadhesive ability should be evaluated. Mucociliary clearance is the main obstacle for better contact between the carrier and the nasal mucosa and, accordingly, for a higher rate of drug absorption [63,64]. Several methods have been developed to study mucoadhesion [65,66]. There is no standard apparatus for determining adhesive strength and there is a great variety of potential techniques [67]. In the present work, the mucoadhesive ability of nanocomposite microspheres as a drug delivery system was investigated ex vivo in direct contact with the nasal mucosa [25,26]. The maximum force required to detach a cylinder of compressed nanocomposite microparticles from native sheep nasal mucosa after different contact times (1, 3, 5, 10, 15, and 25 min) was determined.

The results of the study (Figure 13) showed a high degree of attachment to the nasal mucosa. The chronological change in adhesion strength showed a statistically significant difference at all time points compared to the initial moment. This is an indicator of achieving a high degree of attachment even after one minute of contact with the nasal mucosa. As the contact time increases, the maximum adhesive strength increases and reaches a maximum after five minutes of contact. It was found that a contact time longer than 5 min did not lead to an additional increase in the adhesive strength. On the contrary, a decrease and reaching a stable mechanical tension was registered after 15 min.

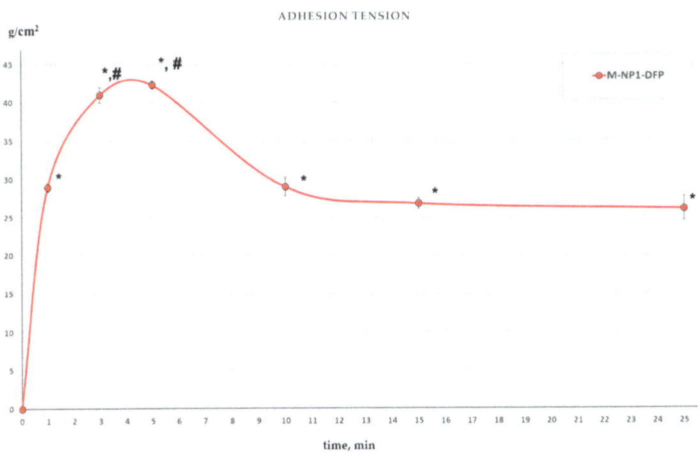


**Figure 13.** Chronological change of the maximal adhesion force in batch M-NP1-DFP. The symbols *, #, indicate the presence of a statistically significant difference compared to the initial moment (*) and after the established steady state of the process 15 min (#).

3.3.7. In Vitro Determination of Fe-Chelating Activity

The study aims to determine whether there is a change in the chelating ability of DFP after its incorporation into the composite structures. The test is based on the fact that in the presence of iron ions, ferrozine forms a complex compound (ferrozine—Fe(II)) with a characteristic red color, which has an absorption maximum of 562 nm. In the presence of other chelating agents in the solution, the formation of the complex is prevented, which leads to a decrease in the absorption. In a water solution, DFP prevented the formation of the ferrozine—Fe(II) complex and demonstrated chelating activity of over 95% (Figure 14). The inclusion of DFP in the nanocomposite microspheres led to a slight decrease in Fe-chelating activity (84.38%), but that was probably due to the incomplete and delayed release of DFP from the composite structures. The placebo nanocomposite microspheres (M-NP-Placebo) also demonstrated some Fe-chelating activity (45.2%) resulting from the formation of a complex between alginate and iron ions. The mechanism of this interaction has been studied for a long time [68].

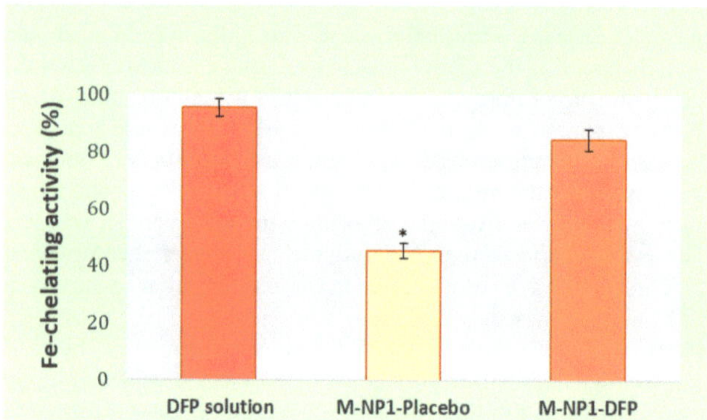


**Figure 14.** Comparison of Fe-chelating activity of DFP solution, nanocomposite microspheres without the drug (M-NP-Placebo), and DFP-loaded nanocomposite microspheres (M-NP1-DFP). Data is presented as mean values ± SD, $n = 3$. * Indicates a statistically significant result ($p < 0.05$).

3.3.8. Determination of the Binding Ability of Nanoparticles Loaded with DFP to Human Serum Albumin (HSA)

Albumin is the major protein in plasma and the cerebrospinal fluid. It is a pliable molecule with the ability to change its structure depending on environmental conditions such as temperature, pH, or ionic strength. It can bind many different molecules and can even act as an antioxidant [69].

Proteins such as HSA, lipoproteins, and globulin can be adsorbed on the surface of drug-loaded nanoparticles, thereby altering the in vivo release behavior and targeting sites of the nanoparticles [70–72].

In the present research, fluorescence spectroscopy was used for in situ investigation of nanoparticle–protein interactions (Figure 15). Quantitative analysis of HSA binding was performed using the reduction of fluorescence emission of albumin with a characteristic peak at about 340 nm. The performed analysis showed a noticeable decrease in fluorescence intensity after the addition of nanosuspension from batch NP1-DFP (Figure 15).

DFP-loaded nanoparticles were found to interact with HSA. A fluorescence study of the HSA solution with placebo nanoparticles was also performed. A negligible reduction in fluorescence was registered compared to that observed in batch M-NP1-DFP when increasing the amount of the ligand (Figure 13).

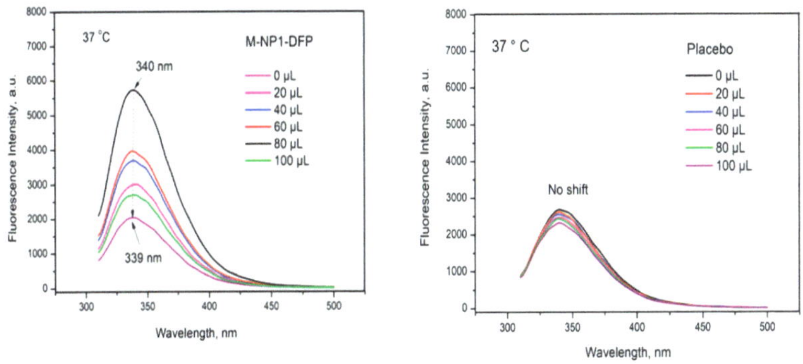


**Figure 15.** Fluorescence spectra of HSA (2.7 mg/mL) upon addition of different volumes of samples containing dispersed particles from batch M-NP1-DFP and placebo particles at 37 °C.

These results reveal a minor interaction of the nanosized carrier with albumin and suggest a preferential interaction of the drug substance DFP with the protein. It is logical to conclude that this effect was due to the interaction between HSA and the drug molecules. However, considering the low release rate of DFP from the nanocarriers (<10%, Figure 6) within 1 h (the duration of the analysis), it can be assumed that the observed decrease in fluorescence spectra is not solely due to the interaction between the active substance with albumin. It can be suggested that the incorporation of DFP into PCL nanoparticles significantly changed their surface properties and geometry because their affinity for binding to the protein increased dramatically.

## 4. Conclusions

In this study, nanocomposite microspheres loaded with DFP were successfully produced by emulsification solvent evaporation method and spray drying. The resulting particles have high mucoadhesive ability and an average size of 6.05 ± 1.78 µm. pH of the aqueous phases influenced the amount of drug incorporated into the nanoparticles. The drug release study confirmed the feasibility of the developed carrier for prolonged delivery of DFP. The inclusion of DFP in PCL nanoparticles and the subsequent incorporation of nanoparticles into composite microspheres did not lead to a change in its Fe-chelating activity. The binding affinity of PCL nanoparticles to human serum albumin was determined. In conclusion, it can be summarized that the loading of polymer nanoparticles with active ingredients is crucial for their behavior, possible bio-nano interactions, and thus their potential application to achieve specific therapeutic goals (targeted delivery, controlled release, etc.).

**Author Contributions:** Conceptualization, R.B. and B.P.; methodology, R.B., P.K., A.H. and P.Z.; software, P.Z.; investigation, R.B., P.K., P.Z., A.H. and S.A.; data curation, P.Z. and S.A.; writing—original draft preparation, R.B.; writing—review and editing, B.P.; visualization, R.B. and B.P.; supervision, B.P.; project administration, B.P.; funding acquisition, B.P and P.Z. All authors have read and agreed to the published version of the manuscript.

**Funding:** This research was funded by the European Union—NextGenerationEU, through the National Recovery and Resilience Plan of the Republic of Bulgaria, project No. BG-RRP-2.004-0007-C01.

**Institutional Review Board Statement:** Not applicable.

**Informed Consent Statement:** Not applicable.

**Data Availability Statement:** The original contributions presented in the study are included in the article, further inquiries can be directed to the corresponding author.

**Conflicts of Interest:** The authors declare no conflicts of interest.

## References

1. De la Torre, C.; Ceña, V. The Delivery Challenge in Neurodegenerative Disorders: The Nanoparticles Role in Alzheimer's Disease Therapeutics and Diagnostics. *Pharmaceutics* **2018**, *10*, 190. [CrossRef] [PubMed]
2. Domínguez-Fernández, C.; Egiguren-Ortiz, J.; Razquin, J.; Gómez-Galán, M.; De las Heras-García, L.; Paredes-Rodríguez, E.; Astigarraga, E.; Miguélez, C.; Barreda-Gómez, G. Review of Technological Challenges in Personalised Medicine and Early Diagnosis of Neurodegenerative Disorders. *Int. J. Mol. Sci.* **2023**, *24*, 3321. [CrossRef] [PubMed]
3. Aragón-González, A.; Shaw, P.J.; Ferraiuolo, L. Blood–Brain Barrier Disruption and Its Involvement in Neurodevelopmental and Neurodegenerative Disorders. *Int. J. Mol. Sci.* **2022**, *23*, 15271. [CrossRef] [PubMed]
4. Xu, H.; Wang, Y.; Song, N.; Wang, J.; Jiang, H.; Xie, J. New Progress on the Role of Glia in Iron Metabolism and Iron-Induced Degeneration of Dopamine Neurons in Parkinson's Disease. *Front. Mol. Neurosci.* **2017**, *10*, 455. [CrossRef]
5. Ward, R.J.; Dexter, D.T.; Crichton, R.R. Neurodegenerative diseases and therapeutic strategies using iron chelators. *J. Trace Elem. Med. Biol.* **2015**, *31*, 267–273. [CrossRef]
6. Long, H.Z.; Zhou, Z.W.; Cheng, Y.; Luo, H.Y.; Li, F.J.; Xu, S.G.; Gao, L.C. The Role of Microglia in Alzheimer's Disease from the Perspective of Immune Inflammation and Iron Metabolism. *Front. Aging Neurosci.* **2022**, *14*, 888989. [CrossRef]
7. Kenkhuis, B.; Somarakis, A.; de Haan, L.; Dzyubachyk, O.; Ijsselsteijn, M.E.; de Miranda, N.F.C.C.; Lelieveldt, B.P.F.; Dijkstra, J.; van Roon-Mom, W.M.C.; Höllt, T.; et al. Iron loading is a prominent feature of activated microglia in Alzheimer's disease patients. *Acta Neuropathol. Commun.* **2021**, *9*, 27. [CrossRef]
8. Wang, M.; Tang, G.; Zhou, C.; Guo, H.; Hu, Z.; Hu, Q.; Li, G. Revisiting the intersection of microglial activation and neuroinflammation in Alzheimer's disease from the perspective of ferroptosis. *Chem. Biol. Interact.* **2023**, *375*, 110387. [CrossRef] [PubMed]
9. Kontoghiorghes, G.J. The Vital Role Played by Deferiprone in the Transition of Thalassaemia from a Fatal to a Chronic Disease and Challenges in Its Repurposing for Use in Non-Iron-Loaded Diseases. *Pharmaceuticals* **2023**, *16*, 1016. [CrossRef]
10. Hoyes, K.P.; Porter, J.B. Subcellular distribution of desferrioxamine and hydroxypyridin-4-one chelators in K562 cells affects chelation of intracellular iron pools. *Br. J. Haematol.* **1993**, *85*, 393–400. [CrossRef]
11. Bellanti, F.; Danhof, M.; Della Pasqua, O. Population pharmacokinetics of deferiprone in healthy subjects. *Br. J. Clin. Pharmacol.* **2014**, *78*, 1397–1406. [CrossRef] [PubMed]
12. Patharapankal, E.J.; Ajiboye, A.L.; Mattern, C.; Trivedi, V. Nose-to-Brain (N2B) Delivery: An Alternative Route for the Delivery of Biologics in the Management and Treatment of Central Nervous System Disorders. *Pharmaceutics* **2024**, *16*, 66. [CrossRef] [PubMed]
13. Gandhi, S.; Shastri, D.H.; Shah, J.; Nair, A.B.; Jacob, S. Nasal Delivery to the Brain: Harnessing Nanoparticles for Effective Drug Transport. *Pharmaceutics* **2024**, *16*, 481. [CrossRef] [PubMed]
14. Jin, Z.; Guo, G.; Yu, A.; Qian, H.; Tong, Z. Comparative Analysis of Micrometer-Sized Particle Deposition in the Olfactory Regions of Adult and Pediatric Nasal Cavities: A Computational Study. *Pharmaceutics* **2024**, *16*, 722. [CrossRef]
15. Cheng, Y.S. Mechanisms of pharmaceutical aerosol deposition in the respiratory tract. *AAPS PharmSciTech* **2014**, *15*, 630–640. [CrossRef]
16. Rassu, G.; Soddu, E.; Cossu, M.; Gavini, E.; Giunchedi, P.; Dalpiaz, A. Particulate formulations based on chitosan for nose-to-brain delivery of drugs. *J. Drug Deliv. Sci. Technol.* **2016**, *32*, 77–87. [CrossRef]
17. Dalpiaz, A.; Gavini, E.; Colombo, G.; Russo, P.; Bortolotti, F.; Ferraro, L.; Tanganelli, S.; Scatturin, A.; Menegatti, E.; Giunchedi, P. Brain uptake of an anti-ischemic agent by nasal administration of microparticles. *J. Pharm. Sci.* **2008**, *97*, 4889–4903. [CrossRef]
18. Maaz, A.; Blagbrough, I.S.; De Bank, P.A. In Vitro Evaluation of Nasal Aerosol Depositions: An Insight for Direct Nose to Brain Drug Delivery. *Pharmaceutics* **2021**, *13*, 1079. [CrossRef]
19. Ugwoke, M.I.; Agu, R.U.; Verbeke, N.; Kinget, R. Nasal mucoadhesive drug delivery: Background, applications, trends and future perspectives. *Adv. Drug Deliv. Rev.* **2005**, *57*, 1640–1665. [CrossRef]
20. Adnet, T.; Groo, A.-C.; Picard, C.; Davis, A.; Corvaisier, S.; Since, M.; Bounoure, F.; Rochais, C.; Le Pluart, L.; Dallemagne, P.; et al. Pharmacotechnical Development of a Nasal Drug Delivery Composite Nanosystem Intended for Alzheimer's Disease Treatment. *Pharmaceutics* **2020**, *12*, 251. [CrossRef]
21. Yarragudi, S.B.; Kumar, H.; Jain, R.; Tawhai, M.; Rizwan, S. Olfactory Targeting of Microparticles through Inhalation and Bi-directional Airflow: Effect of Particle Size and Nasal Anatomy. *J. Aerosol Med. Pulm. Drug Deliv.* **2020**, *33*, 258–270. [CrossRef] [PubMed]
22. Dinis, T.C.; Maderia, V.M.; Almeida, L.M. Action of phenolic derivatives (acetaminophen. salicylate. and 5-aminosalicylate) as inhibitors of membrane lipid peroxidation and as peroxyl radical scavengers. *Arch. Biochem. Biophys.* **1994**, *315*, 161–169. [CrossRef] [PubMed]
23. Peters, T. All about Albumin: Biochemistry. Genetics. and Medical Applications. In 2—*The Albumin Molecule: Its Structure and Chemical Properties*; Academic Press: San Diego, CA, USA, 1995. [CrossRef]
24. Ray, A.; Seth, B.K.; Pal, U.; Basu, S. Nickel(II)-Schiff base complex recognizing domain ii of bovine and human serum albumin: Spectroscopic and docking studies. *Acta Part A Mol. Biomol. Spectrosc.* **2012**, *92*, 164–174. [CrossRef] [PubMed]
25. Davidovich-Pinhas, M.; Harari, O.; Bianco-Peled, H. Evaluating the mucoadhesive properties of drug delivery systems based on hydrated thiolated alginate. *J. Control. Release* **2009**, *136*, 38–44. [CrossRef]

26. Tangri, P.; Khurana, S.; Satheesh, M. Mucoadhesive drug delivery: Mechanism and method of evaluation. *Int. J. Pharma Bio. Sci.* **2011**, *2*, 458–467.
27. Woertz, C.; Preis, M.; Breitkreutz, J.; Kleinebudde, P. Assessment of test methods evaluating mucoadhesive polymers and dosage forms: An overview. *Eur. J. Pharm. Biopharm.* **2013**, *85*, 843–853. [CrossRef] [PubMed]
28. Yang, Y.Y.; Chung, T.S.; Ng, N.P. Morphology, drug distribution, and in vitro release profiles of biodegradable polymeric microspheres containing protein fabricated by double-emulsion solvent extraction/evaporation method. *Biomaterials* **2001**, *22*, 231–241. [CrossRef]
29. Mudrić, J.; Šavikin, K.; Ibrić, S.; Đuriš, J. Double emulsions (W/O/W emulsions): Encapsulation of Plant Biactives. *Lek. Sirovine* **2019**, *39*, 76–83. [CrossRef]
30. Raviadaran, R.; Muthoosamy, K.; Manickam, S. Simple and multiple emulsions emphasizing on industrial applications and stability assessment. In *Food Process Engineering and Quality Assurance*, 1st ed.; Mohan, C.O., Carvajal-Millan, E., Ravishankar, C.N., Haghi, A.K., Eds.; Apple Academic Press: Oakville, ON, Canada, 2018; pp. 179–230. [CrossRef]
31. Alex, A.T.; Joseph, A.; Shavi, G.; Rao, J.V.; Udupa, N. Development and evaluation of carboplatin-loaded PCL nanoparticles for intranasal delivery. *Drug Deliv.* **2016**, *23*, 2144–2153. [CrossRef]
32. Woodruff, M.A.; Hutmacher, D.W. The return of a forgotten polymer—Polycaprolactone in the 21st century. *Prog. Polym. Sci.* **2010**, *35*, 1217–1256. [CrossRef]
33. Mohamed, R.M.; Yusoh, K. A Review on the Recent Research of Polycaprolactone (PCL). *Adv. Mater. Res.* **2015**, *1134*, 249–255. [CrossRef]
34. Bhadran, A.; Shah, T.; Babanyinah, G.K.; Polara, H.; Taslimy, S.; Biewer, M.C.; Stefan, M.C. Recent Advances in Polycaprolactones for Anticancer Drug Delivery. *Pharmaceutics* **2023**, *15*, 1977. [CrossRef] [PubMed]
35. Sinha, V.R.; Bansal, K.; Kaushik, R.; Kumria, R.; Trehan, A. Poly-epsilon-caprolactone microspheres and nanospheres: An overview. *Int. J. Pharm.* **2004**, *278*, 1–23. [CrossRef]
36. Javed, I.; Ranjha, N.M.; Mahmood, K.; Kashif, S.; Rehman, M.; Usman, F. Drug release optimization from microparticles of poly (E-caprolactone) and hydroxypropyl methylcellulose polymeric blends: Formulation and characterization. *J. Drug Deliv. Sci. Technol.* **2014**, *24*, 607–612. [CrossRef]
37. Jeong, J.C.; Lee, J.; Cho, K. Effects of crystalline microstructure on drug release behavior of poly(epsilon-caprolactone) microspheres. *J. Control. Release* **2003**, *92*, 249–258. [CrossRef]
38. Aguilar-De-Leyva, A.; Gonçalves-Araujo, T.; Daza, V.; Caraballo, I. A new deferiprone controlled release system obtained by ultrasound-assisted compression. *Pharm. Dev. Technol.* **2014**, *19*, 728–734. [CrossRef] [PubMed]
39. Lukova, P.; Katsarov, P. Contemporary Aspects of Designing Marine Polysaccharide Microparticles as Drug Carriers for Biomedical Application. *Pharmaceutics* **2023**, *15*, 2126. [CrossRef]
40. Cherait, A.; Banks, W.A.; Vaudry, D. The Potential of the Nose-to-Brain Delivery of PACAP for the Treatment of Neuronal Disease. *Pharmaceutics* **2023**, *15*, 2032. [CrossRef]
41. Ziaee, A.; Albadarin, A.B.; Padrela, L.; Femmer, T.; O'Reilly, E.; Walker, G. Spray drying of pharmaceuticals and biopharmaceuticals: Critical parameters and experimental process optimization approaches. *Eur. J. Pharm. Sci.* **2019**, *127*, 300–318. [CrossRef]
42. Lai, J.; Azad, A.K.; Sulaiman, W.M.A.W.; Kumarasamy, V.; Subramaniyan, V.; Alshehade, S.A. Alginate-Based Encapsulation Fabrication Technique for Drug Delivery: An Updated Review of Particle Type, Formulation Technique, Pharmaceutical Ingredient, and Targeted Delivery System. *Pharmaceutics* **2024**, *16*, 370. [CrossRef]
43. Sundararajan, P.; Moser, J.; Williams, L.; Chiang, T.; Riordan, C.; Metzger, M.; Zhang-Plasket, F.; Wang, F.; Collins, J.; Williams, J. Driving Spray Drying towards Better Yield: Tackling a Problem That Sticks Around. *Pharmaceutics* **2023**, *15*, 2137. [CrossRef] [PubMed]
44. Poozesh, S.; Bilgili, E. Scale-up of pharmaceutical spray drying using scale-up rules: A review. *Int. J. Pharm.* **2019**, *562*, 271–292. [CrossRef]
45. Henriques, P.; Fortuna, A.; Doktorovová, S. Spray dried powders for nasal delivery: Process and formulation considerations. *Eur. J. Pharm. Biopharm.* **2022**, *176*, 1–20. [CrossRef] [PubMed]
46. Katsarov, P.; Pilicheva, B.; Manev, H.; Lukova, P.; Kassarova, M. Optimization of Chitosan Microspheres Spray Drying via $3^2$ Full Factorial Design. *Folia Medica* **2017**, *59*, 310–317. [CrossRef] [PubMed]
47. Bagheri, L.; Madadlou, A.; Yarmand, M.; Mousavi, M.E. Spray-dried alginate microparticles carrying caffeine-loaded and potentially bioactive nanoparticles. *Food Res. Int.* **2014**, *62*, 1113–1119. [CrossRef]
48. Ehrick, J.D.; Shah, S.A.; Shaw, C.; Kulkarni, V.S.; Coowanitwong, I.; De, S.; Suman, J.D. Considerations for the Development of Nasal Dosage Forms. *Sterile Prod. Dev.* **2013**, *6*, 99–144. [CrossRef]
49. Scherließ, R. Nasal formulations for drug administration and characterization of nasal preparations in drug delivery. *Ther. Deliv.* **2020**, *11*, 183–191. [CrossRef]
50. Tiozzo Fasiolo, L.; Manniello, M.D.; Tratta, E.; Buttini, F.; Rossi, A.; Sonvico, F.; Bortolotti, F.; Russo, P.; Colombo, G. Opportunity and challenges of nasal powders: Drug formulation and delivery. *Eur. J. Pharm. Sci.* **2018**, *113*, 2–17. [CrossRef]
51. Maury, M.; Murphy, K.; Kumar, S.; Shi, L.; Lee, G. Effects of process variables on the powder yield of spray-dried trehalose on a laboratory spray-dryer. *Eur. J. Pharm. Biopharm.* **2005**, *59*, 565–573. [CrossRef]

52. Hussein, N.; Omer, H.; Ismael, A.; Albed Alhnan, M.; Elhissi, A.; Ahmed, W. Spray-dried alginate microparticles for potential intranasal delivery of ropinirole hydrochloride: Development, characterization and histopathological evaluation. *Pharm. Dev. Technol.* **2020**, *25*, 290–299. [CrossRef]
53. Dukovski, B.J.; Mrak, L.; Winnicka, K.; Szekalska, M.; Juretić, M.; Filipović-Grčić, J.; Pepić, I.; Lovrić, J.; Hafner, A. Spray-Dried Nanoparticle-Loaded Pectin Microspheres for Dexamethasone Nasal Delivery. *Dry. Technol.* **2019**, *37*, 1915–1925. [CrossRef]
54. Alhalaweh, A.; Andersson, S.; Velaga, S.P. Preparation of zolmitriptan-chitosan microparticles by spray drying for nasal delivery. *Eur. J. Pharm. Sci.* **2009**, *38*, 206–214. [CrossRef] [PubMed]
55. De, A.; Chakraborty, S.; Mukherjee, A.; Chattopadhyay, J. Formulation of the In-Situ Forming Mucoadhesive Nasal Gel of Salbutamol Using Pluronic F-127 as Thermo sensative Gel Forming Polymer. *Int. J. Res. Pharm. Biomed. Sci.* **2014**, *4*, 926–933.
56. Pamlényi, K.; Kristó, K.; Sovány, T.; Regdon, G., Jr. Development and evaluation of bioadhesive buccal films based on sodium alginate for allergy therapy. *Heliyon* **2022**, *8*, 10364. [CrossRef]
57. Ghorab, D.; Refai, H.; Tag, R. Preparation and evaluation of fenoterol hydrobromide suppositories. *Drug Discov. Ther.* **2011**, *5*, 311–318. [CrossRef]
58. Prasanthi, N.L.; Krishna, C.S.; Gupta, M.E.; Manikiran, S.S.; Rao, N.R. Design and development of sublingual fast dissolving films for an antiasthmatic drug. *Der Pharm. Lett.* **2011**, *3*, 382–395.
59. Purushothaman, M.; Dhanapal, R.; Vijayakumar, S.; Ratna, V.J. Development of sustained release matrix tablets of salbutamol sulphate using different polymers. *Int. J. Adv. Pharm.* **2012**, *3*, 5–8.
60. Sivaprakasam, S.; Khatiwada, S.P.; Sivasubramanian, J. Comparative study of desferrioxamine and deferiprone protects against aluminum induced compositional, structural and functional changes in liver tissue of mice (mus musculus) investigated by FT-IR spectroscopy. *Biomed. Prev. Nutr.* **2014**, *4.2*, 231–238.
61. Badri, W.; Miladi, K.; Robin, S.; Viennet, C.; Nazari, Q.A.; Agusti, G.; Fessi, H.; Elaissari, A. Polycaprolactone Based Nanoparticles Loaded with Indomethacin for Anti-Inflammatory Therapy: From Preparation to Ex Vivo Study. *Pharm. Res.* **2017**, *34*, 1773–1783. [CrossRef]
62. Badita, C.R.; Aranghel, D.; Burducea, C.; Mereuta, P. Characterization of sodium alginate based films. *Rom. J. Phys.* **2020**, *65*, 1–8.
63. Gizurarson, S. The effect of cilia and the mucociliary clearance on successful drug delivery. *Biol. Pharm. Bull.* **2015**, *38*, 497–506. [CrossRef] [PubMed]
64. Merkus, F.W.; Verhoef, J.C.; Schipper, N.G.; Marttin, E. Nasal mucociliary clearance as a factor in nasal drug delivery. *Adv. Drug Deliv. Rev.* **1998**, *29*, 13–38. [CrossRef] [PubMed]
65. Chowdary, K.P.; Rao, Y.S. Design and in vitro and in vivo evaluation of mucoadhesive microcapsules of glipizide for oral controlled release: A technical note. *AAPS PharmSciTech.* **2003**, *4*, E39. [CrossRef]
66. Bassi da Silva, J.; Ferreira, S.B.d.S.; Reis, A.V.; Cook, M.T.; Bruschi, M.L. Assessing Mucoadhesion in Polymer Gels: The Effect of Method Type and Instrument Variables. *Polymers* **2018**, *10*, 254. [CrossRef]
67. Singh, I.; Vikas, R. Techniques for the Assessment of Mucoadhesion in Drug Delivery Systems: An Overview. *J. Adhes. Sci. Technol.* **2012**, *26*, 2251–2267. [CrossRef]
68. Sreeram, K.J.; Yamini Shrivastava, H.; Nair, B.U. Studies on the nature of interaction of iron(III) with alginates. *Biochim. Biophys. Acta.* **2004**, *1670*, 121–125. [CrossRef] [PubMed]
69. Picón-Pagès, P.; Bonet, J.; García-García, J.; Garcia-Buendia, J.; Gutierrez, D.; Valle, J.; Gómez-Casuso, C.E.; Sidelkivska, V.; Alvarez, A.; Perálvarez-Marín, A.; et al. Human Albumin Impairs Amyloid β-peptide Fibrillation Through its C-terminus: From docking Modeling to Protection Against Neurotoxicity in Alzheimer's disease. *Comput. Struct. Biotechnol. J.* **2019**, *17*, 963–971. [CrossRef]
70. Yuan, L.; Cao, Y.; Luo, Q.; Yang, W.; Wu, X.; Yang, X.; Wu, D.; Tan, S.; Qin, G.; Zhou, J.; et al. Pullulan-Based Nanoparticle-HSA Complex Formation and Drug Release Influenced by Surface Charge. *Nanoscale Res. Lett.* **2018**, *13*, 317. [CrossRef]
71. Dai, J.; Chen, C.; Yin, M.; Li, H.; Li, W.; Zhang, Z.; Wang, Q.; Du, Z.; Xu, X.; Wang, Y. Interactions between gold nanoparticles with different morphologies and human serum albumin. *Front. Chem.* **2023**, *11*, 1273388. [CrossRef]
72. Maffre, P.; Brandholt, S.; Nienhaus, K.; Shang, L.; Parak, W.J.; Nienhaus, G.U. Effects of surface functionalization on the adsorption of human serum albumin onto nanoparticles—A fluorescence correlation spectroscopy study. *Beilstein J. Nanotechnol.* **2014**, *7*, 2036–2047. [CrossRef]

Journal of
*Functional Biomaterials*

MDPI

*Article*

# Advancing Adult-Acquired Flatfoot Deformity Treatment: Enhanced Biomechanical Support Through Graphene Oxide-Integrated Bioengineered Grafts Tested In Silico

**Sebastián Nieto [1], Mónica Gantiva-Díaz [1], María A. Hoyos [1], Yuliet Montoya [2], Juan C. Cruz [1,*] and Christian Cifuentes-De la Portilla [1,*]**

1 Department of Biomedical Engineering, Universidad de Los Andes, Bogotá 111711, Colombia; s.nieto4@uniandes.edu.co (S.N.); mr.gantiva@uniandes.edu.co (M.G.-D.); ma.hoyosa@uniandes.edu.co (M.A.H.)

2 Grupo de Dinámica Cardiovascular, Línea Ingeniería de Tejidos y Protésica Cardiovascular, Universidad Pontificia Bolivariana, Medellín 050031, Colombia; yulieth.montoya@upb.edu.co

* Correspondence: jc.cruz@uniandes.edu.co (J.C.C.); cc.cifuentes@uniandes.edu.co (C.C.-D.l.P.)

**Abstract:** Adult-Acquired Flatfoot Deformity (AAFD) is a progressive orthopedic condition causing the collapse of the foot's medial longitudinal arch, often linked with injuries to the plantar arch's passive stabilizers, such as the spring ligament (SL) and plantar fascia. Conventional treatment typically involves replacing the SL with synthetic material grafts, which, while providing mechanical support, lack the biological compatibility of native ligaments. In response to this shortcoming, our study developed an electrospun, twisted polymeric graft made of polycaprolactone (PCL) and type B gelatin (GT), enhanced with graphene oxide (GO), a two-dimensional nanomaterial, to bolster biomechanical attributes. The addition of GO aimed to match the native ligamentous tissue's mechanical strength, with the PCL-GT-GO 2.0% blend demonstrating an optimal Young's modulus of 240.75 MPa. Furthermore, the graft showcased excellent biocompatibility, evidenced by non-hemolytic reactions, suitable wettability and favorable platelet aggregation—essential features for promoting cell adhesion and proliferation. An MTT assay revealed cell viability exceeding 80% after 48 h of exposure, highlighting the potential of the graft as a regenerative scaffold for affected ligaments. Computational modeling of the human foot across various AAFD stages assessed the graft's in situ performance, with the PCL-GT-OG 2.0% graft efficiently preventing plantar arch collapse and offering hindfoot pronator support. Our study, based on in silico simulations, suggests that this bioengineered graft holds significant promise as an alternative treatment in AAFD surgery, marking a leap forward in the integration of advanced materials science for enhanced patient care.

**Keywords:** electrospun graft; graphene oxide; polycaprolactone; gelatin; spring ligament; finite element analysis; adult-acquired flatfoot deformity

## 1. Introduction

The pervasive condition known as Adult-Acquired Flatfoot Deformity (AAFD) is marked by the partial or full collapse of the longitudinal medial arch of the foot [1], catalyzing progressive deformities like heel valgus and forefoot abduction [2]. These changes subsequently trigger foot pain, misalignment, and gait dysfunction [1]. Historically, AAFD has been ascribed to the deterioration of the posterior tibial tendon (PTT) [3], but a more comprehensive understanding acknowledges the role of other structures that contribute to plantar arch alignment and stability. These include the plantar fascia (PF), spring ligament (SL), talocalcaneal ligaments, and deltoid ligaments [1].

Recent studies suggest that AAFD often arises secondary to injuries of the spring ligament, either independently or in conjunction with PTT degeneration [4–9]. The spring ligament, a key ligamentous structure extending from the calcaneus to the navicular bone, serves critical functions in supporting the head of the talus, maintaining the medial arch [10], and restraining valgus deformity of the foot [3].

The Bluman–Myerson classification categorizes AAFD into four stages, each corresponding to the level of deformity and the progression of the pathology. Therapeutic interventions vary with each stage, and spring ligament injuries are predominantly associated with grade II AAFD, wherein the flatfoot remains flexible [1]. Available treatment options span from orthoses, tendon transfers, and calcaneal osteotomies to arthrodesis and spring ligament augmentation [1]. Yet certain interventions, such as midfoot fusions, may inadvertently induce secondary effects on the stiffness and flexibility of the foot, potentially exerting additional stress on the spring ligament [11]. Other types of arthrodesis may similarly exert undue strain on the forefoot and rearfoot [11], alongside the possible loss of certain biomechanical foot functions owing to tendon transfers. This underscores the pressing need to innovatively address spring ligament injuries implicated in AAFD and avert these potential complications.

Given their low cell density and restricted oxygen and nutrient supply, tendons and ligaments possess limited regenerative capacity. Hence, it is imperative to circumvent the limitations of conventional surgical techniques by developing synthetic and natural substitutes via advanced materials engineering. These substitutes ought to mimic the intricate structure and mechanical properties of native tissues while demonstrating superior biological performance [12].

Electrospinning has emerged as a promising method for fabricating polymeric nanofibers for material engineering applications, especially in ligament and tendon research. This is largely due to its capacity to replicate the fibrillar microstructure of these tissues [13], facilitating cell adhesion, proliferation, and extracellular matrix production [14,15], while enabling the amalgamation of diverse types of polymers [16]. Electrospinning is a technique used to produce nanofibers through the application of an electric charge to a polymer solution, which is then ejected as fine fibers. In this process, the polymer solution is passed through a metal needle that is connected to the positive terminal of a DC power source. Simultaneously, a target collector with a negative charge is also connected to the power source, resulting in the formation of a cone-shaped jet (referred to as the Taylor cone) that moves towards the area of lower electrical potential. As a result, the solvent evaporates from the polymer solution, leading to the deposition of nanofibers [17].

Nevertheless, one of the critical challenges associated with electrospinning is the limited mechanical strength of the resulting nanofibers, which could potentially hinder their clinical applicability [12–14,16,18]. To counter this, researchers have twisted or coiled electrospun nanofibers to construct more complex 3D structures with appropriate mechanical properties [12]. Moreover, the incorporation of nanocomposites such as carbon nanotubes, graphene, graphene oxide, carbon, and cellulose nanofibers [19,20] has been shown to significantly enhance the strength and longevity of the resultant structures.

The goal of this study was to design electrospun grafts from biodegradable polymers as a novel strategy for reinforcing and augmenting elastic ligament injuries associated with AAFD (see Figure 1). The grafts were synthesized using a blend of synthetic and natural polymers, specifically polycaprolactone (PCL) and gelatine type B (GT), to achieve an optimal balance of strength, durability, and enhanced biocompatibility [12,16]. PCL, a synthetic polymer, offers mechanical resilience and protracted degradation time while retaining biocompatibility. Simultaneously, gelatine enhances cell adhesion, courtesy of its integrin-rich structure, which augments the biocompatibility of the graft and mitigates immunogenic responses [12]. To fortify the mechanical robustness of the graft, graphene oxide (GO), a two-dimensional nanomaterial, was incorporated. Recognized for its improved mechanical properties, increased colloidal stability, and physiologically stable, biocompatible, and antibacterial properties even at lower concentrations, GO represents an ideal component for this application [20,21]. The electrospun graft was then subjected to a battery of tests—physicochemical, morphological, mechanical, and biological—to evaluate its properties.

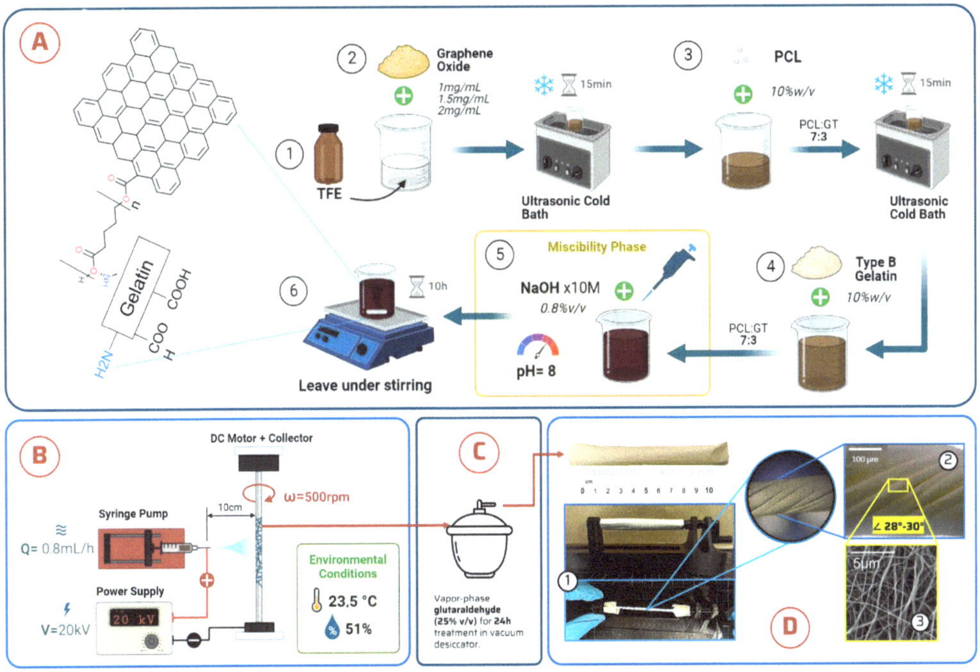


**Figure 1.** Schematic diagram of (**A**) solution preparation; (**B**) electrospinning equipment assembly and operating parameters; (**C**) vapor crosslinking method in vacuum desiccator; and (**D**) electrowinning cylindrical membrane twisting machine. (**D1**) Twisting; (**D2**) macrograph of graft; (**D3**) SEM micrograph of electrospun graft.

Furthermore, to replicate the graft's final application, finite element analysis was undertaken to assess the insertion of the graft in a patient's foot affected by AAFD. A computational model was formulated using CT images of a healthy patient, encompassing all foot bones, plantar fascia, cartilage, and elastic ligaments while preserving their anatomical distribution and mechanical properties. This model has been validated in several previous works, including analyzing plantar soft tissue stresses and applying different traditional surgical methods on the foot [11].

## 2. Materials and Methods

### *2.1. Materials*

Polycaprolactone pellets (PCL, MW 80.000), type B gelatine (porcine skin), 2,2,2-trifluoroethanol (TFE, 99.0%), glutaraldehyde solution (grade II, 25% ($v/v$)), sodium hydroxide (NaOH) pellets (reactive level, >98%), phosphate-buffered saline (PBS), 3-(4,5-Dimethyl-2-thiazolyl)-2,5-diphenyl-2H-tetrazolium bromide (MTT), phosphate-buffered saline (PBS), and Triton X-100 were purchased at Sigma-Aldrich Inc. (Saint Louis, MI, USA, EE.UU). High-glucose Dulbecco's modified Eagle medium (DMEM) was purchased from Gibco (Amarillo, TX, USA). Sodium hydroxide was purchased from PanReac AppliChem (Chicago, IL, USA). L929 P + 13 (mouse connective tissue fibroblasts) were from ATCC® (Manassas, VA, USA).

### *2.2. Polymer Solution Preparation*

In this study, a standardized process was utilized to prepare four distinctive polymer solutions. Initially, trifluoroethanol (TFE) served as the solvent, to which GO was added at concentrations of 1.0 mg/mL, 1.5 mg/mL, and 2.0 mg/mL. GO was synthesized from graphite oxidation/exfoliation according to the Tour Method [22]. Briefly, graphite powder was oxidized using a mixture of $H_2SO_4/H_3PO_4$ (9:1) with $KMnO_4$, followed by the controlled addition of $H_2O_2$ and multiple washing steps with water, HCl, and ethanol. The resulting GO was characterized by FTIR and TGA to confirm successful oxidation and exfoliation. The synthesis protocol followed our previously established methods [20], yielding GO sheets with lateral dimensions in the submicron range. The mixtures underwent cold sonication for 15 min, ensuring dispersion. Then, PCL pellets were added at a concentration of 7% ($w/v$) and sonicated again for 15 min for homogeneity. Gelatine type B (GT) was then added at a 3% ($w/v$) concentration and stirred at 200 rpm for two hours. The pH of GT was adjusted to 8 using 1M NaOH to ensure miscibility. The final solution was left stirring overnight at 200 rpm [23]. A separate solution was prepared without GO for comparison. The resulting solutions were designated as PCL-GT-GO 1.0%; PCL-GT-GO 1.5%; PCL-GT-GO 2.0%; and PCL-GT for control (Figure 1A).

### 2.3. Electrospinning Setup

The electrospinning apparatus consisted of a rotating (500 rpm) cylindrical aluminum collector (20 mm diameter and 160 mm length). A total of 5 mL of the prepared solution was loaded in a syringe with a 21 G needle and pumped at a rate of 0.8 mL/h. A voltage of 20 kV was maintained across a 10 cm gap between the needle and the collector. Ambient conditions were controlled at 23.5 °C with a relative humidity of 51% during the collection process. Electrospinning proceeded until the solution was fully dispensed. Optimal electrospinning parameters were determined by iterating conditions in collector speed, voltage, and flow rate (Figure 1B).

### 2.4. Post Electrospinning Processing

Upon retrieval from the collector, the electrospun membranes exhibited a hollow cylindrical morphology. Due to GT's aqueous solubility and the necessity for crosslinking to ensure stability at physiological temperatures, we used glutaraldehyde vapor exposure in a vacuum desiccator with 25% glutaraldehyde solution [24] for 24 h for crosslinking. For biological assays, the membranes were sterilized under UV light exposure for 40 min, cleansed overnight with 70% ethanol, and extensively rinsed with type I water to ensure suitability for subsequent assays.

### 2.5. Membrane Twisting

To improve the mechanical strength of the nanofiber membranes, we applied a textile twisting technique, manipulating the fiber architecture. The membranes, possessing a hollow cylindrical shape, were placed on a manually operated device custom-made by our 3D-printing team. The apparatus allowed for one end of the membrane to be fixed while the other was rotated to achieve a consistent torsion angle between 28° and 30° [25]. Different levels of twists were applied to create various structures: 20 twists for PCL-GT, 15 for PCL-GT-GO 1.0%, and 12 for PCL-GT-GO 2.0%.

### 2.6. Fourier Transform Infrared Spectroscopy (FTIR)

The chemical characteristics of the membranes were analyzed using Fourier Transform Infrared Spectroscopy (FTIR) on a BRUKER Alpha II A250/D system (Billerica, MA, USA). The spectra were obtained in the wavenumber range of 4000–500 $cm^{-1}$ with a spectral resolution of 2 $cm^{-1}$, enabling us to elucidate the chemical composition and confirm the presence of expected functional groups within the nanofibers.

### 2.7. Thermogravimetric Analysis (TGA) and Differential Scanning Calorimetry

To determine the thermal stability and decomposition profiles, the electrospun membranes were analyzed using Thermogravimetric Analysis (TGA) on an SDT Q600 (TA Instruments, New Castle, DE, USA). This analysis provided detailed information on the mass loss at various temperature thresholds from 0 °C to 650° C. Additionally, Differential

Scanning Calorimetry (DSC) on a DSC Q2000 (TA Instruments, New Castle, DE, USA) was utilized to identify the thermal transitions of the materials within a temperature range of 25 °C to 400 °C. This thermal analysis helped to assess the melting and crystallization behaviors of the polymers, which are indicative of their processing stability and potential performance as graft materials.

### 2.8. Polymer Contact Angle (Wettability)

The wettability of the electrospun membranes was quantified by measuring the contact angles using a Theta Lite optical tensiometer (Biolin Scientific, Hängpilsgatan, Sweden). Employing the sessile drop method, a 3 µL water droplet was carefully placed onto each membrane's surface. The spread of the droplet was recorded, and the contact angles were calculated with Digimizer image analysis software (v. 6.4.0)® (Ostend, Belgium).

### 2.9. Morphological Analysis

The 2D morphology of the electrospun nanofibers was observed under a scanning electron microscope (SEM) (TESCAN LYRA3, Brno, Czechia) at 5 kV. Membranes prepared for SEM were subjected to ion bombardment to make their surfaces conductive. High-resolution micrographs were captured at magnifications of 5 kx, 10 kx, and 20 kx to accurately gauge the nanofiber diameters, which were then analyzed using ImageJ software (v 1.54g)®.

### 2.10. Hemolysis and Platelet Aggregation

The hemolysis assays were conducted following the ISO 10993-4 [26] and ASTM F 756-00 standards [26]. We prepared extracts by incubating 3 mm × 2 mm membrane samples in 2 mL of 1X PBS at 37 °C for 24 h. We drew 4 mL of blood into an EDTA tube from a healthy O+ human donor, which was then centrifuged at 1800 rpm for 5 min. After discarding the plasma and white blood cells, we replenished the tube to its original volume with 1X PBS, repeating this washing step thrice. For hemolysis testing, Triton X-100 and PBS 1X served as the positive and negative controls, representing complete (100%) and no (0%) hemolysis, respectively. We combined the extracts with the erythrocyte suspension in a 96-well plate and incubated them at 37 °C for 1 h. Post centrifugation at 3000 rpm for 5 min, the absorbance of the supernatant, indicative of hemoglobin release, was measured at 540 nm using a Multiskan FC microplate reader (ThermoFisher Scientific, Waltham, MA, USA). The percentage of hemolysis was calculated using the following formula:

$$Hemolysis\ (\%) = \frac{Abs_s - Abs_{(-)}}{Abs_{(+)} - Abs_{(-)}} \times 100\%$$

where $Abs_s$ is the absorbance of the sample, $Abs_{(-)}$ is the absorbance of the negative control (1X PBS), and $Abs_{(+)}$ is the absorbance of the positive control (Triton X-100, 10% ($v/v$)).

Platelet aggregation was assessed by collecting 8 mL of blood from a healthy O+ donor in sodium citrate tubes and centrifuging it at 1000 rpm for 10 min to obtain plasma. Epinephrine and 1X PBS were employed as positive and negative controls to induce strong and weak aggregation, respectively. The assay involved mixing the plasma with our membrane extracts in a 96-well plate. Absorbance readings were taken using a Multiskan FC microplate reader (ThermoFisher Scientific, Waltham, MA, USA) at 610 nm. The platelet aggregation percentage was determined using the following formula:

$$Platelet\ aggregation\ (\%) = \frac{Abs_s - Abs_{(-)}}{Abs_{(+)} - Abs_{(-)}} \times 100\%$$

where $Abs_s$ is the absorbance of the sample, $Abs_{(+)}$ is the absorbance of the positive control (Epinephrine), and $Abs_{(-)}$ is that of the negative control (1X PBS).

### 2.11. Cytotoxicity

To examine the cytotoxicity of the electrospun membranes, L929 P + 13 mouse connective tissue fibroblasts were cultured. A density of $1 \times 10^5$ cells/mL was seeded into a 96-well microplate and incubated for 24 h in standard conditions (37 °C, 5% $CO_2$) in DMEM supplemented with 5% FBS, 1% P/S. Post incubation, the cells were exposed to the various electrospun membrane samples, each providing a contact area of 12.5 $mm^2$ for 24 and 48 h. DMEM served as the positive control (C+) for cellular viability, while DMSO (10% ($v/v$)) functioned as the negative control (C−). The MTT assay was employed to evaluate cell viability. After exposure to the MTT reagent, cells were incubated for an additional 2 h to enable formazan crystal formation (37 °C). Subsequently, these crystals were solubilized with DMSO, and absorbance was measured at 595 nm using a Multiskan FC microplate reader (ThermoFisher Scientific, Waltham, MA, USA).

The L929 mouse fibroblast cell line was selected for cytotoxicity evaluation in accordance with ISO 10993-5 [27] guidelines, which establish this cell line as a standard reference for initial biomaterial biocompatibility assessment. These cells are particularly valuable for standardized testing due to their well-characterized responses to cytotoxic substances and their documented sensitivity in detecting potential material toxicity. Furthermore, L929 fibroblasts represent a primary cellular component of connective tissues, making them particularly relevant for evaluating materials intended for ligament applications. Their use enables standardized comparison with other biomaterial studies in the literature, providing a validated foundation for biocompatibility assessment [28].

### 2.12. Finite Element Analysis Using a Foot Model

To evaluate the use of the graft designed, we performed some simulations using a computational model of the human foot previously used and validated by our research group to study AAFD progression. The model reproduces the foot of a 49-year-old male subject, weighing 720 N and standing 170 cm tall, preserving the natural morphology of the cartilage, cortical and trabecular bone, plantar fascia, and spring ligament [28] (see Figure 2A). The model has been validated for both healthy and pathological conditions. For this study, we positioned graft geometries in various foot regions, aiming for more dorsal locations while preserving the spring ligament's insertion area. We made graft placement decisions based on three criteria: a. the grafts should replace the spring ligament's passive function in preventing medial arch drop; b. the grafts should perform the passive work of the LS in hindfoot pronator stability; and c. the grafts should be located in areas that prevent iatrogenic effects during access and surgical anchoring to bone structures.

We modeled three types of grafts, designed in Fusion360 (Autodesk, Mill Valley, CA, USA), with a double helical morphology to mirror the macroscopic structure of the electrospun grafts post-torsional treatment. The graft placement was guided by the advice of expert foot and ankle surgeons and was based on medical images of surgical procedures from Techniques in Orthopaedic Surgery [29]. The grafts were named and positioned as follows: Calcaneonavicular Graft (CNG): Located between the sustentaculum tail of the medial aspect of the calcaneus and the navicular tuberosity. This graft is closest to the LS's native location (See Figure 2(B1)). Talonavicular Tuberosity Graft (TNTG): Positioned between the navicular tuberosity and the talus. This graft prevents sagging of the medial longitudinal arch and supports the surrounding grafts (See Figure 2(B1)). Talonavicular Dorsal Graft (TNDG): Located in the foot's most dorsal area, between the navicular and the talus. This graft works in tandem with the other grafts to prevent rearfoot pronation and the fall of the medial longitudinal arch (See Figure 2(B1)).

The mesh of the grafts models was generated using linear tetrahedral elements (C3D4) with a maximum size of 0.5 mm in Ansys (Ansys V.2121.R1, Canonsburg, PA, USA) (see Figure 2C). We checked the mesh quality according to the guidelines described by Burkhart [30].

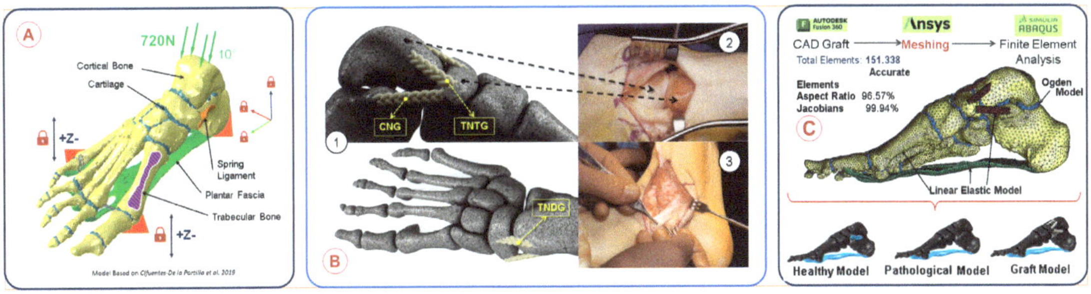


**Figure 2.** Characteristics and parameters of the computational biomechanical foot model. (**A**) Model tissues, structures, static input load, and motion constraints of the foot model [28]. (**B**) Graft placement. (**B1**) Rendering of the foot model with the 3 grafts placed in low iatrogenic surgical access structures. (**B2**) Medial midfoot incision. (**B3**) Incision with large iatrogenic effects starting at the medial malleolus along the internal axis of the foot, towards the cuneometatarsal junction [29]. (**C**) Meshing characteristics of the foot model, implemented models, and software used for graft design. Healthy model: Foot model with SL and PF native properties. Pathological model: Foot model without SL. Graft model: Foot model without SL and hindfoot grafts.

The mechanical characteristics of the tissues included on the computational model are described in Table 1. We modeled the bone (cortical and trabecular), spring ligament, and plantar fascia as elastic–linear (E-L), whereas we considered the cartilage to be nonlinear and hyperelastic [11].

**Table 1.** Mechanical properties of the elastic–linear tissues of the human foot model. * PCL-GT-OG 2.0%. Values from [28,31].

| Tissue | Elasticity Modulus | Poisson Ratio |
|---|---|---|
| Cortical bone | 17,000 MPa | 0.3 |
| Trabecular bone | 700 MPa | 0.3 |
| Spring ligament | 250 MPa | 0.28 |
| Plantar fascia | 240 MPa | 0.28 |
| Grafts * | 240.7 MPa | 0.3 |

The Ogden model assigned to the cartilage material considers the strain energy density function U, described by following equation:

$$U = \frac{\mu}{\alpha^2}(\lambda_1^\alpha + \lambda_2^\alpha + \lambda_3^\alpha) + \frac{1}{D}(J-1)^2$$

where μ is the initial shear modulus, α is the strain hardening exponent, and D is the compressibility parameter. The values used are μ = 4.4, α = 2, and D = 0.45. The model works by applying a load of 720 N, representing the total weight of an adult person in monopodal support. This load is distributed in the tibio-ankle (90%) and peroneal–ankle (10%) contact zone. The constraints for our model were established by locking all the degrees of displacement at the base of the calcaneus and by inhibiting the vertical displacement (Z axis) of the first and fifth metatarsal bases [28].

We carried out the simulation and biomechanical analysis of the computational model using Abaqus (Dassault Sistemes, Velizy-Villacoublay, France). The parameters for evaluation were selected in two directions: a. biomechanical tissue stress: stress on the plantar fascia, and b. structural foot displacements: medial longitudinal arch fall and fore/hind foot displacements (foot abduction/adduction performance).

These were considered across three distinct models: a healthy model (preserves all foot structures and healthy mechanical properties of the native tissues, including the LS), a diseased model (mimics an injured LS scenario, does not consider the work carried out by the LS, other structures maintain their mechanical properties), and the grafted model (an iterative model of the three grafts, disregards the LS, other structures maintain their mechanical properties) (Figure 2C).

We assessed the biomechanical tissue stress under the principal maxima criterion; thus, the tensile loads of the plantar fascia were calculated to identify the contribution of the LS and grafts in the pathological scenario. We measured the structural deformation of the foot at the sagging of the longitudinal medial arch by placing a sensor-node on the medial head of the talus and measuring the vertical displacement (Z axis).

### 2.13. Statistical Analysis

Statistical analysis was performed using GraphPad Prism 8® (GraphPad Software, San Diego, CA, USA). The data, particularly related to the impact of varying graphene oxide concentrations on the properties of electrospun membranes, were presented as mean values with their corresponding standard deviations. One-way ANOVA followed by Tukey's multiple comparison tests were utilized to discern the statistical significance between the groups. This analytical approach ensures a rigorous evaluation of the treatment effects, validating the robustness of the experimental outcomes.

## 3. Results

### 3.1. Synthesis of Electrospun Grafts

The integration of GO into electrospun scaffolds was effectively validated using Fourier Transform Infrared (FTIR) Spectroscopy and thermogravimetric analysis (TGA). The FTIR spectra, displayed in Figure 3A, reveal distinct absorption bands for various PCL-GT-GO formulations alongside a GO control. Hydroxyl group stretching vibrations are evident in the 3000–3500 $cm^{-1}$ range, signifying the presence of GO. Aromatic peaks at 1627 $cm^{-1}$, attributed to C=C bond stretching, along with bands at 1726 $cm^{-1}$ and 1084 $cm^{-1}$ for C=O and C-O bonds, respectively, confirm the synthesis process's efficacy in retaining oxygen-rich functional groups. Amide bonds from gelatin incorporation are discernible at 1640 $cm^{-1}$ (amide I) and 1540 $cm^{-1}$ (amide II), corroborating successful polymer integration [2]. The spectrum also includes peaks that suggest PCL's presence, such as at 1740 $cm^{-1}$ for the carbonyl group's stretching vibration and 2875 $cm^{-1}$ and 2940 $cm^{-1}$ for $CH_2$ bond vibrations, along with other PCL-related bands at 1230 $cm^{-1}$ (asymmetric stress vibration of the C-O-C bond) and 1300 $cm^{-1}$ (stretching vibration of the C-O and C-C bonds) [2,32–34].

The TGA results, depicted in Figure 3C, indicate a prominent weight loss at around 325 °C across all grafts, ascribed to PCL's ester chain cleavage, yielding $H_2O$, $CO_2$, and 5-hexenoic acid. A secondary weight reduction, approximately 9%, concludes around 450–460 °C, linked to ε-caprolactone production from depolymerization [35]. Incorporating GO alters this behavior; GO-containing grafts undergo earlier mass loss due to GO decomposition at about 163 °C, where carboxyl groups break down to release $CO_2$ [36]. DSC analyses show a consistent melting temperature near 59.36 °C for all grafts, suggesting GO's addition does not significantly alter the thermal properties of the electrospun material (Figure 3D).

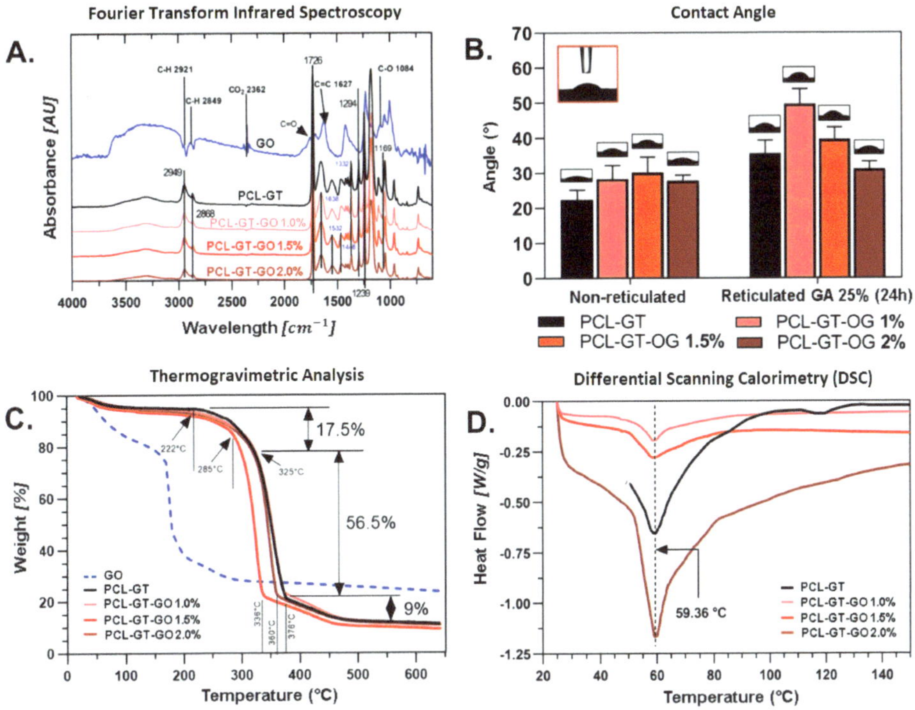


**Figure 3.** (**A**) Absorbance FTIR spectra for graphene oxide and electrospun grafts in each of their treatments and (**B**) evaluation of wettability in all electrospun membranes by means of contact angle test with deionized water and optical images associated with each graft. (**C**) Thermal analysis results TGA (0–650 °C). (**D**) Thermal analysis results DSC (25–400 °C) for all electrospun grafts.

### 3.2. *Polymer Contact Angle (Wettability)*

The wettability of the electrospun graft surfaces was evaluated by measuring contact angles, as depicted in Figure 3B. Contact angles less than 90° typically denote hydrophilic materials, while angles greater than 90° suggest hydrophobic properties. Following glutaraldehyde vapor crosslinking treatment, a marked decrease in hydrophilicity was noted among the grafts, likely as a result of chemical crosslinking within gelatin's polymeric chains. However, it is noteworthy that none of the graft samples exhibited contact angles exceeding the 90° threshold.

In samples containing GO, the post-crosslinking increase in contact angle was mitigated. For example, the contact angle of the PCL-GT graft diminished from 35.6° to 31.1° upon the addition of 2% GO (PCL-GT-GO 2%). This suggests that GO contributes to preserving the wettability of the grafts even after undergoing chemical crosslinking.

### 3.3. *Mechanical Evaluation*

Mechanical characterization of our electrospun grafts indicated compaction within the fibers corresponding to the helical orientation of polymer chains under mechanical stress. In samples with increased GO concentration, we observed a reduction in ultimate stress but an increase in stiffness. The mechanical properties were evaluated at two critical stages of graft preparation: the initial electrospun mat and the final twisted yarn configuration. The electrospun mat in its untwisted form (length = 12.38 mm; height = 5.7 mm; thickness = 0.28 mm) showed average tensile strengths of 1.375 MPa, with Young's moduli between 6.8 and 40.5 MPa across different GO concentrations. Following the twisting process, which was designed to better mimic the hierarchical structure of native ligament tissue, the mechanical properties were significantly enhanced. The twisted yarn configuration exhibited increased tensile strengths (ranging from 7.7 to 16.8 MPa) and higher Young's moduli (125 to 275 MPa), with the PCL-GT-GO 2.0% formulation achieving the optimal value of 240.75 MPa, closely aligning with the mechanical properties of native tissues among all tested samples. These properties made this sample a prime candidate for grafting model simulations aimed at flatfoot pathology applications. This enhancement can be attributed to the compaction and alignment of fibers during the twisting process, leading to more efficient load distribution throughout the structure. The dramatic improvement in mechanical properties after twisting underscores the importance of this processing step in achieving properties suitable for ligament applications.

Figure 4A illustrates the mechanical properties of the grafts, including the modulus of elasticity and ultimate stress at break. The inclusion of GO across all grafts resulted in enhanced mechanical performance relative to samples comprising solely PCL and GT. The most significant improvement was observed in the PCL-GT-GO 1% graft, which displayed an ultimate tensile strength increase of 112% over the PCL-GT control.

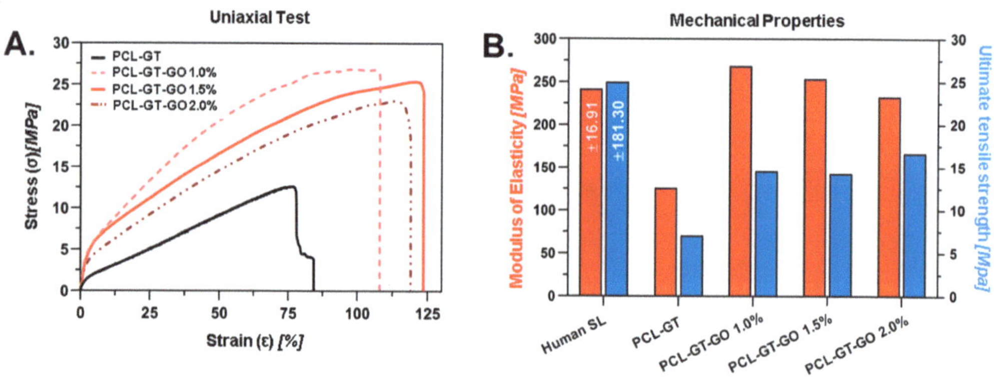


**Figure 4.** Characterization of the mechanical properties of electrospun grafts. (**A**) Stress–strain curves in a tensile test. (**B**) Elastic modulus and tensile stress at break.

Our findings suggest that the methodical integration of GO within the polymeric matrix and the strategic fiber twisting process contribute substantially to the observed mechanical enhancements. This improvement is crucial for the potential use of these grafts as temporary reinforcement structures and as scaffolds for tissue regeneration in ligament injuries.

### 3.4. Biocompatibility

In assessing the biocompatibility of electrospun grafts, hemolytic behavior and cytotoxicity were crucial parameters. The hemolysis tests, adhering to ASTM F 756-00 standards, revealed that while PCL-GT grafts were slightly hemolytic, grafts with any concentration of GO were deemed non-hemolytic. Specifically, the PCL-GT-GO 1.5% variant demonstrated a notable reduction in hemolytic activity compared to PCL-GT grafts, suggesting improved compatibility with blood (Figure 5A) [37].

Platelet aggregation assays indicated that all grafts, regardless of GO concentration, function as medium aggregators, with no substantial differences in aggregation behavior across different GO treatments. Such a medium level of aggregation is beneficial for supporting tissue healing processes (Figure 5B) [38].

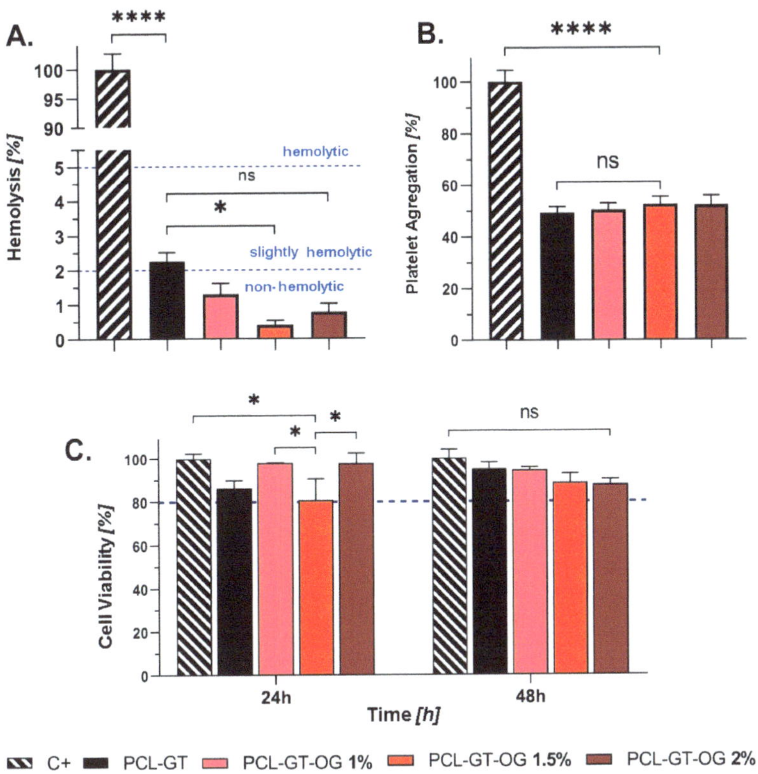


**Figure 5.** Biocompatibility results: (**A**) Hemolytic behavior, (**B**) platelet aggregation, and (**C**) cell viability for PCL-GT, PCL-GT-GO 1%, PCL-GT-GO 1.5%, and PCL-GT-GO 2%. The symbol * corresponds to a statistically significant difference with a $p$-value in the range of $0.01 \leq p\text{-value} \leq 0.05$, **** to $p$-value < 0.0001.

Cell viability assays utilizing the L929 P + 13 mouse fibroblast cell line showed promising results. Within the first 24 h, all grafts maintained over 80% viability. There were significant viability differences noted between the control group and the PCL-GT-GO grafts, especially the 1.5% concentration, indicating a possible concentration-dependent effect of GO on cell viability. By 48 h, cell viability had improved across all samples, with no significant differences noted among them, indicating good cytocompatibility (Figure 5C).

### 3.5. Morphological Analysis

Scanning electron microscopy revealed the surface morphology of the electrospun grafts, showcasing stable nanofibers with minimal defects and a largely random orientation that mimics the natural architecture of connective tissue [39]. The measured average fiber diameters ranged from 161 nm to 115 nm across the different graft formulations. Specifically, the diameters for PCL-GT, PCL-GT-GO 1%, PCL-GT-GO 1.5%, and PCL-GT-GO 2% specimens were quantified, with the smallest diameter observed in grafts with the highest GO concentration.

Notably, a trend of decreasing fiber diameter with increasing GO content was observed, except for the PCL-GT-GO 2.0% sample which, counterintuitively, showed larger fiber diameters than the grafts with lower GO concentrations [40]. This unexpected result was consistently replicated across multiple observations and measurements, indicating a potential variation in the dispersion of GO within the samples.

Figure 6 presents a series of micrographs that visually document these findings, with the stable fiber formation and uniformity clearly displayed. These images are integral for validating the consistency of the electrospinning process and ensuring the reproducibility of the scaffold's nanofibrous structure.

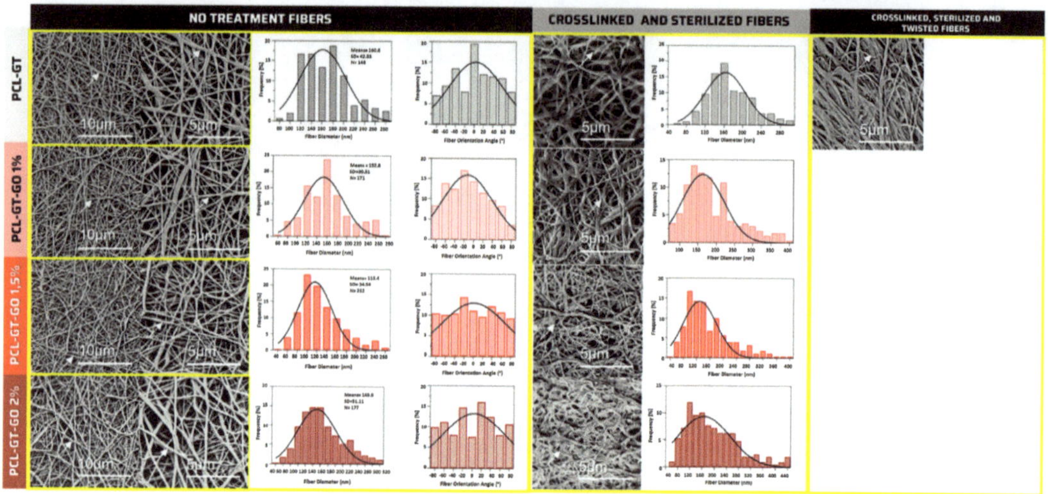


**Figure 6.** Measurement of nanofiber diameters after crosslinking from the surface morphology of electrospun membranes using SEM micrographs. From top to bottom, the order of grafts is PCL-GT, PCL-GT-GO 1.0%, PCL-GT-GO 1.5%, and PCL-GT-GO 2.0%. From left to right, the images show no treatment fibers (fiber diameter and fiber orientation angle), crosslinked and sterilized fibers, and crosslinked (fiber diameter), sterilized, and mechanically twisted fiber treatment (fiber orientation angle). Insert plots: histograms and Gaussian fit of fiber diameters.

### 3.6. Finite Element Analysis

Adult-Acquired Flatfoot Deformity is typically marked by the progressive weakening and subsequent collapse of the foot's medial longitudinal arch [40]. The condition is complex and often impairs the individual's gait and balance. Through computational modeling, the vertical displacement of the talus—a critical indicator of arch integrity—was meticulously evaluated. Results can be seen in Figure 7.

In the healthy foot model, the talus node experienced a displacement of −4.32 mm. By contrast, the model representing the diseased state exhibited a more pronounced collapse, with a 10% increase in displacement, measuring −4.75 mm. This metric clearly illustrates the mechanical compromise associated with AAFD. Yet when the model was adjusted to incorporate the proposed grafts, there was a notable correction in the pathological drop, with a reduction to −4.44 mm, indicating a 6% improvement.

It is essential to consider the interconnected nature of the foot's arches; the failure of one arch can precipitate a cascade of biomechanical dysfunctions throughout the structure [1]. Despite this, the lateral longitudinal arch's collapse, another potential area of concern, did not significantly differ across the analyzed models (See Table 2). This finding could indicate that the corrective measures primarily influence the medial arch, leaving the lateral arch relatively unaffected, or that the model's scope did not extend to detectable changes in the lateral arch. This nuanced understanding of AAFD progression and the correction potential of grafts offers valuable insights for clinical interventions aimed at restoring foot stability and function.

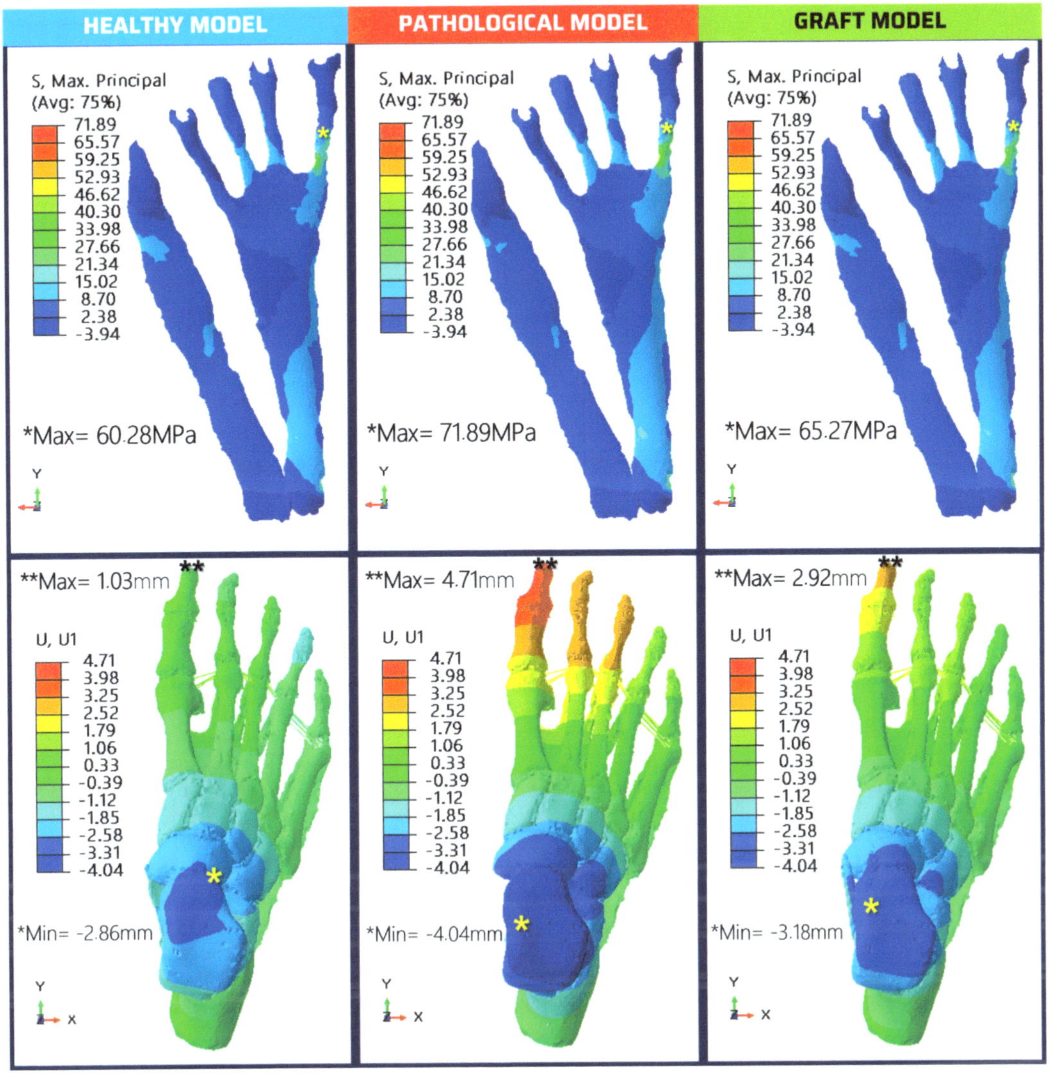


**Figure 7.** Top: Results of the evaluation of principal maxima in the plantar fascia for the three models. Bottom: Analysis of foot displacements in the X axis (evaluation of lateral displacements in the rearfoot and forefoot) for the three models. Asterisks mark the location of the maxima (**) and minima (*).

**Table 2.** Results of the foot model simulations, using the healthy model (SL + PF), pathological model (PF only), and all iterations in all combinations of the three grafts. The results of the healthy model are given in physical magnitudes; all other values are represented in percentages (%). These percentages represent the differential increase compared to the healthy model (SL + PF).

| Foot Model | Medial Long Arch Fall (mm) | Foot Displacement (mm) | | Plantar Fascia Stress (MPa) |
|---|---|---|---|---|
| | Displacement | Forefoot | Hindfoot | Max. Principal |
| SL + PF (healthy) | 4.32 | 1.03 | 2.86 | 60.28 |
| PF only (pathological) | 9.80 | 357.78 | 41.20 | 19.26 |

Table 2. *Cont.*

| Foot Model | Medial Long Arch Fall (mm) | Foot Displacement (mm) | | Plantar Fascia Stress (MPa) |
|---|---|---|---|---|
| | Displacement | Forefoot | Hindfoot | Max. Principal |
| CNG + PF | 5.49 | 183.95 | 19.80 | 10.57 |
| TNTG + PF | 9.49 | 343.48 | 39.98 | 18.64 |
| TNDG + PF | 7.14 | 368.29 | 32.46 | 17.40 |
| CNG + TNTG + PF | 5.36 | 180.74 | 19.03 | 10.36 |
| CNG + TNDG + PF | 2.78 | 192.80 | 11.33 | 8.56 |
| TNTG + TNDG + PF | 6.87 | 347.08 | 31.76 | 16.63 |
| CNG + TNTG + TNDG + PF | 2.68 | 184.44 | 11.12 | 8.27 |

## 4. Discussion

In the quest to address AAFD, a complex condition characterized by the breakdown of the foot arch's structural integrity, this study embarks on an innovative approach. Traditional interventions, such as the reinforcement or replacement of the spring ligament, often utilize synthetic material grafts for mechanical support, yet these lack the biological affinity inherent to native tissues. To bridge this gap, our research has homed in on a novel graft fabrication methodology. We have engineered a composite, twisted polymeric graft that integrates PCL and type B gelatin (GT) with GO, a reinforcement agent, aimed at amplifying the graft's biomechanical properties.

This graft is meticulously designed to emulate the biomechanical support furnished by the natural spring ligament, which plays a pivotal role in maintaining the arch structure. The inclusion of GO not only enhances the mechanical strength of the graft but also contributes to its overall stability and longevity—traits imperative for an effective treatment modality for AAFD. Through this synergy of PCL's robustness, GT's biocompatibility, and GO's structural enhancement, we present a promising therapeutic alternative that may transcend the limitations of current synthetic grafts. The results showed that the incorporation of GO into polymeric scaffolds enhances both mechanical and biological properties, which is pivotal for their successful application in tissue engineering and regenerative medicine, particularly for surgical interventions such as those for AAFD. This study's electrospun grafts, augmented with GO, displayed improved mechanical strength and a commendable biological compatibility profile. The synthesis process preserved the intricate structures of both the polymeric matrix and the embedded GO, as substantiated by the characteristic absorption bands and peaks in the FTIR spectra, which are in line with the oxygen-rich functional groups' resonances resulting from the synthesis of GO [41]. The sustained mechanical integrity of the grafts after GO integration is of particular relevance given that the mechanical support is critical for replacing ligaments in AAFD.

Furthermore, the TGA data confirm that our electrospun materials exhibit appropriate thermal degradation points, similar to native ligamentous tissue, suggesting that the structural integrity of the grafts would be maintained under physiological conditions [42]. The consistent melting temperatures reported in the DSC curves reaffirm that the integration of GO into the scaffolds does not adversely affect their thermal stability, echoing findings from other works that have explored the incorporation of GO into various polymeric matrices for biomedical applications [41]. Together, these results affirm the potential of these GO-enhanced electrospun grafts to serve as suitable candidates for ligament replacement in AAFD surgeries. Their physicochemical attributes promise a graft that can withstand biomechanical forces while fostering favorable cellular interactions, a necessary condition for the long-term success of implantable devices [43].

The observed wettability of the electrospun grafts in this study is of paramount importance, as it influences the material's interaction with biological fluids and cells. Contact angle measurements yielded results that highlight the hydrophilic nature of our grafts, even after glutaraldehyde vapor crosslinking, with angles consistently below 90°. This hydrophilicity is crucial for biomedical applications, particularly those involving direct contact with cells and tissue, as it promotes better adhesion and proliferation of cells. The chemical crosslinking of gelatin's polymeric chains seems to induce a decrease in hydrophilicity, which is counteracted by the inclusion of GO. Notably, the PCL-GT-GO 2% demonstrated a significant retention of hydrophilicity post crosslinking, which can be attributed to the nanoscale roughness and high density of oxygen-containing functional groups on GO. This result aligns with previous studies indicating that GO's unique structure and chemistry can influence surface wettability and enhance biomolecule adsorption [44,45].

Furthermore, the addition of GO to the grafts likely contributes to the biomaterial's bioactivity. GO is known for its ability to adsorb biomolecules, owing to its functional groups, which provide binding sites for proteins and other cellular components. This interaction is not just a passive physical adsorption but can lead to bioactive conformational changes in the adsorbed biomolecules, thus impacting cellular responses [46–48]. In the context of muscle cell adhesion, GO's surface properties are hypothesized to enhance muscle cell binding capacity, potentially through the adsorption of extracellular matrix proteins that mediate cell–material interactions. Such properties are invaluable in tissue engineering applications where promoting cell–material interactions is pivotal for the integration and functionality of the implanted material [49].

The implications of these findings are twofold. Firstly, the maintenance of hydrophilicity and bioactivity in graft materials post crosslinking is instrumental for their use in vivo, where they must interact favorably with the host environment. Secondly, the nuanced understanding of how GO modifies these properties can inform the design of future biomaterials that leverage these interactions to enhance cell adhesion and proliferation, leading to improved outcomes in tissue engineering and regenerative medicine.

As the GO concentration within a polymer matrix increases, our findings reveal that ultimate stress tends to decrease, whereas stiffness, a critical factor for robust biomaterials, augments. Such an increase in stiffness was observed in the PCL-GT-GO 2% sample, which boasted a stiffness value of 240.75 MPa, closely resembling the mechanical characteristics of native ligamentous tissue. This underscores the potential of GO-reinforced polymers in tissue engineering, particularly for applications demanding high-strength materials such as ligament scaffolds for AAFD. The improved mechanical properties, including the modulus of elasticity and the ultimate stress at break observed in the PCL-GT-GO 1% graft, indicate a 112% enhancement over the PCL-GT sample alone [50]. This substantial improvement is largely attributed to the homogeneous dispersion of GO within the fibers, which is a critical aspect in the reinforcement of polymers [51]. Furthermore, the twisting process applied to the fibers plays an integral role in achieving the desired stiffness properties, making the developed graft a viable temporary reinforcement solution as well as a scaffold for tissue regeneration.

The development of biocompatible grafts, particularly for integration with human tissues, is complex and requires balancing mechanical attributes with biological compatibility. The current study's findings indicate that incorporating GO into electrospun grafts substantially affects these aspects, promoting an environment suitable for tissue regeneration. For hemocompatibility assessment, the PCL-GT-GO 1.5% grafts showed significantly reduced hemolytic behavior compared to PCL-GT, aligning with the standards of ASTM F 756-00. This reduction in hemolysis is crucial as the rupture of erythrocytes and the resulting release of hemoglobin can have adverse clinical effects. The role of GO in reducing hemolytic activity has been affirmed by its success in various biomedical applications, as highlighted in a study on graphene oxide-polymer aerogels for their hemostatic potential [52]. Additionally, blood-compatible properties of GO have been demonstrated in a superhydrophobic graphene/titanium dioxide coating study, emphasizing its non-cytotoxicity and compatibility with blood-contacting applications [53].

In terms of platelet aggregation, the medium aggregation profile of our grafts is of particular importance, as this is crucial for healing. GO's introduction did not significantly alter the aggregation behavior, ensuring that the grafts support chemotactic gradients essential for the migration and differentiation of stem cells. Such aggregation is optimal for stem cell migration and differentiation, as it helps in tissue regeneration—a vital aspect emphasized by the work on graphene oxide's impact on anticoagulation and the hemolytic properties of human blood [54].

The L929 P + 13 mouse fibroblast cell line was utilized for cytotoxic assays due to fibroblasts being the main cellular component of dense connective tissues [55]. Cell viability above 80% across all grafts after 48 h indicates the favorable interaction of cells with the material, a result that aligns with other studies which discuss graphene-based materials as keys for successful application in blood-contacting devices [38]. The selection of a 48 h timeframe for cell viability assessment follows ISO 10993-5 guidelines and captures the critical initial period of cell–material interaction. During this period, cells are particularly susceptible to any cytotoxic effects from material degradation products or leachable components [56]. The maintained cell viability above 80% throughout this period, coupled with our material stability data from thermal and mechanical analyses, suggests favorable long-term biocompatibility prospects. While extended in vitro and subsequent in vivo studies would provide additional insights into sustained biocompatibility, our current results establish a strong foundation for the material's biological safety. This is particularly relevant given that the initial 48 h represent a crucial window for cell survival and attachment, which are prerequisites for successful long-term tissue integration.

Regarding the long-term biological implications of GO in our composite, several factors contribute to its expected safety profile. The GO in our system is firmly integrated within the PCL-GT polymer matrix, rather than existing as free nanoparticles, which significantly reduces potential systemic distribution. Recent studies have shown that matrix-bound GO primarily remains localized at the implantation site, with minimal risk of particle dissemination [38]. Furthermore, the gradual degradation of PCL allows for controlled exposure of GO components, while the presence of cellular machinery capable of biodegrading graphene-based materials through peroxidase-mediated mechanisms has been documented [49]. The concentration of GO used in our system (maximum 2.0%) is well within the range demonstrated to be safe in long-term implantation studies. Additionally, our biocompatibility results showing negligible hemolytic activity and sustained cell viability support the material's biological safety. Nevertheless, we acknowledge that comprehensive long-term in vivo studies would provide valuable additional information about the material's degradation patterns and potential systemic effects.

Overall, the addition of GO contributes not only to the mechanical robustness of the grafts but also enhances their biological performance [57]. The ability of GO to maintain hydrophilicity post chemical crosslinking is a notable finding, reinforcing the idea that GO can facilitate biomolecule retention and cell-binding capacity—this adaptability of GO is instrumental in encouraging favorable cellular behavior. The potential for GO-enhanced electrospun grafts in clinical applications for ligament repair and tissue engineering has been further validated through in vivo studies on the toxicity and blood compatibility of GO nanoparticles [57].

The morphological intricacies of electrospun grafts are pivotal for their biological and mechanical performance. Our analysis revealed stable, defect-minimized nanofibers that effectively mimic the dimensions of natural connective tissue fibrils. A notable reduction in nanofiber diameter was observed with increasing GO concentrations. This reduction aligns with findings on the effects of graphene oxide on electrical conductivity and attraction forces during electrospinning, which are essential for creating biomimetic structures [58].

However, disparities in fiber size within the PCL-GT-GO 2.0% sample suggest a non-uniform dispersion of GO, a phenomenon that has been investigated for its impact on the uniformity of nanofiber properties [59]. The implications of this non-uniformity are significant, as uniform dispersion is crucial for achieving consistent performance, especially in biomedical applications where scaffold architecture can affect cell adhesion and growth.

The optimal nanofiber diameter for wound dressing materials, as highlighted by [60], emphasizes the importance of these findings. Moreover, the challenge of achieving a balanced fiber morphology is discussed by [61], who demonstrate the complex relationship between electrospinning parameters and the resultant nanofiber structure.

The mechanical behavior of foot structures under stress, particularly the plantar fascia (PF), is crucial for understanding foot dynamics and pathologies. The PF's role as a primary passive stabilizer of the plantar arch makes it a focal point in biomechanical studies and simulations. In this context, our study's computational model, as illustrated in Figure 7, quantified the tensile stress in the PF, revealing a baseline stress of 60.28 MPa against a pathological model. This metric is in line with observations from previous studies, such as those conducted by McDonald et al. (2016), where the significance of PF stress in running mechanics was investigated, indicating similar baselines for healthy tissue [62].

The diseased state, characterized by a compromised spring ligament, showed an excess stress of 19% (11.61 MPa) transferred to the PF, highlighting the ligament's integral support role. This corroborates the findings presented by Pontious et al. (1996), which emphasized the critical stabilizing function of the spring ligament and its influence on adjacent structures [63]. Incorporating the proposed graft in our model resulted in an 11% reduction in excess stress on the PF, thereby validating the graft's mechanical effectiveness. This mirrors the biomechanical implications discussed in research presented by Gu et al. (2013), where the role of the PF in distributing plantar stress was explored, reinforcing the benefits of targeted interventions [64].

Lateral deformation assessments provided insights into the foot's pronation and abduction patterns. In healthy models, the left lateral displacement (*Min) at the talus-navicular joint depicted the pronatory movements of the hindfoot. Displacement shifts in diseased models toward the medial region highlighted the altered biomechanical lever arm, reflecting findings by Beltran (2022), which discussed the implications of medial shifts on foot stability [8,65]. Maximum right lateral displacements (**Max) observed in distal phalanges indicated abduction motions. The grafted model's correction of this displacement by 112% indicated a restorative effect, closely aligning with simulations performed by McDonald et al. (2016), demonstrating the corrective capabilities of biomechanical interventions on foot deformation. Collectively, these results not only showcase the mechanical resilience of the graft in simulating healthy foot mechanics but also its potential as a clinically viable option for AAFD management in its early stages. Such potential is corroborated by recent advancements in biomaterials and tissue engineering that emphasize the importance of mimicking natural biomechanics in synthetic grafts, as discussed previously [15,62].

While our mechanical characterization focused primarily on tensile properties, which represent the predominant physiological loads experienced by the spring ligament, we acknowledge that fatigue and creep behavior are also relevant for long-term ligament applications. The recent literature on graphene oxide-reinforced composites suggests that materials demonstrating enhanced tensile properties, particularly those achieving native tissue-like elastic moduli, typically exhibit favorable fatigue resistance and creep behavior [50,51]. The achievement of a Young's modulus of 240.75 MPa in our PCL-GT-GO 2.0% formulation, matching native ligament tissue properties, suggests promising mechanical durability. This is further supported by our computational modeling results, which demonstrate the graft's ability to withstand physiological loads while maintaining structural integrity.

As shown in Table 3, our developed PCL-GT-GO graft offers several advantages compared to current clinical solutions for AAFD treatment. While traditional tendon transfers provide excellent biocompatibility, they are limited by donor site morbidity and availability. Synthetic grafts, though offering high initial strength, often lack optimal biological integration. Allografts present immunological concerns and availability limitations. Our PCL-GT-GO graft addresses these limitations by providing mechanical properties matching native tissue (240.75 MPa), excellent biocompatibility (>80% cell viability), and controlled degradation properties, without the constraints of donor site morbidity or tissue availability.

Furthermore, the customizable nature of our graft's properties through GO concentration adjustment offers potential advantages for patient-specific treatment approaches.

**Table 3.** Comparison of current clinical solutions with the developed PCL-GT-GO graft for AAFD treatment.

| Treatment Approach | Mechanical Properties | Biological Response | Clinical Considerations |
|---|---|---|---|
| Tendon Transfer [1] | Native tissue properties (150–300 MPa) | Excellent biocompatibility | Risk of donor site morbidity; Limited availability |
| Synthetic Grafts (e.g., LARS) [51] | High initial strength (>400 MPa) | Limited cell adhesion; Risk of foreign body response | No donor site morbidity; Risk of long-term failure |
| Allograft [13] | Similar to native tissue (150–250 MPa) | Good integration; Risk of immune response | Limited availability; Cost considerations |
| PCL-GT-GO Graft (Current Study) | 240.75 MPa | >80% cell viability; Non-hemolytic; Controlled degradation | No donor site morbidity; Customizable properties |

The degradation profile of our composite graft is expected to be advantageous for ligament tissue engineering applications. PCL, our primary polymer component, exhibits a degradation timeline of 18–24 months through hydrolytic degradation of ester linkages [16], which aligns well with typical ligament healing and remodeling timeframes. The incorporation of GO has been shown to modulate polymer degradation rates, with studies indicating that GO can enhance the hydrolytic stability of polymer matrices while maintaining biocompatibility [49]. Additionally, the presence of gelatin in our composite introduces enzymatically degradable components, potentially creating a more biomimetic degradation profile. This combination of materials is designed to provide sustained mechanical support during the critical healing period while allowing for gradual tissue ingrowth and matrix remodeling. While specific degradation studies would provide valuable additional information, the established degradation characteristics of our constituent materials suggest a favorable profile for ligament tissue engineering applications.

One of the limitations of this study is that we did not include experimental data about the presence of GO as raw material once in the electrospun material. However, we have provided comprehensive characterization of GO integration through complementary analytical techniques, building upon our established expertise in GO characterization as demonstrated in our previous works [20,66]. It is important to acknowledge that while our study provides comprehensive in vitro characterization and computational modeling of the graft's performance, future in vivo investigations would offer valuable additional insights into its behavior in a physiological environment. Our current approach combining in vitro testing and computational modeling represents an essential first step in the development pipeline, aligning with established protocols in biomaterial development. The robust mechanical, biocompatibility, and simulation data presented here establish a strong foundation for subsequent in vivo studies, which could further validate the graft's potential for clinical applications. The promising results from our hemolysis, platelet aggregation, and cell viability assays, coupled with the favorable mechanical properties and computational predictions, suggest that the graft warrants further investigation in physiological conditions.

## 5. Conclusions

Our study presents a novel GO integrated polymeric graft, revealing quantitatively superior mechanical and biological properties compared to traditional PCL-GT scaffolds. The PCL-GT-GO 2% formulation exhibited a significant stiffness value of 240.75 MPa, mirroring the mechanical robustness of native spring ligaments and suggesting potential applicability in reinforcing larger ligaments, such as the ACL, which are subject to substantial mechanical loads. For ligaments bearing less mechanical stress, like those in grade I or II injuries, our grafts not only provide temporary structural support but also show promising results as scaffolds for cellular growth and tissue regeneration. The biocompatibility of these grafts is underscored by negligible hemolytic activity (hemolysis < 2%) and favorable platelet aggregation, which are critical for facilitating the natural healing process through chemotactic signaling and cellular migration. Furthermore, the grafts maintained high cell viability, with more than 80% of cells remaining viable after 48 h in an MTT assay. This is largely attributed to the hydrophilic nature of the natural polymer GT in the graft composition, which significantly enhances cell adhesion—a finding confirmed by wettability measurements, where the PCL-GT-OG 2% formulation demonstrated a contact angle conducive to cellular interaction (31.1°). Biomechanical simulations provided quantitative evidence of the grafts' efficacy in situ. Within the mechanically demanding environment of the medial longitudinal arch, the PCL-GT-OG 2% graft commendably mimicked the biomechanical behavior of native structures, with only an 11% deviation in talus displacement compared to the healthy model.

In the larger context of ligament repair and tissue engineering, our findings suggest that PCL-GT-GO grafts have a strong potential as both temporary reinforcement for acute ligament injuries and as a scaffold for sustained tissue regeneration. Their mechanical resilience combined with exceptional biocompatibility and favorable cell interaction characteristics could herald a new era in the treatment of ligament-related pathologies. Our study advocates for further research to explore the full potential of these advanced biomaterial grafts across a spectrum of biomechanical applications. This work provides a compelling proof-of-concept that could pave the way for the development of next-generation ligament repair strategies, potentially improving outcomes for patients worldwide.

**Author Contributions:** Conceptualization, S.N., C.C.-D.l.P. and J.C.C.; methodology, S.N., M.G.-D., Y.M. and M.A.H.; software, S.N.; validation, S.N., M.G.-D. and M.A.H.; formal analysis, S.N. and M.G.-D.; investigation, S.N., M.G.-D., Y.M. and M.A.H.; resources, C.C.-D.l.P., Y.M. and J.C.C.; data curation, S.N., Y.M. and M.G.-D.; writing—original draft preparation, S.N. and M.G.-D.; writing—review and editing, S.N., M.G.-D., C.C.-D.l.P. and J.C.C.; visualization, S.N. and M.G.-D.; supervision, C.C.-D.l.P. and J.C.C.; project administration, C.C.-D.l.P. and J.C.C.; funding acquisition, C.C.-D.l.P. and J.C.C. All authors have read and agreed to the published version of the manuscript.

**Funding:** This work was supported by the funding for assistant professors of the Engineering school at Universidad de Los Andes (FAPA: PR.3.2020.7427) and by the graduate teaching assistant funds from the Biomedical Engineering Department of the same University.

**Institutional Review Board Statement:** Not applicable.

**Informed Consent Statement:** Not applicable.

**Data Availability Statement:** The original contributions presented in the study are included in the article, further inquiries can be directed to the corresponding authors.

**Acknowledgments:** All authors acknowledge financial provided by the Vice Presidency for Research & Creation publication fund at the Universidad de los Andes and the members of the Dinámica Cardiovascular group of the Universidad Pontificia Bolivariana that providing us access to their electrospinning instrument.

**Conflicts of Interest:** The authors declare that the research was conducted without any commercial or financial relationships that could be construed as a potential conflict of interest.

## References

1. Flores, D.V.; Gómez, C.M.; Hernando, M.F.; Davis, M.A.; Pathria, M.N. Adult Acquired Flatfoot Deformity: Anatomy, Biomechanics, Staging, and Imaging Findings. *RadioGraphics* **2019**, 39, 1437–1460. [CrossRef] [PubMed]
2. Yang, M.; Gao, X.; Shen, Z.; Shi, X.; Lin, Z. Gelatin-assisted conglutination of aligned polycaprolactone nanofilms into a multilayered fibre-guiding scaffold for periodontal ligament regeneration. *RSC Adv.* **2019**, 9, 507–518. [CrossRef] [PubMed]
3. Abousayed, M.M.; Alley, M.C.; Shakked, R.; Rosenbaum, A.J. Adult-Acquired Flatfoot Deformity. *JBJS Rev.* **2017**, 5, e7. [CrossRef] [PubMed]
4. Orr, J.D.; Nunley, J.A. Isolated Spring Ligament Failure as a Cause of Adult-Acquired Flatfoot Deformity. *Foot Ankle Int.* **2013**, 34, 818–823. [CrossRef]

5. Balen, P.F.; Helms, C.A. Association of Posterior Tibial Tendon Injury with Spring Ligament Injury, Sinus Tarsi Abnormality, and Plantar Fasciitis on MR Imaging. *Am. J. Roentgenol.* **2001**, *176*, 1137–1143. [CrossRef]
6. Tryfonidis, M.; Jackson, W.; Mansour, R.; Cooke, P.H.; Teh, J.; Ostlere, S.; Sharp, R.J. Acquired adult flat foot due to isolated plantar calcaneonavicular (spring) ligament insufficiency with a normal tibialis posterior tendon. *Foot Ankle Surg.* **2008**, *14*, 89–95. [CrossRef]
7. Deland, J.T.; Asla, R.J.; Sung, I.H.; Ernberg, L.A.; Potter, H.G. Posterior Tibial Tendon Insufficiency: Which Ligaments are Involved? *Foot Ankle Int.* **2005**, *26*, 427–435. [CrossRef]
8. Corentin, P.; Palierne, S.; Mathon, D.; Lintz, F.; Ancelin, D. Which tendon graft to choose for anatomical ligament reconstruction in chronic lateral ankle instability? A biomechanical study. *Orthop. Traumatol. Surg. Res.* **2024**, 104017. [CrossRef]
9. Hintermann, B.; Ruiz, R. Balancing and Stabilizing the Ankle. In *Total Ankle Replacement: A Practical Guide to Surgical Management*; Springer International Publishing: Cham, Switzerland, 2024; pp. 105–153.
10. Steginsky, B.; Vora, A. What to Do with the Spring Ligament. *Foot Ankle Clin.* **2017**, *22*, 515–527. [CrossRef]
11. Cifuentes-De la Portilla, C.; Larrainzar-Garijo, R.; Bayod, J. Analysis of biomechanical stresses caused by hindfoot joint arthrodesis in the treatment of adult acquired flatfoot deformity: A finite element study. *Foot Ankle Surg.* **2020**, *26*, 412–420. [CrossRef]
12. Silva, M.; Ferreira, F.N.; Alves, N.M.; Paiva, M.C. Biodegradable polymer nanocomposites for ligament/tendon tissue engineering. *J. Nanobiotechnol.* **2020**, *18*, 23. [CrossRef] [PubMed]
13. Brennan, D.A.; Conte, A.A.; Kanski, G.; Turkula, S.; Hu, X.; Kleiner, M.T.; Beachley, V. Mechanical Considerations for Electrospun Nanofibers in Tendon and Ligament Repair. *Adv. Healthc. Mater.* **2018**, *7*, 1701277. [CrossRef] [PubMed]
14. Pauly, H.M.; Kelly, D.J.; Popat, K.C.; Trujillo, N.A.; Dunne, N.J.; McCarthy, H.O.; Donahue, T.L. Mechanical properties and cellular response of novel electrospun nanofibers for ligament tissue engineering: Effects of orientation and geometry. *J. Mech. Behav. Biomed. Mater.* **2016**, *61*, 258–270. [CrossRef] [PubMed]
15. Kelly, M.; Dean, D.; Hussaini, S.; Neufeld, S.; Cuttica, D. Safety profile of synthetic elastic degradable matrix for soft tissue reconstruction in foot & ankle surgery. *Foot Ankle Spec.* **2024**, *17*, 201–207. [PubMed]
16. Saatcioglu, E.; Ulag, S.; Sahin, A.; Yilmaz, B.K.; Ekren, N.; Inan, A.T.; Palaci, Y.; Ustundag, C.B.; Gunduz, O. Design and fabrication of electrospun polycaprolactone/chitosan scaffolds for ligament regeneration. *Eur. Polym. J.* **2021**, *148*, 110357. [CrossRef]
17. Ramakrishna, S.; Fujihara, K.; Teo, W.E.; Lim, T.C.; Ma, Z. *An Introduction to Electrospinning and Nanofibers*; World Scientific: Singapore, 2005.
18. Olvera, D.; Schipani, R.; Sathy, B.N.; Kelly, D.J. Electrospinning of highly porous yet mechanically functional microfibrillar scaffolds at the human scale for ligament and tendon tissue engineering. *Biomed. Mater.* **2019**, *14*, 035016. [CrossRef]
19. Kausar, A. Polymeric nanocomposite via electrospinning: Assessment of morphology, physical properties and applications. *J. Plast. Film Sheet.* **2020**, *37*, 70–92. [CrossRef]
20. Céspedes-Valenzuela, D.N.; Sánchez-Rentería, S.; Cifuentes, J.; Gantiva-Diaz, M.; Serna, J.A.; Reyes, L.H.; Ostos, C.; Cifuentes-De la Portilla, C.; Muñoz-Camargo, C.; Cruz, J.C. Preparation and Characterization of an Injectable and Photo-Responsive Chitosan Methacrylate/Graphene Oxide Hydrogel: Potential Applications in Bone Tissue Adhesion and Repair. *Polymers* **2021**, *14*, 126. [CrossRef]
21. Aldana, A.A.; Abraham, G.A. Current advances in electrospun gelatin-based scaffolds for tissue engineering applications. *Int. J. Pharm.* **2017**, *523*, 441–453. [CrossRef]
22. Marcano, D.C.; Kosynkin, D.V.; Berlin, J.M.; Sinitskii, A.; Sun, Z.; Slesarev, A.; Alemany, L.B.; Lu, W.; Tour, J.M. Improved Synthesis of Graphene Oxide. *ACS Nano* **2010**, *4*, 4806–4814. [CrossRef]
23. Feng, B.; Tu, H.; Yuan, H.; Peng, H.; Zhang, Y. Acetic-Acid-Mediated Miscibility toward Electrospinning Homogeneous Composite Nanofibers of GT/PCL. *Biomacromolecules* **2012**, *13*, 3917–3925. [CrossRef] [PubMed]
24. Campiglio, C.E.; Negrini, N.C.; Fare, S.; Draghi, L. Cross-Linking Strategies for Electrospun Gelatin Scaffolds. *Materials* **2019**, *12*, 2476. [CrossRef] [PubMed]
25. *ISO 10993-4*; Biological Evaluation of Medical Devices. Part 4—Selection of Tests for Interactions with Blood. International Organization for Standardization: Geneva, Switzerland, 2017.
26. *ASTM F756-00*; Standard Practice for Assessment of Hemolytic Properties of Materials. American Society for Testing and Materials: Philadelphia, PA, USA, 2000.
27. *ISO 10993-5:2009*; Biological Evaluation of Medical Devices. Part 5: Tests for In Vitro Cytotoxicity. International Organization for Standardization: Geneva, Switzerland, 2009.
28. Cifuentes-De la Portilla, C.; Larrainzar-Garijo, R.; Bayod, J. Biomechanical stress analysis of the main soft tissues associated with the development of adult acquired flatfoot deformity. *Clin. Biomech.* **2019**, *61*, 163–171. [CrossRef] [PubMed]
29. Chang, T.J. *The Foot and Ankle*; Lippincott Williams & Wilkins: Philadelphia, PA, USA, 2005.
30. Burkhart, T.A.; Andrews, D.M.; Dunning, C.E. Finite element modeling mesh quality, energy balance and validation methods: A review with recommendations associated with the modeling of bone tissue. *J. Biomech.* **2013**, *46*, 1477–1488. [CrossRef]
31. Siegler, S.; Block, J.; Schneck, C.D. The Mechanical Characteristics of the Collateral Ligaments of the Human Ankle Joint. *Foot Ankle* **1988**, *8*, 234–242. [CrossRef]
32. Azizi, M.; Azimzadeh, M.; Afzali, M.; Alafzadeh, M.; Mirhosseini, S.H. Characterization and optimization of using calendula offlcinalis extract in fabrication of polycaprolactone-gelatin electrospun nanofibers for wound dressing applications. *J. Adv. Mater. Process.* **2018**, *6*, 34–46.

33. Sudesh; Kumar, N.; Das, S.; Bernhard, C.; Varma, G.D. Effect of graphene oxide doping on superconducting properties of bulk $MgB_2$. *Supercond. Sci. Technol.* **2013**, *26*, 095008. [CrossRef]
34. Ickecan, D.; Zan, R.; Nezir, S. Eco-Friendly Synthesis and Characterization of Reduced Graphene Oxide. *J. Phys. Conf. Ser.* **2017**, *902*, 012027. [CrossRef]
35. Longo, R.; Catauro, M.; Sorrentino, A.; Guadagno, L. Thermal and mechanical characterization of complex electrospun systems based on polycaprolactone and gelatin. *J. Therm. Anal. Calorim.* **2022**, *147*, 5391–5399. [CrossRef]
36. Najafi, F.; Rajabi, M. Thermal gravity analysis for the study of stability of graphene oxide–glycine nanocomposites. *Int. Nano Lett.* **2015**, *5*, 187–190. [CrossRef]
37. Coimbra, P.; Santos, P.; Alves, P.; Miguel, S.P.; Carvalho, M.P.; Sa, K.D.; Correia, I.J.; Ferreira, P. Coaxial electrospun PCL/Gelatin-MA fibers as scaffolds for vascular tissue engineering. *Colloids Surf. B Biointerfaces* **2017**, *159*, 7–15. [CrossRef] [PubMed]
38. Pereira, A.T.; Henriques, P.C.; Schneider, K.H.; Pires, A.L.; Pereira, A.M.; Martins, M.C.L.; Magalhães, F.D.; Bergmeister, H.; Gonçalves, I.C. Graphene-based materials: The key for the successful application of pHEMA as a blood-contacting device. *Biomater. Sci.* **2021**, *9*, 3362–3377. [CrossRef] [PubMed]
39. Jull, G.; Moore, A.; Falla, D.; Lewis, J.; McCarthy, C.; Sterling, M. *Grieve's Modern Musculoskeletal Physiotherapy*; Elsevier Health Sciences: Amsterdam, The Netherlands, 2015.
40. Aboamera, N.M.; Mohamed, A.; Salama, A.; Osman, T.A.; Khattab, A. Characterization and mechanical properties of electrospun cellulose acetate/graphene oxide composite nanofibers. *Mech. Adv. Mater. Struct.* **2017**, *26*, 765–769. [CrossRef]
41. Razzaghi, D.; Rezaei, M.; Babaie, A. The effect of incorporating graphene and polycaprolactone-grafted graphene oxide nanosheets on thermal and physico-mechanical properties, microstructure and biocompatibility of electrospun polyurethane nanocomposite mats. *Compos. Part B Eng.* **2021**, *224*, 109210. [CrossRef]
42. Shen, C.; Liu, J.; Lu, Q.; Wang, G.; Wang, Z.; Liu, L. Pre-vascularized electrospun graphene oxide–gelatin chamber for intestinal wall defect repair. *Int. J. Nanomed.* **2022**, *17*, 681–695. [CrossRef]
43. Ou, Y.R.; Yin, J.; Xiao, M.; Cui, H.; Huang, K.S.; Li, Y.; Ke, Y. Preparation of antibacterial PHBV/GO nanocomposite membranes via electrospinning. *Mater. Today Commun.* **2023**, *35*, 106370. [CrossRef]
44. Das, A.; Deka, J.; Rather, A.M.; Bhunia, B.K.; Saikia, P.P.; Mandal, B.B.; Raidongia, K.; Manna, U. Strategic formulation of graphene oxide sheets for flexible monoliths and robust polymeric coatings embedded with durable bioinspired wettability. *ACS Appl. Mater. Interfaces* **2017**, *9*, 42354–42365. [CrossRef]
45. Golda-Cepa, M.; Kumar, D.; Bialoruski, M.; Lasota, S.; Madeja, Z.; Piskorz, W.; Kotarba, A. Functionalization of graphenic surfaces by oxygen plasma toward enhanced wettability and cell adhesion: Experiments corroborated by molecular modelling. *J. Mater. Chem. B* **2023**, *11*, 4946–4957. [CrossRef]
46. Laurenti, M.; Lamberti, A.; Genchi, G.G.; Roppolo, I.; Canavese, G.; Vitale-Brovarone, C.; Ciofani, G.; Cauda, V. Graphene oxide finely tunes the bioactivity and drug delivery of mesoporous ZnO scaffolds. *ACS Appl. Mater. Interfaces* **2018**, *11*, 449–456. [CrossRef]
47. Son, J.; Lee, J.Y.; Han, N.; Cha, J.; Choi, J.; Kwon, J.; Nam, S.; Yoo, K.H.; Lee, G.H.; Hong, J. Tunable wettability of graphene through nondestructive hydrogenation and wettability-based patterning for bioapplications. *Nano Lett.* **2020**, *20*, 5625–5631. [CrossRef]
48. Sun, L.; Bian, F.; Wang, Y.; Wang, Y.; Zhang, X.; Zhao, Y. Bioinspired programmable wettability arrays for droplets manipulation. *Proc. Natl. Acad. Sci. USA* **2020**, *117*, 4527–4532. [CrossRef] [PubMed]
49. Rostami, F.; Tamjid, E.; Behmanesh, M. Drug-eluting PCL/graphene oxide nanocomposite scaffolds for enhanced osteogenic differentiation of mesenchymal stem cells. *Mater. Sci. Eng. C* **2020**, *115*, 111102. [CrossRef] [PubMed]
50. Kesarwani, S.; Verma, R.K.; Jayswal, S.C.; Khare, P. Investigation of physiochemical and mechanical properties of reduced graphene oxide (rGO) modified carbon fiber polymer composites. *J. Text. Inst.* **2024**, *115*, 188–200. [CrossRef]
51. Lodhi, R.S.; Kumar, P.; Achuthanunni, A.; Rahaman, M.; Das, P. Mechanical properties of polymer/graphene composites. In *Polymer Nanocomposites Containing Graphene*; Elsevier: Amsterdam, The Netherlands, 2022; pp. 75–105.
52. Borges-Vilches, J.; Figueroa, T.; Guajardo, S.; Carmona, S.; Mellado, C.; Melendrez, M.; Aguayo, C.; Fernández, K. Novel and effective hemostats based on graphene oxide-polymer aerogels: In vitro and in vivo evaluation. *Biomater. Adv.* **2022**, *139*, 213007. [CrossRef]
53. Wu, X.H.; Liew, Y.K.; Lim, W.M.; Mai, C.W.; Then, Y.Y. Blood compatible and noncytotoxic superhydrophobic graphene/titanium dioxide coating with antibacterial and antibiofilm properties. *J. Appl. Polym. Sci.* **2023**, *140*, e53629. [CrossRef]
54. Kamenska, T.; Abrashev, M.; Georgieva, M.; Krasteva, N. Impact of polyethylene glycol functionalization of graphene oxide on anticoagulation and haemolytic properties of human blood. *Materials* **2021**, *14*, 4853. [CrossRef]
55. Bhatia, S.K.; Yetter, A.B. Correlation of visual in vitro cytotoxicity ratings of biomaterials with quantitative in vitro cell viability measurements. *Cell Biol. Toxicol.* **2007**, *24*, 315–319. [CrossRef]
56. Sharma, A.; Luthra, G. Significance of ISO 10993 Standards in ensuring biocompatibility of medical devices: A review. *J. Pharm. Res. Int.* **2023**, *8*, 23–24. [CrossRef]
57. Imarah, A.A.; Abood, A.H.; Jabir, M.S. Toxicity and blood compatibility of graphene oxide nanoparticles: In-vivo study. *AIP Conf. Proc.* **2022**, *2398*, 040050.

58. Abdullah, Z.; Anwar, A.W.; Haq, I.U.; Arslan, Z.; Mubashar, A.; Ahmad, S.; Waheed, A.; Ajmal, M.; Baig, I.I.A. Synthesis of Graphene Oxide/Poly (Vinyl Alcohol) Composite and Investigation of Graphene Oxide Effect on Diameter and Pore Size of Poly (Vinyl Alcohol) Nanofibers. *J. Nano Res.* **2023**, *78*, 23–30. [CrossRef]
59. Sangani, N.; Eslahi, N.; Varsei, M.; Ghanbari, H. Electrospinning of cellulose acetate/graphene/nanoclay nanocomposite for textile wastewater filtration. *J. Text. Inst.* **2023**, *115*, 647–655. [CrossRef]
60. Khorshidi, S.; Mohebbali, M.; Imani, R.; Mahmoodi, M.; Solouk, A. Electrospun fibroin/graphene oxide nanocomposite mats: An optimization for potential wound dressing applications. *Fibers Polym.* **2020**, *21*, 480–488. [CrossRef]
61. Abdollahi, S.; Ehsani, M.; Morshedian, J.; Khonakdar, H.A.; Aram, E. Application of response surface methodology in assessing the effect of electrospinning parameters on the morphology of polyethylene oxide/polyacrylonitrile blend nanofibers containing graphene oxide. *Polym. Bull.* **2019**, *76*, 1755–1773. [CrossRef]
62. McDonald, K.A.; Stearne, S.M.; Alderson, J.A.; North, I.; Pires, N.J.; Rubenson, J. The role of arch compression and metatarsophalangeal joint dynamics in modulating plantar fascia strain in running. *PLoS ONE* **2016**, *11*, e0152602. [CrossRef]
63. Pontious, J.; Flanigan, K.P.; Hillstrom, H.J. Role of the plantar fascia in digital stabilization. A case report. *J. Am. Podiatr. Med. Assoc.* **1996**, *86*, 43–47. [CrossRef]
64. Gu, Y.D.; Li, Z.Y.; Shen, W.W.; Ma, J.B. Mechanical analysis of foot plantar fascia during normal walking condition. In *World Congress on Medical Physics and Biomedical Engineering May 26–31, 2012, Beijing, China*; Springer: Berlin/Heidelberg, Germany, 2013; pp. 242–244.
65. Beltran, L.S. Presurgical Perspective and Postsurgical Evaluation of the Plantar Fascia. *Semin. Musculoskelet. Radiol.* **2022**, *26*, 684–694. [CrossRef]
66. Céspedes-Valenzuela, D.; Sánchez-Rentería, S.; Cifuentes, J.; Gómez, S.; Serna, J.; Rueda-Gensini, L.; Ostos, C.; Muñoz-Camargo, C.; Cruz, J.C. Novel photo-and thermo-responsive nanocomposite hydrogels based on functionalized rGO and modified SIS/Chitosan polymers for localized treatment of malignant cutaneous melanoma. *Front. Bioeng. Biotechnol.* **2022**, *10*, 947616. [CrossRef]

Journal of
*Functional Biomaterials*

MDPI

*Article*

# Evaluation of the Degradation Properties of Plasma Electrolytically Oxidized Mg Alloy AZ31 Using Fluid Dynamic Accelerated Tests for Biodegradable Implants

**Muhammad Saqib [1,*], Kerstin Kremmer [2], Joerg Opitz [1], Michael Schneider [2] and Natalia Beshchasna [1,*]**

1 Department of Bio and Nanotechnology, Fraunhofer Institute for Ceramic Technologies and Systems IKTS, Maria-Reiche-Strasse 2, 01109 Dresden, Germany; joerg.opitz@ikts.fraunhofer.de

2 Department of Electrochemistry, Fraunhofer Institute for Ceramic Technologies and Systems IKTS, Winterbergstrasse 28, 01277 Dresden, Germany; kerstin.kremmer@ikts.fraunhofer.de (K.K.); michael.schneider@ikts.fraunhofer.de (M.S.)

* Correspondence: muhammad.saqib@ikts.fraunhofer.de (M.S.); natalia.beshchasna@ikts.fraunhofer.de (N.B.)

**Abstract:** Magnesium alloys are promising biodegradable implant materials due to their excellent biocompatibility and non-toxicity. However, their poor corrosion resistance limits their application in vivo. Plasma electrolytic oxidation (PEO) is a powerful technique to improve the corrosion resistance of magnesium alloys. In this study, we present the accelerated degradation of PEO-treated AZ31 samples using a fluid dynamic test. The samples were prepared using different concentrations of KOH as an electrolyte along with $NaSiO_3$. The anodizing time and the biasing time were optimized to obtain the increased corrosion resistance. The analysis of the degraded samples using microscopy, SEM EDX measurements, and by calculating mass loss and corrosion rates showed a significant increase in the corrosion resistance after the polymer (Resomer© LG 855 S) coating was applied to the anodized samples. The results confirm (or convince) that PEO treatment is an effective way to improve the corrosion resistance of AZ31 magnesium alloy. The fluid dynamic test can be used as an accelerated degradation test for biodegradable alloys in simulated body fluids at a physiological temperature. The polymer coating further improves the corrosion resistance of the PEO-treated AZ31 samples.

**Keywords:** plasma electrolytic oxidation; biodegradable implant; corrosion; accelerated degradation test; fluid dynamic test; resomer; Mg alloy

## 1. Introduction

We are living in the age of the scientific revolution, where most body parts can be replaced or supported by implants. According to the patient's medical condition, a permanent or a temporary implant can be used. In recent decades, biodegradable implants have attracted more attention from researchers due to the issues associated with permanent metallic implants (e.g., thrombosis, physical irritation, restenosis, etc.) and also their inability to adapt to the growth of and changes in the human body [1–3].

Recently, as biodegradable materials for implantation, magnesium and its alloys have gained popularity because of their improved biocompatibility and virtually no toxicity [4–11]. Notably, among all the magnesium alloys, researchers were particularly interested in AZ31, AZ91D, Mg–Li–Ca, and WE43, and efforts have been made to employ these as bio-absorbable stents [12] and orthopedic implants [13].

Because of its lower aluminum content, improved microstructure, low fatigue, and corrosion resistance comparable to other magnesium alloys, AZ31 has received more attention [7,11,14–17]. In vivo experiments reveal that magnesium alloys have low corrosion resistance, despite their promising material features [12]. Due to their inability to adequately support the blood vessel wall, magnesium alloys are therefore not suitable for use as biodegradable stent materials. In order to improve the corrosion properties of existing magnesium alloys, it is crucial to alter their surface properties.

Various surface modification techniques have been applied to control the corrosion of Mg alloys, e.g., chemical conversion coating, physical vapor deposition, laser surface treatment, and anodic oxidation, to name a few [1].

A very powerful technique to improve the corrosion behavior of magnesium and its alloys is plasma electrolytic oxidation [18]. The process is also known under various labels, e.g., micro arc oxidation (MAO) or anodic oxidation by spark discharge (ANOF) [19]. The process is related to conventional anodizing, but the operating voltage is significantly above the breakdown potential of the passive anodic oxide layer [20]. The high operating voltage briefly ionizes the oxygen gas that is simultaneously formed at the anode. The recombination of the same appears as micro-sparks that are randomly distributed over the anode surface. The energy released in this process leads to the growth of the anodic layer, which partly consists of the crystalline high-temperature modification of magnesium oxide. Štrbák et al. reported the clearly improved corrosion stability of plasma electrolytic anodized AZ91 in chloride solution [21].

The targeted variation in the process parameters, e.g., time, voltage, and electrolytes, allows for tuning of the resulting oxide layer and its properties.

To evaluate the degradation properties of the biodegradable materials, several in vitro tests are performed (e.g., static immersion test, fluid dynamic test, and the electrochemical corrosion test) before any in vivo tests. Each in vitro test has its pros and cons and provides the different corrosion rates of the same sample. This is because of the presence and absence of influencing factors (e.g., fluid flow, electric potential, etc.) in each method. For instance, Xue et al. 2012 [22] reported that the corrosion rate of AZ31 is about five times higher for the in vitro static immersion environment than the in vivo environment. Furthermore, the corrosion rate was two times higher in PBS, whereas it was 5 times higher when they used SBF.

Koo et al., 2017 [23] compared the corrosion rates of biodegradable magnesium pins (as-drawn pure Mg, as-cast Mg-Zn-Mn, and extruded Mg-Zn-Mn) in static and dynamic conditions. They reported a corrosion rate of $1.915 \pm 0.062$ mm/year in the fluid dynamic conditions at 1.5 mL/min (1.6 mm/s), whereas the CR was $0.236 \pm 0.022$ mm/year in the static test for pure Mg. This shows the 8.1 times greater corrosion rate in the given dynamic conditions. Similarly, for as-cast Mg-Zn-Mn, the corrosion rate was $2.251 \pm 0.288$ mm/year and $0.527 \pm 0.118$mm/year in dynamic and static conditions, respectively, and for extruded Mg-Zn-Mn, the corrosion rates of $2.113 \pm 0.139$ mm/year and $0.188 \pm 0.068$ mm/year in dynamic and static conditions, respectively. The aforementioned results by Koo et al. 2017 showed the 4.3 times and 11.2 times increment in the corrosion rates of As-cast and extruded Mg-Zn-Mn, respectively, in dynamic conditions as compared to the static immersion tests. Therefore, using fluid dynamic conditions, the corrosion rates of Mg alloys can be accelerated further. Thus, this is a suitable choice for accelerated degradation tests of biodegradable alloys in the simulated body fluids at physiological temperature.

In this work, we present the accelerated degradation of the PEO-treated AZ31 samples using the fluid dynamic test. The samples were prepared using two different concentrations of KOH as an electrolyte along with $NaSiO_3$. In order to achieve greater corrosion resistance, the anodizing and biasing times were also adjusted. The anodized surfaces were impregnated with Resomer©, a polymer known for its controlled degradation and non-toxic properties, offering advantages over other polymers such as PLA and PCL. The analysis of the degraded samples using microscopy and SEM-EDX measurements and by calculating mass loss and corrosion rates showed a significant increase in corrosion resistance after the polymer (resomer) coating was applied to the anodized samples.

## 2. Materials and Methods

### 2.1. Sample Preparation

The magnesium alloy AZ31 was used in this investigation. Its nominal chemical composition is shown in Table 1. The sheets were degreased and pickled with Gardoclean® 5165 and Gardoclean® 5491 from Chemetall (Frankfurt/M., Germany). Between the degreasing and the pickling, the sheets were cleaned with deionized water. For the handling of the sheets during the PEO process, we used a specially designed sample holder.

**Table 1.** Chemical composition in Wt% according to DIN 1729-1 [24].

| Al | Zn | Mn | Si | Fe | Cu | Ni | Mg |
|---|---|---|---|---|---|---|---|
| 2.5–3.5 | 0.5–1.5 | 0.05–0.4 | ≤0.1 | ≤0.03 | ≤0.1 | ≤0.0005 | Balance |

### 2.2. Plasma Electrolytic Oxidation Process

The PEO process was carried out in a tempered glass beaker. The anodizing process was carried out in aqueous potassium hydroxide electrolytes of varying concentrations and a fixed content of sodium silicate (see Table 2). The electrolyte conductivity was measured with 33 mS $cm^{-1}$ (electrolyte A) and 50 mS $cm^{-1}$ (electrolyte B). The pH value of the electrolyte was 14. The temperature was adjusted with a cryostat and was 20 °C for all experiments. The bath temperature was monitored with a thermocouple during the process. The bath was stirred during the process. An EA PS8720-15 (Elektroautomatik, Viersen, Germany) was used as a power supply. The PEO was carried out as a current-controlled pulse regime with a linear current ramp from 0 to 20 $mA/cm^2$ for the first 10 s. Afterwards, the pulse regime worked with a pulse-on amplitude of 20 $mA/cm^2$ and a pulse-on time of 0.5 s. The pulse-off current density was 0 $mA/cm^2$ with a pulse-off time of 1 s. The total process time was 1000 s.

**Table 2.** Composition of the electrolytes.

| Electrolyte | KOH (g/L) | $Na_2SiO_3$ (g/L) |
|---|---|---|
| A | 5 | 10 |
| B | 10 | 10 |

### 2.3. Impregnation Process

For the impregnation, a dispersion was used consisting of dichloromethane and the commercial Resomer© LG 855 S (Evonik Nutrition and Care GmbH, Essen, Germany). A total of 3% of the Resomer© was dissolved in the dichloromethane. The dip-coating parameters were as follows: withdrawing rate 4 mm/s, dipping time 1 s, room temperature. Following this, the samples were dried in a furnace at 35 °C/72 h and 80 °C/2 h. For better readability and clarity, the samples were designated as follows: Sample R (reference sample, i.e., untreated AZ31 surface), Sample 1 (anodized with electrolyte A), Sample 2 (anodized with electrolyte A and impregnated with Resomer), Sample 3 (anodized with electrolyte B), and Sample 4 (anodized with electrolyte B and impregnated with Resomer).

### 2.4. Contact Angle and Surface Wettability

The term "wettability" describes a liquid's capacity to spread out or adhere to a solid surface. Surface wettability can have an impact on four key biological processes: (1) the adhesion of proteins and other macromolecules to the surface (conditioning); (2) the interactions between the cells of hard and soft tissues and the pre-conditioned surfaces; (3) bacterial adhesion and subsequent biofilm formation; and (4) the rate of osseointegration in the body (in vivo) [25]. The wettability is directly proportional to the contact angle. The Dataphysics OCA20 system, which makes use of industry-standard optical contact angle measuring and contour analysis techniques, was used to evaluate CAs. By using a syringe with a 0.52 mm diameter to dispense 1 L of distilled water, static water CAs were calculated. The stated CAs are averages based on a minimum of five readings per sample.

### 2.5. Optical Microscopy

A Zeiss Axioscope with brightfield and darkfield capabilities was used to capture microscopic images. A steady, vibration-free surface was used for the microscope, which was set up in a controlled lab setting. To make sure that the specimens were properly lit, the halogen light source of the microscope was adjusted to the required intensity and direction. To obtain consistent illumination, the Köhler illumination was adjusted. The proper objective lenses with 2.5× and 20× magnifications were applied. Images were taken using the Zeiss imaging program AxioVision Rel. 4.8.

### 2.6. SEM-EDX Measurements

The surface morphologies of the pure PEO layer and the impregnated PEO layer were investigated by scanning electron microscopy (Carl Zeiss Microscopy GmbH, Oberkochen, Germany).

The Environmental Scanning Electron Microscope XL30 ESEM FEG (Philips, Amsterdam, The Netherlands) was used to capture all SEM pictures and EDX measurements for fluid dynamic-accelerated degradation testing, unless otherwise noted. For SEM measurements, the accelerating voltage was adjusted to 3.0 kV with a spot size of 3 nm and 5.0 kV with a spot size of 5 nm. SEM pictures were taken before and after the degradation points of 1, 2, 4, 7, 14, 21, and 30 days for all samples. EDX measurements were also taken to determine the elemental makeup of the samples before and after degradation. For 3–5 min, the corroded samples were cleaned in ultrapure water in an ultrasonic water bath.

### 2.7. Electrochemical Measurements

The electrochemical measurements were carried out in two different solutions. The first was Hanks' Balanced Salt Solution (HBSS) with a pH of 7.1 and the second was 0.1 M NaOH pH 12.9. For the electrochemical measurements, a common three-electrode flat cell was used at room temperature. The electrochemical tests consisted of open circuit potential measurements (ocp) over different times (0 h, 1 h and 10 h) and, afterwards, potentiostatic measurements at a potential of −1.7 V vs. SCE for 24 h. The pH value was measured at the end of each experiment. The electrochemical measurements were carried out on two different areas of the layer surfaces.

### 2.8. Fluid Dynamic Experimental Setup for In Vitro Degradation Studies

The fluid dynamic experimental setup presented in [26,27] was modified for this research. Figure 1 depicts the modified fluid dynamic experimental test setup to simulate a physiological environment with pH control and parameter monitoring. The experimental setup consisted of: (1) a peristaltic pump (to mimic the heart's pumping action); (2) puriflex tubes (as an artificial blood vessel); (3) sensors (for pressure, temperature, flow velocity, and pH); (4) a circulating water bath (to maintain a constant temperature); (5) a fluid reservoir; (6) a solenoid valve; (7) a dilute acid container; (8) a microcontroller unit box; (9) a pH controlling unit; and (10) a computer (LabVIEW program or VI to control and monitor the parameters and display the results); and (11) a flow chamber containing the samples.

With the pH being controlled, our experimental setup can offer the physiological conditions for the parameters indicated. Since the pH is crucial in the Mg's and its alloys' degradation and it increases with the degradation time, there is a need to regulate the pH during the experiment.

In the presented testing setup, when the pH value changes, the pH control unit of the setup begins to work and adds diluted HCl (to decrease the pH) or any other buffering solution to the fluid until it reaches the setpoint, i.e., 7.4, in our case. Depending on the needs of the experiment, the amount of buffering solution can be adjusted.

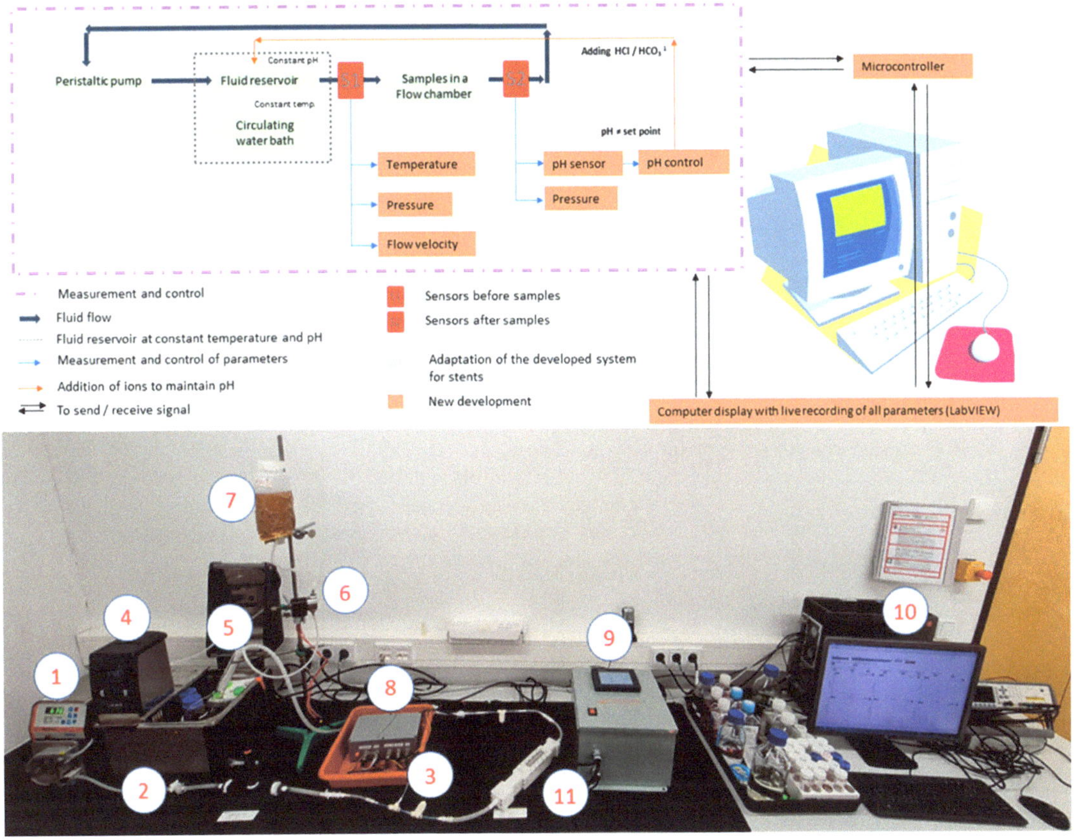


**Figure 1.** Schematic diagram of the fluid dynamic circulation setup.

### 2.9. In Vitro Fluid Dynamic Degradation Test

All samples were degraded in HBSS for 30 days utilizing a fluid dynamic system, as shown in Figure 1, with measurement time points at 1, 2, 7, 14, 21, and 30 days. The degradation of all samples was accelerated by applying a flow velocity of 20 cm/s and a shear stress of 2 dyn/cm$^2$. To ensure the samples' initial cleanliness, they were cleansed in ultrapure water in an ultrasonic bath before the initial fluid dynamic exposure to remove any dust residues. The uncoated AZ31 samples were cleaned in two steps after each exposure to the fluid. They were first cleaned for 5 min in a chromic acid solution to effectively remove the degradation products. They were then cleaned again with ultrapure water in an ultrasonic bath. However, coated samples were cleaned completely in ultrapure water to avoid potential coating degradation caused by the acidic environment of the chromic acid solution.

To ensure precise results, the materials were rigorously dried using a nitrogen flush prior to mass measurements.

## 3. Results and Discussion

### 3.1. Plasma Electrolytic Oxide Formation

Figure 2 shows the voltage-time response to the applied current controlled pulse regime of AZ31 in electrolytes A and B. The pulse time on was 0.5 s and the pulse time off was 1 s, therefore Figure 2 shows a compressed view of the pulse regime and not the single pulses. The electrode partially depolarized during the pulse time off.

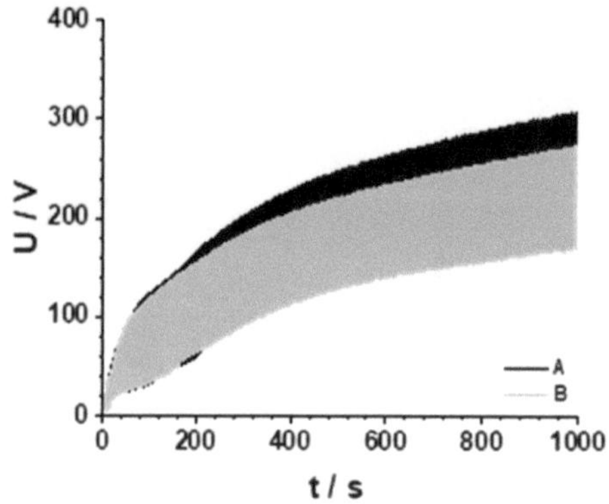


**Figure 2.** Voltage-time response during PEO for electrolytes A and B.

The necessary overvoltage for plasma electrolytic oxidation is higher in electrolyte A in comparison with electrolyte B. One reason for this could be the different voltage drop across the electrolytes due to their different conductivities. Otherwise, the voltage across the oxide is more than 95%, which means that small differences in oxide thickness must have a higher impact on overvoltages. The PEO process in electrolytes with different KOH contents was described in detail in [28].

### 3.2. Surface Morphology

The surface morphologies of PEO layers anodized in electrolyte A and B are shown in Figure 3. The layers show a ceramic-like porous surface structure due to the microdischarges during the PEO process. The pore size varies by a range of few micrometers. On the left side, the PEO layers anodized in electrolyte A show smaller pores, which are partially closed. With increasing KOH concentration, a greater number of pores are opened and the pore size increases. This fact corresponds with the results published in [28].

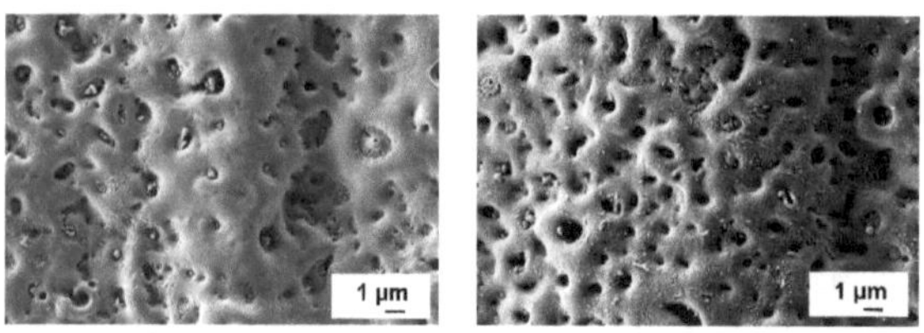


electrolyte A electrolyte B

**Figure 3.** SEM images of PEO layers produced in different electrolytes.

Figure 4 shows the surface morphology of all the samples before any degradation testing. The reference specimen (Sample R) without degradation, as expected, displayed only signs of mechanical processing even under high magnification and showed no unusual unevenness. Samples treated with PEO had larger pore size and fewer pores per unit area when KOH (rather than NaOH) was used as the electrolyte in the preparation with $NaSiO_3$. Pores can be observed in Samples 1 and 3, but not in Samples 2 and 4 due to the polymer coating over the oxide layer. Sample 3 was prepared similarly to Sample 1, with only the concentration of KOH in the anodization process differing. SEM analysis revealed a greater number of pores in Sample 3 compared to Sample 1, which is due to the lower concentration of KOH used in its preparation. It can be determined that pore size is directly proportional to KOH concentration, while the number of pores is inversely proportional to KOH concentration. Additionally, the porosity of the anodized sample is influenced not just by the type of electrolyte, but also by the quantity of the electrolyte.

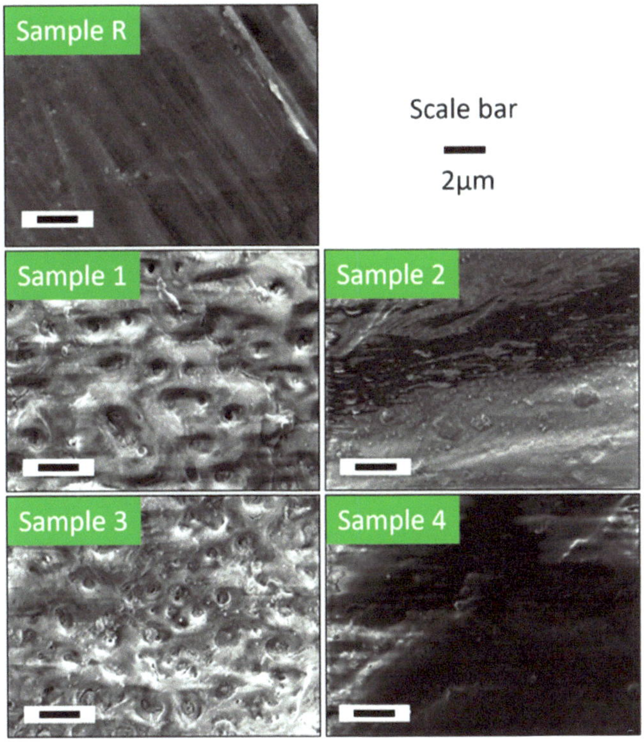


**Figure 4.** Surface morphology of all samples before degradation test.

Figure 5a shows the surface morphology of all samples after 2, 14, and 30 days in fluid dynamic circulation.

Sample R began to corrode early on and showed degradation products on the surface. The degradation products were chip-like structures that were smaller after two days of deterioration and changed to larger chips after 14 days. The degradation products covered a significant part of the sample's surface in both time intervals, but after 30 days of degradation, the regions with and without corrosion products were detected with large and deep pits.

Sample 1 showed that half of the surface was still covered with the cracked PEO layer after two days of fluid dynamic circulation, which was fully removed within the first week. The degradation was similar to that of Sample R after the removal of the oxide layer. Interestingly, white circular traces were observed due to the removal of corrosion products from the surface, which were not present in Sample R.

Sample 2 showed minimal signs of degradation after 2 days due to the polymer coating. The polymer coating was gradually being removed from the beginning, and after 14 days, about half of the polymer coating was removed and a cracked oxide layer was shown. A similar phenomenon was observed, but with less polymer coverage, after the full 30 days of degradation.

Sample 3 showed less resistance to shear stress in a fluidic environment, the coating was removed heavily within the first two days, and the corrosion products were also visible. The coating was removed completely during the first week, and degradation products similar to those appearing on Sample R appeared throughout the degradation period after that, with smaller pits as compared to Sample R.

Sample 4 showed a similar morphology, except with more damage to the polymer coating in the first two days. However, after 14 days of the degradation period, degradation products were also seen where the parts of the cracked PEO layer were removed. After the completion of 30 days, minimal traces of the polymer coating were found on the surface of Sample 4, with the presence of both the PEO layer and corrosion products.

(a)

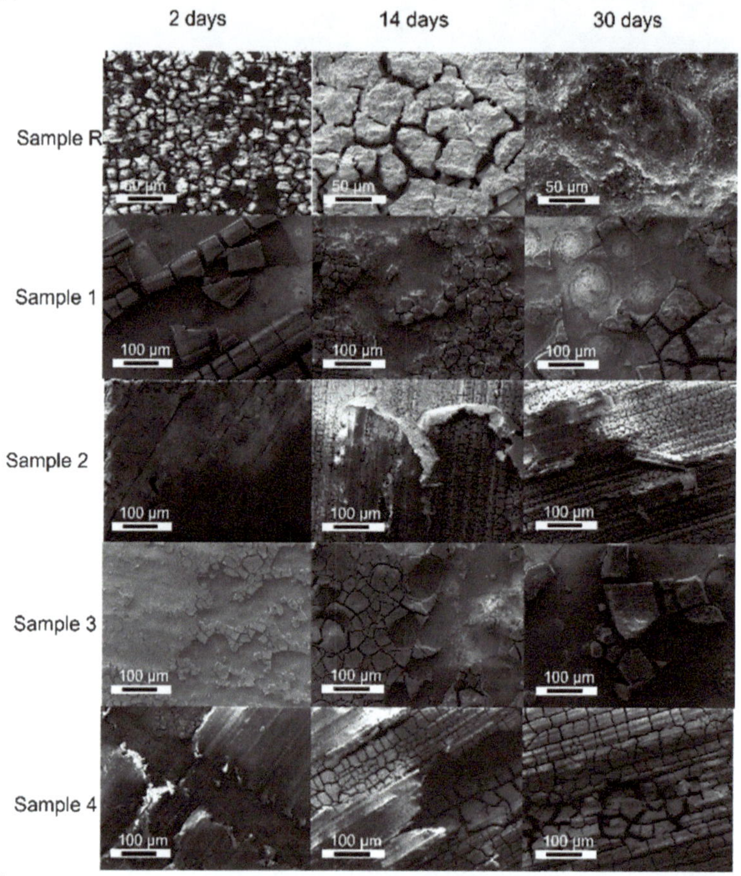


(b)

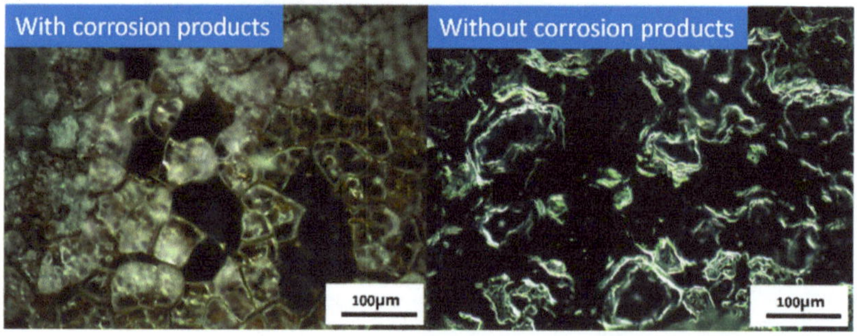


**Figure 5.** (**a**) Surface morphology of all samples after 2, 14, and 30 days of fluid dynamic degradation test using HBSS. (**b**) Optical microscopic image of Sample R after 14 days of fluid dynamic degradation testing using HBSS at magnification 20×. Only one sample surface is shown here, considering similar crystalline degradation products.

Figure 5b shows the surface of Sample R after 14 days of fluid dynamic degradation in HBSS with and without the degradation products. The crystalline, chip-like degradation products can be seen on the sample's surface, which were removed after cleaning, leaving pits on the surface.

### 3.3. Electrochemical Behavior

After the PEO, the samples which were produced in two different electrolytes (A and B) were electrochemically tested. The samples were exposed to an electrolyte under open circuit (ocp) conditions over various times. After this exposure, the samples were polarized at −1.7 V in the same electrolyte over 24 h. The polarization was negative from the ocp, resulting in a negative current density, because the cathodic part reaction dominates under the chosen conditions. Since the PEO layer normally has no electronic conductivity, electron transfer reactions like oxygen reduction or hydrogen evolution should not be possible. Only at weak points of the PEO layer, where an electron transfer is possible, can such a reduction take place. Consequently, the consumed negative charge caused by such a reduction is a measurement of the protection level of the PEO layer.

A clear tendency of the consumed charge depending on the exposure time at the OCP is only observed for electrolyte A (Table 3). However, the consumed charge is not strictly proportional to the exposition time. Electrolyte B does not show a clear relation of the consumed charge depending on the exposition time at prior ocp (Table 3). Therefore, the authors assume that the consumed charge depends more on the individual quality of the PEO layer after anodizing, and that this quality dominates the degradation characteristic. Nevertheless, some reduction takes place and also results in a slight increase in the pH after the test.

**Table 3.** Parameters of the electrochemical tests consist of ocp and potentiostatic measurement in HBSS of the pure PEO layer anodized in electrolyte A and B.

| Electrolyte | A | B | A | B | A | B |
|---|---|---|---|---|---|---|
| exposition time at ocp/h | 0 | | 1 | | 10 | |
| consumed charge over 24 h at −1.7 V/mAs | −10.7 | −17.2 | −11.2 | −6.8 | −19.7 | −2.1 |
| pH measured at the start | 7.1 | | | | | |
| pH measured at the end | 8.1 | 7.9 | 8.3 | 8.3 | 8.2 | 8.1 |

The same test procedure was carried out on a sample with a PEO layer produced in electrolyte B which was additionally impregnated or coated, respectively, by a polymer (see 2.7. Electrochemical Measurements). In this case, the test solution was HBSS as well as NaOH (see Table 4). In HBSS, the consumed charge is significantly smaller in comparison with the uncoated sample discussed before, which can be explained by the additional protection provided by the polymer film. However, the film was not stable in an alkaline solution, as demonstrated by an increase in the consumed charge.

**Table 4.** Parameters of the electrochemical test consist of ocp and potentiostatic measurement in HBSS and 0.1 M NaOH of the impregned PEO layer anodized in electrolyte B.

| | HBSS | NaOH | HBSS | NaOH | HBSS | NaOH |
|---|---|---|---|---|---|---|
| exposition time at ocp/h | 0 | | 1 | | 10 | |
| consumed charge over 24 h at −1.7 V/mAs | −4.6 | −35.3 | −5.4 | −47.4 | −3.6 | −55.7 |
| pH measured at the start | 7.1 | 12.9 | 7.1 | 12.9 | 7.1 | 12.9 |
| pH measured at the end | 7.4 | 12.8 | 7.8 | 12.8 | 7.9 | 12.4 |

*3.4. Degradation Behavior*

PEO treated specimens (Sample 1 and 3): Samples 1 and 3 had substantially higher degradation levels at the start of the test, which stabilized to rather steady levels after 7 days (Figure 5). Meanwhile, the corrosion rate of Sample 3 was much higher when compared to the specimens of Sample 1. This is because of the different degradation properties of the anodized layers obtained with electrolytes A and B. When the pH falls below 11.5, the anodized layer becomes porous and chemically unstable, making it susceptible to the corrosive medium. Furthermore, the higher density of magnesium oxide and hydroxide (density MgO: 3.58 g/cm$^3$; density $Mg(OH)_2$: 2.38 g/cm$^3$; density Mg: 1.7 g/cm$^3$) than Mg may contribute to anodized layer stress [29], which promotes cracks and corrosion. Moreover, the resulting corrosion of the AZ31 alloy results in local hydrogen evolution, which accelerates the breakdown of the oxide/hydroxide layer [30].

Figure 6 shows the surface morphology with the EDX analysis of the coated samples. All of the samples had similar degradation products following the removal of the PEO layer. The elemental mapping and spectra with the quantification of elements after a two-day degradation period are displayed below. It can be seen that the corrosion product layer is dominated by O and P, whereas the degradation products include less magnesium. Additionally, these corrosion products demonstrate that the oxide layer has already been eliminated from these areas during the first two days.

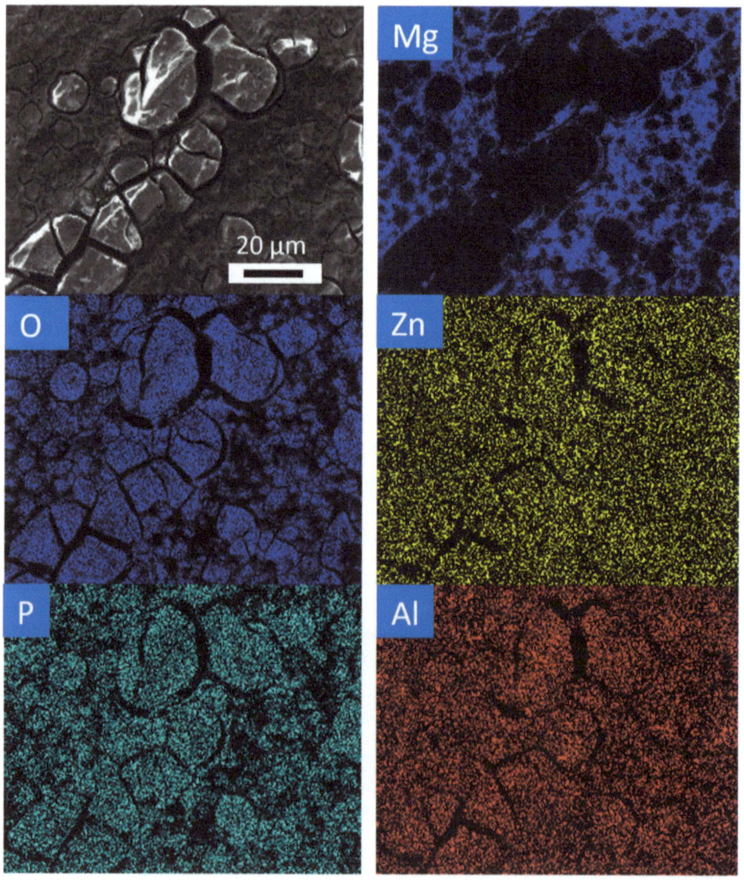


**Figure 6.** *Cont.*

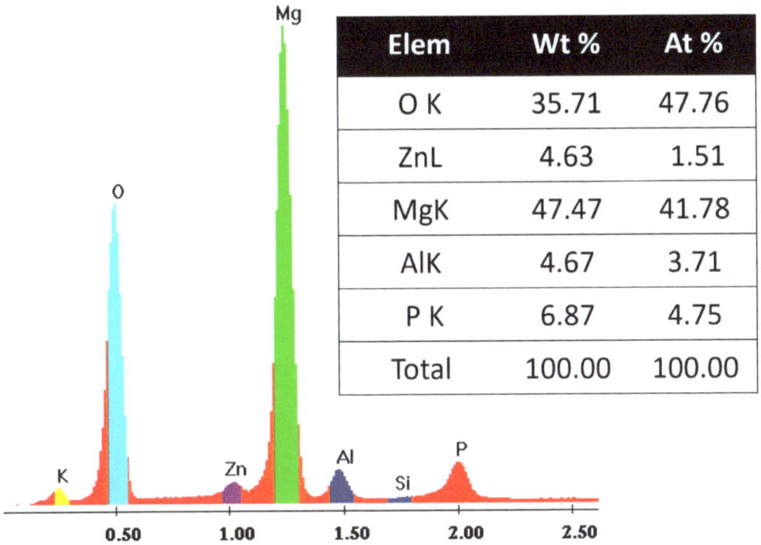


| Elem | Wt % | At % |
|---|---|---|
| O K | 35.71 | 47.76 |
| ZnL | 4.63 | 1.51 |
| MgK | 47.47 | 41.78 |
| AlK | 4.67 | 3.71 |
| P K | 6.87 | 4.75 |
| Total | 100.00 | 100.00 |

**Figure 6.** Surface morphology of PEO-treated specimens after the removal of the PEO layer after 2 days of fluid dynamic degradation testing in HBSS. Only one sample surface is presented here considering the similar degradation products in all samples.

Figure 7 shows the surface morphology and point analysis with the EDX spectra and elemental quantification of the Sample R after 14 days, where the degradation products were observed in two different layers. Point 1 shows the topmost layer of the degradation products, where O was higher in the degradation products as compared to at Points 2 and 3. That means the oxygen is becoming less prevalent as we go deeper into the corroded surface. A similar fact was observed for the Zn, Al, and P for Points 1 and 2. After reaching the third layer, i.e., Point 3, the percentage composition of all these elements is reduced significantly. It can be seen that P is not present at the layer of Point 3, demonstrating the absence of any phosphates at this layer. Similar kinds of degradation products were observed in PEO-treated samples as well after the removal of the oxide layer from the surface. On the other hand, the Mg level was lesser at Point 1 as compared to the levels at Points 2 and 3. The Wt% and At% values of Mg demonstrate that, if we go deeper onto the surface, the Mg will become higher.

PEO-treated specimens with polymer coating (Sample 2 and 4): Samples 2 and 4 showed a slower degradation rate as compared to Samples 1 and 3 due to the polymer coating. This served as a barrier between the corrosive medium and the oxide layer of the sample. Initially, only the hydrolysis of the resomer, which is made up of the PLGA, was the reason for the degradation, as the PLGA's chemical characteristics allow for hydrolytic decomposition by de-esterification [31].

Figure 8 shows the degradation pattern in the polymer-coated samples, where Point 1 shows the polymer on the surface and Point 2 shows the anodized AZ31 surface after the removal of the polymer coating from this part of the sample. With the passage of degradation time, more and more of the sample's surface was free from the polymer and the anodized layer was exposed. Then, this anodized layer cracked, as explained above, gradually removing itself from the sample's surface. After the bulk material is exposed, the degradation products were formed, which were similar to those in Figure 4. In general, Sample 2 had more traces of polymer coating after the 30 days of fluid dynamic degradation, whereas both Samples 2 and 4 have a cracked anodized layer that is still present (Figure 9) and rarely presented with corrosion products due to the removal of this oxide layer.

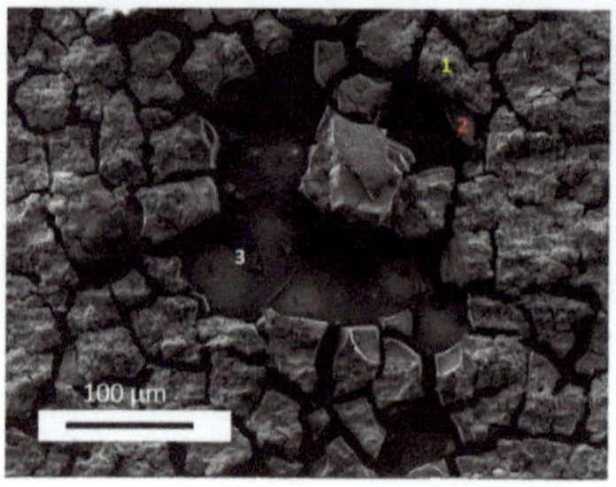


| Elem | Point 1 | | Point 2 | | Point 3 | |
|---|---|---|---|---|---|---|
| | Wt % | At % | Wt % | At % | Wt % | At % |
| O K | 56.92 | 69.91 | 46.54 | 60 | 5.13 | 7.71 |
| ZnL | 5.54 | 1.67 | 5.77 | 1.82 | 2.27 | 0.83 |
| MgK | 23.05 | 18.63 | 30.17 | 25.6 | 90.65 | 89.71 |
| AlK | 6.44 | 4.69 | 9.3 | 7.11 | 1.96 | 1.75 |
| P K | 8.05 | 5.11 | 8.22 | 5.47 | 0 | 0 |
| Total | 100.00 | 100.00 | 100.00 | 100.00 | 100.00 | 100.00 |

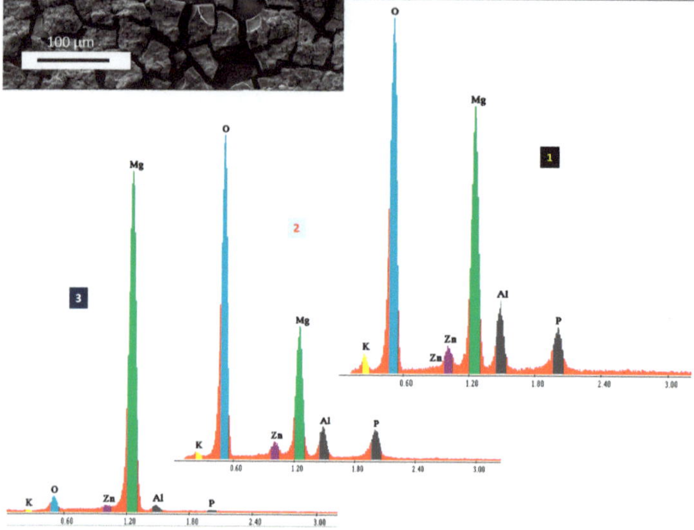


**Figure 7.** Surface morphology of sample R after 14 days of fluid dynamic degradation testing. The three layers of degraded surface are labeled as Points 1 (topmost layer), 2 (middle layer) and 3 (lowest layer). The elemental quantifications of the elements are shown as At% and Wt%.

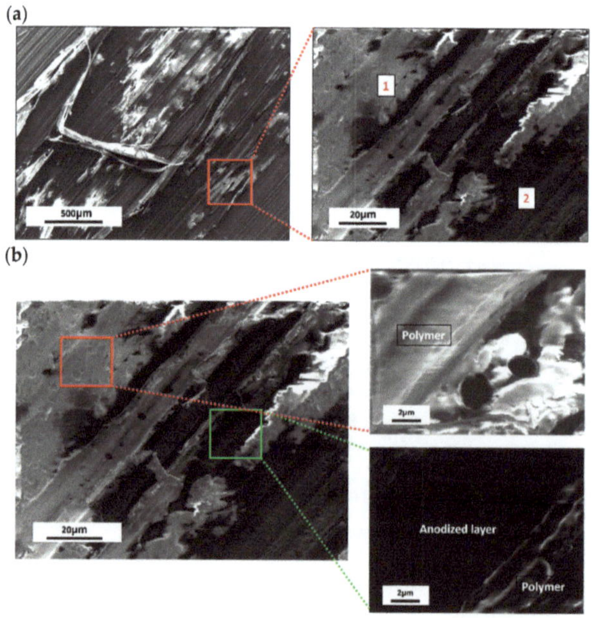


**Figure 8.** *Cont.*

(c)

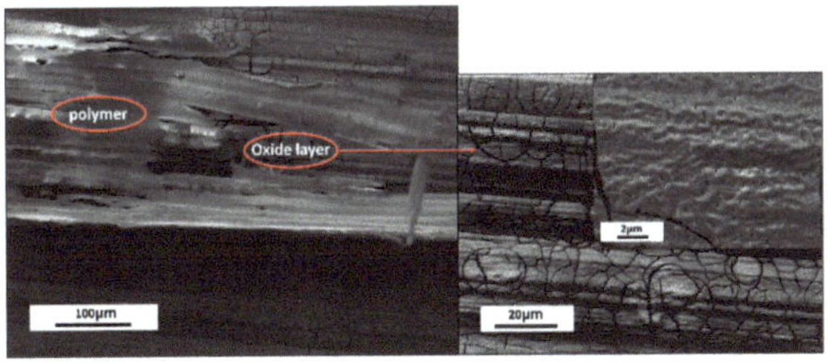


**Figure 8.** Degradation behavior of polymer-coated samples: (**a**) Degradation behavior after 2 days; (**b**) Magnified images of Points 1 and 2 shown in (**a**); (**c**) Degradation behavior after 7 days.

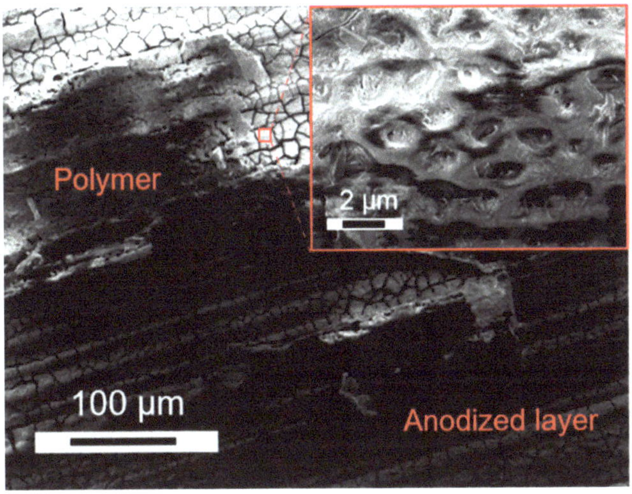


**Figure 9.** Surface morphology of Sample 2 after 30 days of degradation test.

*3.5. Surface Wettability*

Figure 10 shows the static water contact angles of all samples, including treated and untreated samples. The PEO treatment changed the surface wettability of the AZ31 surface as expected. However, the electrolytes also had an influence on the shift in the wettability towards hydrophobic and hydrophilic regions. Electrolyte A shifted the wettability towards being hydrophilic by increasing the contact angle to 73.4° (±8.5), whereas electrolyte B shifted the wettability towards the hydrophilic region, making Sample 3 more wettable by decreasing the contact angle to 62.0° (±11.5). Samples 2 and 4 (the polymer-coated forms of Samples 1 and 3, respectively) showed the increased contact angles because of the polymer coating, i.e., 84.2° (±10.7) and 88.8° (±4.7), respectively. The resomer coating demonstrated similar behavior on anodized samples. The water contact angle of PLGA in the composition of the used polymer has been reported as 88.5° [32], which is close to the values of the contact angles of Sample 2 (84.2°) and Sample 4 (88.8°).

*3.6. Mass Loss and Corrosion Rates*

Figure 11 depicts the MLRs and CRs of AZ31 samples during the 30-day fluid dynamic experiment. The results show that both anodizing time and the drying process have an effect on degradation. For example, among non-polymer-coated anodized samples, Sample 3 exhibited higher MLR and CR after 30 days than Sample 1.

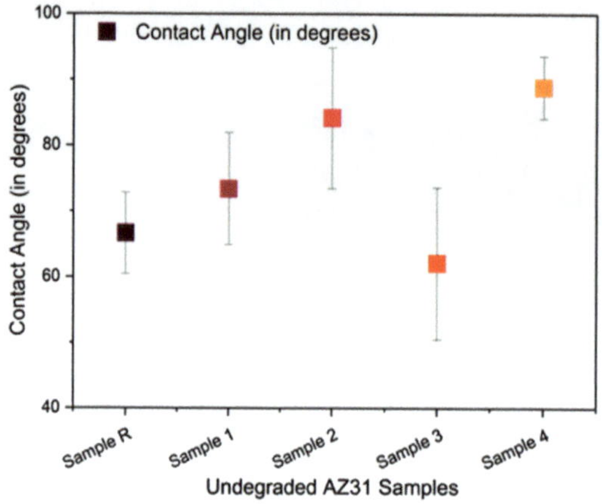


**Figure 10.** CAs of all samples.

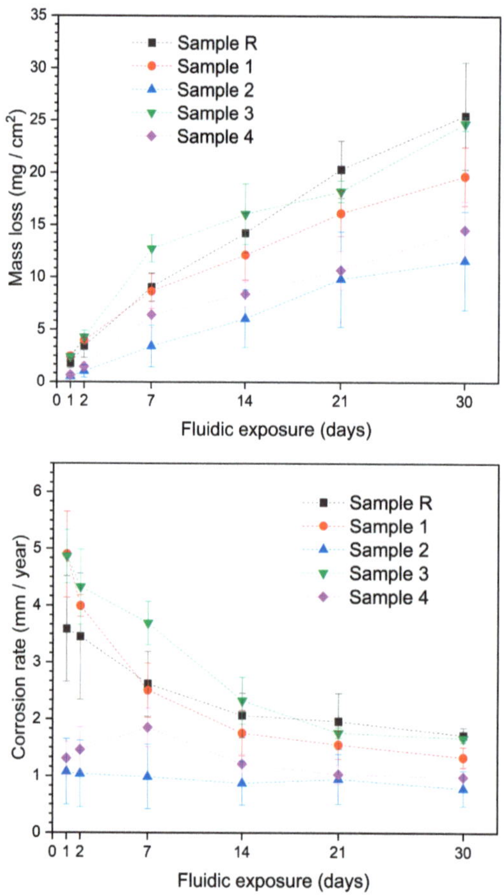


**Figure 11.** Mass loss and corrosion rates of all samples.

Initially, the anodized samples (Samples 1 and 3) showed somewhat higher MLRs than the standard AZ31 surface. This is attributed to the partial removal of the anodized coating over the initial two days. Throughout the experiment, the MLRs of the polymer-coated anodized samples (Samples 2 and 4) were lower than those of any other sample. The anodized layer could not be removed because of the polymer coating. The removal of the oxide layer from the AZ31 surface is the main reason for the elevated ML in anodized samples devoid of a polymer coating.

MLRs and CRs were decreased in both polymer-coated samples, with Sample 2 showing the lowest levels of both among the samples. Polymer-coated samples exhibited consistent behavior and did not exhibit as much fluctuation in MLRs as anodized samples (with the exception of Sample 4's first week of degradation). The consistent corrosion resistance of Samples 1 and 2 shows that electrolyte A is better suited for obtaining higher corrosion-resistant oxide layers on the AZ31's surface by PEO treatment. This also conforms to the fact that, for the best results, KOH and $Na_2SiO_3$ should be used in a 1:2 ratio.

## 4. Conclusions

Plasma electrolytic oxidation is a powerful method for increasing the corrosion resistance of magnesium and its alloys. Using a fluid dynamic test, we investigated the accelerated deterioration of PEO-treated AZ31 samples in this study. The results revealed that PEO-treated AZ31 samples were substantially more corrosion-resistant than untreated ones. The best corrosion resistance was demonstrated by samples that were treated using 5 g/L KOH and 10 g/L $NaSiO_3$. This result also suggests that the optimum concentrations of the two electrolytes are 1:2. Moreover, the corrosion resistance of the PEO-treated samples was increased even more by applying a polymer (resomer) coating to the anodized surface.

According to the findings of this study, PEO-treated AZ31 with a polymer coating is a promising candidate for biodegradable implant applications. However, more research is needed to assess the long-term performance of this material in vivo. Additionally, it is important to investigate how PEO treatment affects the mechanical characteristics of AZ31 samples.

**Author Contributions:** Conceptualization, M.S. (Muhammad Saqib), K.K., J.O., M.S. (Michael Schneider) and N.B.; data curation, M.S. (Muhammad Saqib) and K.K.; formal analysis, M.S. (Muhammad Saqib) and K.K.; funding acquisition, M.S. (Michael Schneider) and N.B.; investigation, M.S. (Muhammad Saqib) and K.K.; methodology, M.S. (Muhammad Saqib), K.K., M.S. (Michael Schneider) and N.B.; project administration, J.O., M.S. (Michael Schneider) and N.B.; resources, J.O., M.S. (Michael Schneider) and N.B.; supervision, J.O., M.S. (Michael Schneider) and N.B.; validation, M.S. (Muhammad Saqib) and K.K.; visualization, M.S. (Muhammad Saqib) and K.K.; writing—original draft, M.S. (Muhammad Saqib) and K.K.; writing—review and editing, M.S. (Muhammad Saqib), K.K., J.O., M.S. (Michael Schneider) and N.B. All authors have read and agreed to the published version of the manuscript.

**Funding:** This research was funded in the frame of internal Fraunhofer funding program "SME" in 2019–2021.

**Institutional Review Board Statement:** Not applicable.

**Informed Consent Statement:** Not applicable.

**Data Availability Statement:** The raw data supporting the conclusions of this article will be made available by the authors on request.

**Conflicts of Interest:** The authors declare no conflicts of interest.

## References

1. Zaffora, A.; Di Franco, F.; Virtù, D.; Carfì Pavia, F.; Ghersi, G.; Virtanen, S.; Santamaria, M. Tuning of the Mg Alloy AZ31 Anodizing Process for Biodegradable Implants. *ACS Appl. Mater. Interfaces* **2021**, *13*, 12866–12876. [CrossRef] [PubMed]
2. Liu, X.; Yue, Z.; Romeo, T.; Weber, J.; Scheuermann, T.; Moulton, S.; Wallace, G. Biofunctionalized Anti-Corrosive Silane Coatings for Magnesium Alloys. *Acta Biomater.* **2013**, *9*, 8671–8677. [CrossRef] [PubMed]

3. Shaw, B.A.; Sikora, E.; Virtanen, S. Fix, Heal, and Disappear: A New Approach to Using Metals in the Human Body. *Electrochem. Soc. Interface* **2008**, *17*, 45–49. [CrossRef]
4. Ascencio, M.; Pekguleryuz, M.; Omanovic, S. An Investigation of the Corrosion Mechanisms of WE43 Mg Alloy in a Modified Simulated Body Fluid Solution: The Influence of Immersion Time. *Corros. Sci.* **2014**, *87*, 489–503. [CrossRef]
5. Ascencio, M.; Pekguleryuz, M.; Omanovic, S. An Investigation of the Corrosion Mechanisms of WE43 Mg Alloy in a Modified Simulated Body Fluid Solution: The Effect of Electrolyte Renewal. *Corros. Sci.* **2015**, *91*, 297–310. [CrossRef]
6. Witte, F.; Hort, N.; Vogt, C.; Cohen, S.; Kainer, K.U.; Willumeit, R.; Feyerabend, F. Degradable Biomaterials Based on Magnesium Corrosion. *Curr. Opin. Solid State Mater. Sci.* **2008**, *12*, 63–72. [CrossRef]
7. Witte, F.; Kaese, V.; Haferkamp, H.; Switzer, E.; Meyer-Lindenberg, A.; Wirth, C.J.; Windhagen, H. In Vivo Corrosion of Four Magnesium Alloys and the Associated Bone Response. *Biomaterials* **2005**, *26*, 3557–3563. [CrossRef]
8. Mao, L.; Shen, L.; Chen, J.; Zhang, X.; Kwak, M.; Wu, Y.; Fan, R.; Zhang, L.; Pei, J.; Yuan, G.; et al. A Promising Biodegradable Magnesium Alloy Suitable for Clinical Vascular Stent Application. *Sci. Rep.* **2017**, *7*, 46343. [CrossRef]
9. Song, G.; Song, S. A Possible Biodegradable Magnesium Implant Material. *Adv. Eng. Mater.* **2007**, *9*, 298–302. [CrossRef]
10. Xiong, H.; Liang, Z.; Wang, Z.; Qin, C.; Zhao, W.; Yu, H. Mechanical Properties and Degradation Behavior of Mg(100−7x)Zn6xYx(x = 0.2, 0.4, 0.6, 0.8) Alloys. *Metals* **2018**, *8*, 261. [CrossRef]
11. Veleva, L.; Fernández-Olaya, M.G.; Feliu, S. Initial Stages of AZ31B Magnesium Alloy Degradation in Ringer's Solution: Interpretation of EIS, Mass Loss, Hydrogen Evolution Data and Scanning Electron Microscopy Observations. *Metals* **2018**, *8*, 933. [CrossRef]
12. Liu, L.; Gebresellasie, K.; Collins, B.; Zhang, H.; Xu, Z.; Sankar, J.; Lee, Y.-C.; Yun, Y. Degradation Rates of Pure Zinc, Magnesium, and Magnesium Alloys Measured by Volume Loss, Mass Loss, and Hydrogen Evolution. *Appl. Sci.* **2018**, *8*, 1459. [CrossRef]
13. Staiger, M.P.; Pietak, A.M.; Huadmai, J.; Dias, G. Magnesium and Its Alloys as Orthopedic Biomaterials: A Review. *Biomaterials* **2006**, *27*, 1728–1734. [CrossRef] [PubMed]
14. Duygulu, O.; Kaya, R.A.; Oktay, G.; Kaya, A.A. Investigation on the Potential of Magnesium Alloy AZ31 as a Bone Implant. *Mater. Sci. Forum* **2007**, *546–549*, 421–424. [CrossRef]
15. Srinivasan, A.; Shin, K.S.; Rajendran, N. Influence of Bicarbonate Concentration on the Conversion Layer Formation onto AZ31 Magnesium Alloy and Its Electrochemical Corrosion Behaviour in Simulated Body Fluid. *RSC Adv.* **2016**, *6*, 49910–49922. [CrossRef]
16. Zhang, L.; Zhang, J.; Chen, C.; Gu, Y. Advances in Microarc Oxidation Coated AZ31 Mg Alloys for Biomedical Applications. *Corros. Sci.* **2015**, *91*, 7–28. [CrossRef]
17. Gray-Munro, J.E.; Seguin, C.; Strong, M. Influence of Surface Modification on the in Vitro Corrosion Rate of Magnesium Alloy AZ31. *J. Biomed. Mater. Res. Part A* **2009**, *91A*, 221–230. [CrossRef] [PubMed]
18. Ghasemi, A.; Raja, V.S.; Blawert, C.; Dietzel, W.; Kainer, K.U. Study of the Structure and Corrosion Behavior of PEO Coatings on AM50 Magnesium Alloy by Electrochemical Impedance Spectroscopy. *Surf. Coat. Technol.* **2008**, *202*, 3513–3518. [CrossRef]
19. Jiang, B.L.; Wang, Y.M. 5-Plasma Electrolytic Oxidation Treatment of Aluminium and Titanium Alloys. In *Surface Engineering of Light Alloys*; Elsevier: Amsterdam, The Netherlands, 2010; pp. 110–154. [CrossRef]
20. Blawert, C.; Bala Srinivasan, P. 6-Plasma Electrolytic Oxidation Treatment of Magnesium Alloys. In *Surface Engineering of Light Alloys*; Woodhead Publishing Limited: Cambridge, UK, 2010; pp. 155–183. [CrossRef]
21. Štrbák, M.; Kajánek, D.; Knap, V.; Florková, Z.; Pastorková, J.; Hadzima, B.; Goraus, M. Effect of Plasma Electrolytic Oxidation on the Short-Term Corrosion Behaviour of AZ91 Magnesium Alloy in Aggressive Chloride Environment. *Coatings* **2022**, *12*, 566. [CrossRef]
22. Xue, D.; Yun, Y.; Tan, Z.; Dong, Z.; Schulz, M.J. In Vivo and In Vitro Degradation Behavior of Magnesium Alloys as Biomaterials. *J. Mater. Sci. Technol.* **2012**, *28*, 261–267. [CrossRef]
23. Koo, Y.; Lee, H.B.; Dong, Z.; Kotoka, R.; Sankar, J.; Huang, N.; Yun, Y. The Effects of Static and Dynamic Loading on Biodegradable Magnesium Pins in Vitro and in Vivo. *Sci. Rep.* **2017**, *7*, 14710. [CrossRef] [PubMed]
24. *DIN 1729-1: 1982-08*; Magnesiumlegierungen. Knetlegierungen. Beuth-Verlag: Berlin, Germany, 1982.
25. Gittens, R.A.; Scheideler, L.; Rupp, F.; Hyzy, S.L.; Geis-Gerstorfer, J.; Schwartz, Z.; Boyan, B.D. A Review on the Wettability of Dental Implant Surfaces II: Biological and Clinical Aspects. *Acta Biomater.* **2014**, *10*, 2907–2918. [CrossRef]
26. Beshchasna, N.; Ho, A.Y.K.; Saqib, M.; Kraśkiewicz, H.; Wasyluk, Ł.; Kuzmin, O.; Duta, O.C.; Ficai, D.; Trusca, R.D.; Ficai, A.; et al. Surface Evaluation of Titanium Oxynitride Coatings Used for Developing Layered Cardiovascular Stents. *Mater. Sci. Eng. C* **2019**, *99*, 405–416. [CrossRef] [PubMed]
27. Saqib, M.; Kuzmin, O.; Kraskiewicz, H.; Wasyluk, L.; Cuniberti, G.; Ficai, A.; Pichugin, V.; Opitz, J.; Beshchasna, N. Evaluation of in Vitro Corrosion Behavior of Titanium Oxynitride Coated Stainless Steel Stents. *IEEE Access* **2021**, *9*, 59766–59782. [CrossRef]
28. Schneider, M.; Kremmer, K.; Höhn, S. Corrosion Protection of Thickness Reduced Plasma Electrolytic Layers on AZ31. *Mater. Corros.* **2016**, *67*, 921–928. [CrossRef]
29. Goubaidoulline, I. Untersuchung von Grenzflächen-Reaktionen in Magnesium/Polymer-Verbundsystemen Mittels Schwingquarz-Mikrowaage Und Infrarot-Spektroskopie. Ph.D. Thesis, der Technischen Universität Clausthal, Clausthal, Germany, 2004.
30. Schlüter, K. Untersuchung von Biodegradierbaren Dünnschicht-Magnesiumlegierungen. Ph.D. Thesis, Christian-Albrechts-Universität zu Kiel, Kiel, Germany, 2012.

31. Gentile, P.; Chiono, V.; Carmagnola, I.; Hatton, P.V. An Overview of Poly(Lactic-Co-Glycolic) Acid (PLGA)-Based Biomaterials for Bone Tissue Engineering. *Int. J. Mol. Sci.* **2014**, *15*, 3640. [CrossRef]
32. Zhang, J.; Liu, Y.; Luo, R.; Chen, S.; Li, X.; Yuan, S.; Wang, J.; Huang, N. In Vitro Hemocompatibility and Cytocompatibility of Dexamethasone-Eluting PLGA Stent Coatings. *Appl. Surf. Sci.* **2015**, *328*, 154–162. [CrossRef]

Journal of
*Functional Biomaterials*

MDPI

*Review*

# 3D Bioprinting in Limb Salvage Surgery

**Iosif-Aliodor Timofticiuc [1], Serban Dragosloveanu [2,3,*], Ana Caruntu [4,5], Andreea-Elena Scheau [6,*], Ioana Anca Badarau [1], Nicolae Dragos Garofil [7,8], Andreea Cristiana Didilescu [9], Constantin Caruntu [1,10] and Cristian Scheau [1,11,*]**

1 Department of Physiology, The "Carol Davila" University of Medicine and Pharmacy, 050474 Bucharest, Romania
2 Department of Orthopaedics and Traumatology, The "Carol Davila" University of Medicine and Pharmacy, 050474 Bucharest, Romania
3 Department of Orthopaedics, "Foisor" Clinical Hospital of Orthopaedics, Traumatology and Osteoarticular TB, 021382 Bucharest, Romania
4 Department of Oral and Maxillofacial Surgery, "Carol Davila" Central Military Emergency Hospital, 010825 Bucharest, Romania
5 Department of Oral and Maxillofacial Surgery, Faculty of Dental Medicine, Titu Maiorescu University, 031593 Bucharest, Romania
6 Department of Radiology and Medical Imaging, Fundeni Clinical Institute, 022328 Bucharest, Romania
7 Department of General Surgery, The "Carol Davila" University of Medicine and Pharmacy, 050474 Bucharest, Romania
8 Department of General Surgery, "Dr. Carol Davila" Clinical Hospital of Nephrology, 010731 Bucharest, Romania
9 Department of Embryology and Microbiology, Faculty of Dentistry, The "Carol Davila" University of Medicine and Pharmacy, 050474 Bucharest, Romania
10 Department of Dermatology, "Prof. N.C. Paulescu" National Institute of Diabetes, Nutrition and Metabolic Diseases, 011233 Bucharest, Romania
11 Department of Radiology and Medical Imaging, "Foisor" Clinical Hospital of Orthopaedics, Traumatology and Osteoarticular TB, 021382 Bucharest, Romania
* Correspondence: serbandrago@gmail.com (S.D.); andreea.ghergus@gmail.com (A.-E.S.); cristian.scheau@umfcd.ro (C.S.)

**Abstract:** With the development of 3D bioprinting and the creation of innovative biocompatible materials, several new approaches have brought advantages to patients and surgical teams. Increasingly more bone defects are now treated using 3D-bioprinted prostheses and implementing new solutions relies on the ability of engineers and medical teams to identify methods of anchoring 3D-printed prostheses and to reveal the potential influence of bioactive materials on surrounding tissues. In this paper, we described why limb salvage surgery based on 3D bioprinting is a reliable and effective alternative to amputations, and why this approach is considered the new standard in modern medicine. The preliminary results of 3D bioprinting in one of the most challenging fields in surgery are promising for the future of machine-based medicine, but also for the possibility of replacing various parts from the human body with bioactive-based constructs. In addition, besides the materials and constructs that are already tested and applied in the human body, we also reviewed bioactive materials undergoing in vitro or in vivo testing with great potential for human applications in the near future. Also, we explored the recent advancements in clinically available 3D-bioprinted constructs and their relevance in this field.

**Keywords:** 3D bioprinting; limb salvage surgery; biocompatible; prostheses; electron beam melting

## 1. Introduction

In the last decade, medical and bioengineering teams aimed to find a better solution for salvaging limbs affected by various diseases or trauma while avoiding amputation. As presented in a study on lower-limb amputations, approximately 79% of the individuals who underwent amputations suffered from a vascular disease [1]. Pathology of the vessels may affect the surrounding tissues, inducing inflammation and oxidative stress, and reducing the protective mechanisms of the surrounding cells [2]. In severe cases of extensive destruction of muscles, bones, connective tissue, nerves, arteries, and veins, the classical amputation remains the optimal approach unless one or more of these components can be replaced. Moreover, various traumas of the limbs or some systemic diseases such as malignancies lead to limb amputations [3,4]. With the fast development of 3D printing, followed by the emergence of a new branch-3D bioprinting, as well as a parallel advancement in biocompatible materials, the distance has shortened to the point where the need for amputations can be replaced with saving limbs. Limb salvage surgery is an innovative approach in medicine that appeared with the emerging field of microvascular surgery around the 1960s, and it has flourished due to the development of different 3D bioprinting techniques and the possibility to create unique and functional builds [5]. As long as a revascularization of the affected area is possible and a reconstruction or a replacement of the affected body part can be performed, the necessity for amputation is very low to none [5]. In addition, limb salvage surgery aims to reduce the high mortality associated with amputations [6]. Standard limb salvage surgery is very effective in maintaining the function and quality of life; however, it faces several unmet clinical needs. Most importantly, traditional approaches often rely on modular prostheses, allografts, or metallic implants, which may not be adequate for complex bone defects. This may lead to poor implant fit, limited integration with host tissues, or higher risk of complications such as infection, implant loosening, or mechanical failure [7–9]. Additionally, conventional materials are not able to mimic the biomechanical and bioactive properties of natural bone, leading to longer recovery times and worse functional outcomes [10,11]. Moreover, for the majority of patients who suffer from vascular disease, a solution for optimal revascularization to perform such salvaging surgeries has not yet been identified. However, there are reported studies about 3D bioprinting vessels, so once the optimal balance between viable cells and other biomaterials that offer integrity to the blood vessels is found, this challenge could be approached [12,13]. Also, if two or more different tissues of the limb are affected, salvage surgery is not a solution due to the difficulty of predicting how two different scaffolds of materials with different purposes interact with each other [5] (Figure 1).

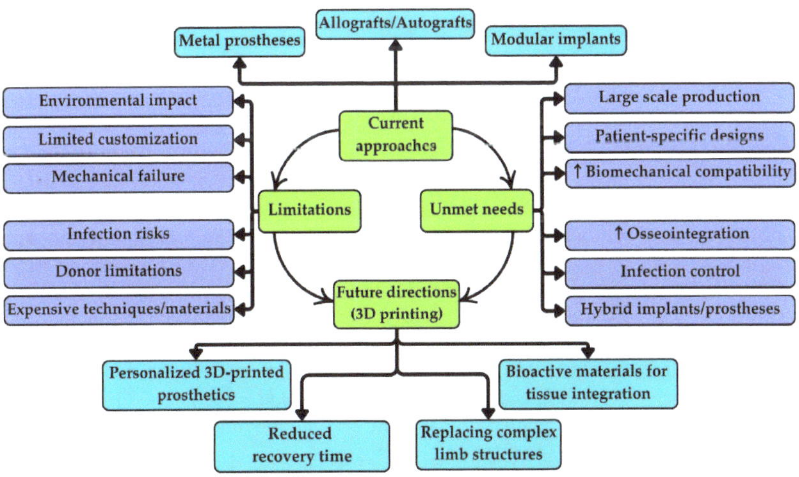


**Figure 1.** Roadmap of limb salvage surgery approaches, limitations, unmet needs, and the perspectives of 3D printing in improved personalized patient care. ↑ = increased/enhanced.

In recent studies on 3D bioprinting, some researchers define the technique as the use of 3D printing for building three-dimensional components for use in the human body or for medical research or simply tissue engineering. However, more rigorous studies consider 3D bioprinting as the field where 3D printing techniques are used to print with viable cells or bioinks [14,15]. Yet, from our point of view, a more accurate definition of 3D bioprinting would be of a field that emerged as a 3D-printing medical branch that aims to use viable cells and nonviable materials or mixes between the two to build a construct to be used in the human body from a functional or strictly structural perspective while also including constructs such as tissue engineering scaffolds that support the development of treatments and new medical or surgical approaches [15–18]. However, to avoid confusion and keep the rigor of the studies, for the purpose of this paper we refer to bioprinting as a 3D-printed construct that includes viable cells.

Following the emerging field of microvascular surgery, the development of limb salvage surgery was supported by new approaches based on constructs created using 3D-bioprinting technologies, such as entire bones, ligaments, and muscles with a key part represented by the properties that these biomaterials show, such as angiogenesis and osteogenesis [19].

In contemporary vision, the only solution to rebuild an entire limb is using 3D-printed biomaterials. As long as an optimal balance is found between the bioactive properties of different materials, we can expect great advancements in the future of regenerative medicine, where in extreme cases, entire limbs are 3D printed and attached to the body in functional harmony.

The purpose of our paper is to highlight the recent approaches and innovations in 3D bioprinting applicable to limb salvage surgery. However, many of the studies that approach 3D printing in limb salvage surgery do not focus on the interaction between the prostheses with the rest of the native tissues. Therefore, considering the limited number of studies found regarding the bioactive properties of the materials used in bioprinting and 3D printing limb parts, we believe that any approach that considers the biological activity and functionality of the builds is innovative in limb salvage surgery. We addressed the current state of development of the field, ranging from recent discoveries and in vitro tests on compounds with potential in bone regeneration and growth to research on animal models that offered solutions for the future of 3D bioprinting in limb salvage surgery. Also, we comprehensively reviewed the recent advancements in clinically available 3D-bioprinted constructions and the promising results of these studies for patients and surgical teams tackling major limb surgery.

## 2. 3D Bioprinting in Orthopedics

The increasing interest in the emerging field of 3D printing is doubled by the necessity for new approaches in limb salvage surgery. As such, extensive research is performed in this area to find solutions for patients with bone defects that normally require amputations [20]. Initially, the main approach was to identify designs and materials that mimic the mechanical behavior of the bone; therefore, metal prostheses made of titanium or tantalum were designed as a new solution for limb salvage surgeons [21,22]. However, with the rapid development of this field, the aim went beyond fulfilling the mechanical characteristics of the bone. An innovation in bone 3D printing is creating a 3D-printed build that can behave as a physiological bone, an active tissue that renews itself, interacts with the surrounding tissues, and influences the homeostasis of the body [23]. To aid in this problem, many biocompatible materials were designed to behave as active tissue in light of their bioactive properties, capacity to promote the activation of the surrounding cells, and limited effect in generating inflammation or being harmful to the body in the long term [24].

### 2.1. In Vitro Studies

Through in vitro testing of different materials, new compounds were identified or designed that can closely mimic the mechanical behavior and bioactivity of the bone, promoting osteogenesis, angiogenesis, and proliferation of the adjacent tissues [25,26].

Only a small fraction of the biomaterials tested on animal models can be clinically implemented; therefore, metal prostheses still represent a reliable solution in orthopedics [27]. However, even though many materials are still in the phase of in vitro testing, they represent a promising solution for the future of 3D bioprinting in limb salvage surgery in light of the recent and innovative results regarding their bioactivity. After the rapid implementation of the classical 3D-printed limb parts in the field of limb salvage surgery, with the development of 3D bioprinting, the main focus switched to finding optimal materials that can promote cell differentiation, thus ensuring an enhanced integration of the prostheses created, in patients [28].

Silk fibroin (SF), a natural protein extracted from silkworms, was tested in vitro and in vivo to assess its potential effects on bony tissue [29,30]. It was concluded that SF presents heightened biocompatibility and does not produce immunological responses when transferred in vivo. In vitro, testing showed low cytotoxicity along with bioresorbability and biodegradability, properties that are mandatory for a material that is required to mimic the bone tissue [31]. The similarities with bone tissue functionality and structure are not sufficient to create a construct that presents unique characteristics for specific patients' needs, but in our opinion, a material needs to present a minimum of bioactive properties to be a potential candidate for bioprinting and for future integration with other scaffolds or native tissues.

Even though many forms of SF were created, such as films, hydrogels, and even nanoparticles, that can be 3D-printed in different scaffolds with bioactive properties and great mechanical resistance (strength of 300–740 MPa and toughness similar to the cortical bone) [31,32], it was also shown that SF can induce the differentiation of human mesenchymal stem cells (MSCs) and promote VEGF synthesis. Thus, SF represents a material optimal for the induction of bone cell proliferation and regeneration while also promoting angiogenesis [33]. Interpreting these results, we can conclude that SF has great compatibility with human cells, which means that integrating any other viable cells with SF in bioinks is an optimistic possibility for the future of bioprinting in limb salvage surgery.

Similar bioactivity with SF can be observed in natural polysaccharides, such as alginates, that were also used in building scaffolds mimicking bone activity. Alginates are substances that can be 3D printed as bioinks, and stem cells can therefore be added to these compounds for optimal promotion of cell growth and low cytotoxicity [34]. Not different from SF, alginates promote the differentiation of MSC and can perform as well as cortical bone in mixtures with bone morphogenetic proteins. However, due to the lack of mechanical properties of alginates, building a prosthesis showcasing alginate's properties requires methods of integrating these polysaccharides with metal or other rigid material structures [35]. These drawbacks of integrating soft materials in 3D-bioprinted limb parts can be frequently observed throughout the studies mentioned in this review. For now, an accessible solution to this challenge is to create hybrid builds. A solution could be 3D printing solid parts, to offer integrability and mechanical properties to the constructs, and then coating them with various classical 3D-printed bioactive coats or applying bio-printed scaffolds to the surfaces or inside the structure.

Many materials, especially biopolymers such as PLLA (Poly-L-Lactic Acid), PCL (Polycaprolactone), PLA (Polylactic Acid), PEEK (Polyetheretherketone), HA (Hydroxyapatite), and β-TCP (β-Tricalcium Phosphate) present bioactive properties in the range of cell proliferation, osteoblast proliferation, osteoinductivity, osteoconductivity, and even angiogenesis [24]. However, various in vitro activities can be stimulated in different compounds; for instance, collagen was observed to deliver proportionally different substances in the surroundings such as active compounds or antibiotics. This property can be classified as a 4D activity, i.e., during the slow degradation in time, the material gradually releases the substances with which it was loaded [36].

Bone morphogenetic proteins are clinically approved and used as loads in 3D-printing constructs to promote bone cell proliferation. In a recent study, a replacement for this classic method of osteoblast induction was researched on ST2 bone marrow-derived cells placed in a scaffold made of PCL and GelMA in which a few nanograms of Wnt3a (osteoinductive protein) were included. It was shown that in the areas where this protein was added, the quantity of alkaline phosphate was high, a marker showing osteoblast differentiation. This promising result could represent a future possibility of treating small bone defects or even usage for healing critical bone defects [37]. Considering these promising results, we believe scaffolds or implants based on this composition can also be created and applied in patients with less severe cases of bone trauma, especially in those who do not necessarily need limb salvage surgery.

Considering that the majority of innovative compounds that can now be 3D printed are biopolymers [38], those with great structural integrity are useful when porosity areas are vast. A relevant example is hydroxyapatite, which presents enhanced metabolic activity and induction of osteoblast differentiation.

However, it is the responsibility of the research teams to find optimal balances in mixtures that may represent a concrete solution in limb salvage surgery and other clinical applications.

### 2.2. In Vivo Animal Models

Total or partial bone replacement in animal models represents a great solution for the transition to the implementation of these 3D-printed prostheses in humans. Alongside the in vitro tests conducted on these materials, animal models allow for the observation of the interaction of the material with the surrounding tissue [39]. This encourages research for methods to fixate the prostheses in the affected limb. Thus, a smoother transition can be made to clinical practice, especially with prostheses designed from already approved and biocompatible materials.

There is paucity of clinical information regarding the interactions of the patient's surrounding tissue with the prostheses. In this issue, a research team performed tests on animal models for radius/ulna-scaffold complexes with biologically active coatings composed of substances such as dipyridamole used as an enhancer for bone formations or collagen [40].

Unique in this radius/ulna scaffold is the use of calcium phosphate-based alloplastic materials, which are known as one of the best bone substitutes, but with challenges in 3D printing due to their fragility and underperforming mechanical properties [24]. In a rabbit model, it was concluded that β-Tricalcium Phosphate scaffolds coated with high concentrations of dipyridamole (1000 μM) very precisely mimic the compact bone [40].

In another animal model testing of ulnar bone replacement, a 3D-printed PLLA model was built with an active and osteogenic compound, bone morphogenetic protein 2 (BMP2) for enhancing bone regeneration [41]. In addition, the PLLA scaffold was also coated with an alginate catechol and collagen to ensure optimal speed and regulation in the release kinetics of the osteogenic compound for 2 months, enough to facilitate the full incorporation and adaptation of the prosthesis in the animal model [41].

Regarding the lower limb, femoral defects may be one of the most extensively researched topics regarding 3D printing solutions, with a major focus on solutions for promoting osteogenesis and angiogenesis [42]. While metal prostheses still represent the majority, the use of polymer-based prostheses is increasing [43]. As already mentioned, polymers are similar when discussing the mechanical properties and superior in terms of the bioactivity of the material in the human body [24].

Another future perspective in medical 3D printing is the attempt to build polymeric prostheses with different compounds that can be added in the process of 3D printing, such as cell-proliferation-inducing substances or even stem/stem-based cells, thus creating bioinks. However, these solutions are underdeveloped for patient applications, and not all test substances have been approved as safe.

A research team tested the functionality of a PCL scaffold, 3D printed with FDM technology in a rat model of a femoral defect, in which stromal-derived factor 1 was added [44]. It was concluded that PCL combined with this bioactive compound was essential for optimal induction of osteogenesis, which led to the perfect healing of the femur. In addition, no cytotoxicity or other side effects were reported [44]. Many other combinations of substances such as PCL and β-TCP, PCL/Nanoparticulate Willemite composite, PCL/hydroxyapatite, porous tantalum with polydopamine, or quaternized chitosan-grafted polylactide-co-glycolide/hydroxyapatite were reported for the induction of osteogenesis for healing large bone defects, and the best mixture is yet to be identified; however, continued testing on the animal models is needed for the future transfer and application of these methods to humans [45–48]. Besides trying to integrate these results into the human surgery field, introducing human viable cells should also be considered. Observing the low cytotoxicity of the biopolymers, viable cells could not only resist inside the 3D-bioprinted scaffolds, but could also potentiate the mentioned bioactive properties.

Tumoral pathology has a serious and damaging evolution when occurring in the limbs, and in more severe cases may affect multiple compartments to a various extents [49–52]. These cases are frequently the subject of limb salvage surgery, and solutions are presently researched on animal models. These include the development of prostheses that fulfill the mechanical roles of the affected bones while behaving as real, bioactive tissue, in continuous communication with the adjacent structures. Substances such as cerium oxide, hydrogels, stem cells BMP-2 and hMSC, and natural collagen were introduced in polymer-based prostheses (PCL, PEEK, HA) for the promotion of proliferation and differentiation of osteoblasts and angiogenesis. They have shown promising results in terms of possible future application in human orthopedics and are expected to be perfected to become the next gold standard in limb salvage surgeries [53–59].

### 2.3. *In Vivo—Clinically Available Approaches*

Three-dimensional bioprinting emerged as a novel and innovative branch of the 3D-printing industry and was rapidly developed with the desire to obtain patient-specific treatments with near to no inflammatory response and rapid healing with fewer complications. The first materials used as scaffolds in 3D bioprinting were rigid and exhibited suboptimal mechanical properties, and this could be one of the reasons why orthopedics was a suitable medical sector for the initiation of bioprinting and its development [60].

Metal-based 3D-printed prostheses represent the vast majority of the clinically approved and applied constructs in today's surgery practice. Polymer-based 3D-printed prostheses (or non-metal prostheses) represent a good future perspective for limb salvage surgery, with significant research still in progress, and a series of materials to be approved for use in the human body. The advent of digital 2D and especially 3D planning has made it possible to create excellent fitting of patient-specific implants concerning the recipient anatomy [61].

As mentioned in the introduction, some studies define bioprinting as 3D printing with materials that incorporate viable cells. In the case of bones, the data regarding 3D printing with mixes that contain viable cells are scarce. However, extensive research can be found about 3D-printed builds that mimic the biological and mechanical properties of the bone tissue.

#### 2.3.1. Metal-Based 3D-Bioprinted Constructs

Defects in the bones of the upper limb represent a great challenge for patients due to function deprivation, and it is the role of medical teams to support fast patient recovery while also considering aesthetics as well as the full recovery of all the functions that were lost due to trauma, infections, tumor growth, or other diseases.

The clavicle is the most frequently fractured bone of the scapular girdle, with a reported incidence of up to 5% of clinically presented fractures in adults [62,63]. According to the Orthopaedic Trauma Association and Canada Orthopedic Trauma Society, approximately 80% of clavicle fractures are located in the midshaft of the bone [64,65]. While some of these fractures may be treated by immobilization alone, many clavicle fractures cannot be healed without surgical intervention, which often implies fixation with plates [66], requiring intraoperative manual adjustments. In the early stages of 3D printing development for orthopedic applications, a large number of prints were used for building bone models for accurate preoperative patient-specific prostheses or plate adjustments. It was concluded that using these new 3D printing technologies was helpful for the surgical teams by way of reducing the incision dimensions and time of the operation [67], especially for patients who reported less discomfort, since it resulted in fewer interventions for implant removals [68]. Three-dimansional printing is a great solution for limb salvage, as shown in the case of a 21-year-old female patient with clavicle Ewing's sarcoma, where a 3D-printed titanium clavicle was manufactured for total bone replacement. Even though it is known that titanium is not an ideal material, it can lead to great results and can save patients from amputations [69]. Titanium can easily achieve the mechanical requirements for total bone replacement. While using metal-based prostheses replaced the need of amputation in patients, metal-based constructs could be coated or integrated with bioprinted scaffold to promote osteogenesis and angiogenesis for better integration of the entire bone with the surrounding tissues [70]. Furthermore, it can also be loaded with antibiotics to reduce the risk of infections or with human viable cells that present great characteristics in vitro but were not yet approved for clinical use, such as ST2 bone marrow cells [37,71].

Scapular bone fractures are infrequently compared with clavicular bones, representing under 5% of shoulder girdle fractures and insignificant among all clinically presented adult fractures [72]. However, in a few cases of the malignancies present in the shoulder girdle area, the scapula may be affected [73]. The most common type of bone sarcoma in adults is chondrosarcoma; however, Ewing's sarcoma can also represent a significant percentage of scapular sarcomas, presenting a great risk of undergoing amputation or total removal of the bone [69,74].

In extreme cases of scapular bone disease, solutions from the 3D bioprinting area are under development for the creation of biological active prostheses that can spare the patients from the inflammatory rejections or the discomfort generated by more classical approaches. Some other defects that the scapular bone can suffer from, such as scapular bone fractures and scapular aneurysmal bone cysts, have already been resolved using 3D-printing instrumentations or medical accessories that assist the surgical teams in a patient-specific treatment; this leads to a reduction in intraoperative time and complications, as shown in Figure 2 [75–78].

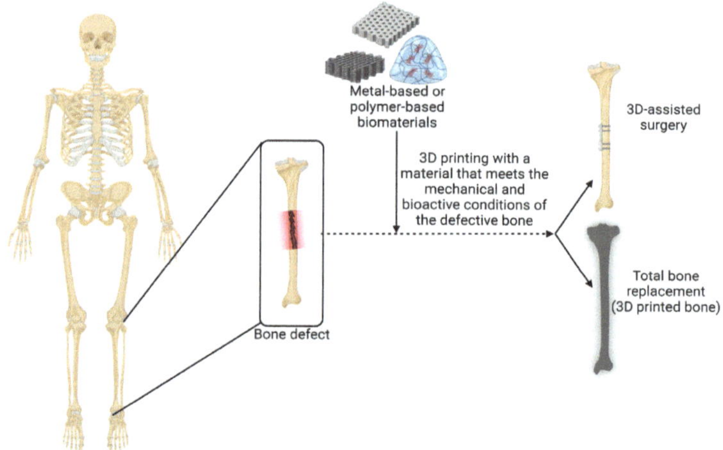


**Figure 2.** Three-dimensional printing constructs can serve as accessories in various orthopedic surgeries or as the main components in limb salvage surgery where 3D bioprinting is used to create entire bone prostheses. Created in BioRender. Timofticiuc, I. (2024) BioRender.com/w87n517, date of last access—12 October 2024.

In the case of a 35-year-old woman diagnosed with right scapular Ewing's sarcoma [69], a technical 3D-printed solution was found, showcasing the vast possibilities of molding the titanium powder in different shapes and sizes. In this manner, the built prostheses do not have any specific requirements to be suitable for 3D printing; however, some drawbacks can appear when designing fixation methods for preserving the majority of the functions of the removed bone.

In a case study of four patients presenting with chondrosarcoma, it was determined that they required partial scapulectomy and reconstruction of the glenoid fossa, the neck of the scapula, and the humeral head. In this regard, a solution using 3D-bioprinted builds made of titanium alloy of the glenoid prosthesis and reverse shoulder prosthesis was identified, resulting in a short-term follow-up with no complications, no advancements of the malignancy, and great mobility recovery [79]. This success revealed the rapid and efficient evolution of the patients when they are treated using 3D-printing methods over a traditional approach, which may result in implant rejection or, in more severe cases, limb amputation.

One of the most serious challenges in orthopedics remains total or partial replacements of the bones affected by tumors or infections. Both primary and metastatic lesions may significantly affect the structural integrity of the bone and expand to adjacent soft tissue structures [80–83]. As mentioned, 3D bioprinting offers promising initial results [84–94]. In the case of a 5-year-old female patient presenting with advanced osteosarcoma of the proximal humerus, partial removal of the bone was necessary. The early age of the patient represented a challenge and a solution was found by building a 3D-printed titanium alloy prosthesis to replace the affected part of the bone. In this particular groundbreaking case, after a 3-year follow-up, the patient was tumor-free, pain-free, and had partial functionality of the arm. These results are very encouraging for the pediatric orthopedic and oncologic sectors, demonstrating that alternative treatments can be found to avoid amputation, providing great contribution to limb rescue operations [95]. Given the cause of the trauma in this patient, future approaches should also include bioprinting these prostheses with viable cells that promote controlled cell differentiation.

Compared to patients under somatic development, adult patients present fewer challenges and more compliance for postoperative medical recovery; also, they require fewer revisions for adjusting the prosthesis size to the dimensions of the bone [96,97]. Relatively few cases were reported for total elbow replacement; however, in the case of a 60-year-old patient who lost the range of motion in the elbow due to distal humerus fractures, a solution with a prosthesis made of titanium alloy was found, and after the surgery and a few weeks of recovery the patient regained initial functionality, showing once again the promising results of 3D-printed prostheses in ensuring the mobility of the limbs or in more serious cases, even saving them [98]. For elbow replacement, salvage surgery might resort to the initial use of megaprotheses; however, this may imply difficult later revisions and possible limited functionality, so fitting a patient-specific 3D-printed implant is ideal in this category of patients [99].

Forearm bone defects can have multiple causes, and similar to previous examples, these defects can be caused by trauma resulting in fractures that may require surgical treatment [100]. In forearm defects caused by infections, traumas, sarcomas, or hereditary conditions, one challenge is restoring the mechanical behavior that the ulna and radius ensure; therefore, 3D bioprinting shows good potential in the functional recovery of the elbow and the wrist after replacements with total or partial prostheses. An easy solution to approach small bone defects is by bioprinting scaffolds made of silk bioinks and alginate bioinks that promote osteogenesis [101,102]. Furthermore, combining the builds with antibiotic coatings or nanoparticles coating could help reduce the infections that initially caused the bone trauma [103].

Due to a leiomyosarcoma of the radius, a 53-year-old man underwent total resection of the radius along with the radial nerve, and a 3D-printed biological prosthesis was designed and built for replacement based on CT scans of the healthy radius [95]. The titanium alloy prosthesis of the entire radial bone allowed the patient to regain basic functionality after 3 years, despite the postoperatively dropped hand caused by the resection of the radial nerve.

One of the most complex biomechanical behaviors of the human body is represented by hand movements [104]. Thus, 3D printing hand components represents a greater challenge than other long-bone prostheses because of the need to maintain the functional and aesthetic purposes of the segment. Several applications in hand surgery using 3D printing were reported. Designing plates for fracture treatment as well as surgical guides are some examples, and they were employed using methods adapted from procedures on larger and longer bones [105–113].

Alongside fractures, a greater risk of hand-associated diseases and defects is represented by giant cell tumors, which can often lead to infection or amputation [114,115]. The treatment of giant cell tumors is complex, with numerous therapeutic options; however, production costs and the multitude of recurrent cases represent a significant drawback in the implementation of 3D-printed approaches. Tissue engineering, especially the 3D-bioprinting branch, provides solutions not only for the production cost and time of design, but also for the lack of highly experienced prostheses specialists.

In 2 years, seven patients presented with scaphoid and lunate fractures, and due to osteonecrosis of the carpal bones, total bone replacement was mandatory. There are few reported studies using titanium alloys as biocompatible materials for bony structures dated before 2020 [116,117]; however, in this particular study, the prostheses were built using porous tantalum, a metal considered to have better mechanical properties than titanium and more efficient integration in the patient's limb [118]. As mentioned later in this article, porous surfaces promote an enhanced interaction of the 3D-printed build with the surrounding cells and proteins. Creating a hybrid construct by adding a coating over metal prostheses that presents porous surfaces but also bioactive properties would therefore greatly increase the functionality of these prostheses in patients.

There is a trend in advancing from metal prostheses to polymer prostheses. However, in the case of metacarpals, the literature on metal prostheses is scarce. In the case of three patients presenting with metacarpal giant cell tumors, total bone removal was mandatory [119]. Titanium alloys known for their mechanical strength and biocompatibility were used in building metacarpal prostheses for these patients, and a satisfactory recovery was reached [119]. Similarly, in the case of a 64-year-old man with a giant cell tumor of the proximal phalanx of the fourth finger, a 3D-printed titanium prosthesis was designed in an attempt to salvage the finger after the patient refused amputation [120].

The bones of the upper and lower limb do not present significant differences in morphology, and pathologies such as tumors, infections, or fractures are similar in terms of pathogenesis [121–124]. However, the biomechanics of the lower body bony structures are different due to the requirement of sustaining the body weight; therefore, resistance, support, and strength of the lower limbs overcome the mobility and complexity of the functions of the upper limbs [125,126]. The bones of the lower limb are also subjected to load-bearing-related deformity, and specific surgical corrective procedures with adequate materials and techniques may be required [127,128]. Restoration of alignment plays a major role in functional recovery and sustained load-bearing leads to better outcomes in terms of implant integration and bone quality [129,130].

However, femoral defects can produce extensive lesions which frequently lead to unwanted limb immobilization associated with severe pain [131,132]. Due to the novel 3D-bioprinting techniques developed in the last decade, such as extrusion-based 3D bioprinting, inkjet-based 3D bioprinting, laser-assisted 3D bioprinting, and stereolithographic-based 3D bioprinting [133], more solutions are available for patients, ensuring a partial or even total rendering of certain functions of the limb. While osteosarcoma is a serious disease with a high risk of metastasis, significant issues are also present in the case of giant cell tumors and even fractures, which often require total or partial replacement of the affected bone [131,132]. In a comparative study of 10 patients with giant cell tumors of the distal femur, the differences in disease evolution and healing were observed. Five patients were treated with cement packing with extra fixation reconstruction of the distal femur while the other five patients were treated using an innovative 3D-bioprinting method [134]. It was concluded that the 3D-printed strut-type prostheses made from titanium alloy in different models performed better in terms of mechanical stress on the knee joint. In addition, the capacity of the prosthesis is superior to cement reconstruction due to the osteoinduction and cell proliferation with curative effect. An innovation in this field could be represented by enhancing these properties of porous metals through integrating the builds with bioprinted scaffolds. Imitating the cancellous bone structure at the site of the distal femur, the titanium 3D-printed prostheses did not promote the disease recurrence nor metastases, despite their effects on cell proliferation [134]. The post-operative knee joint alignment is essential in restoring functionality but is also related to mechanical stress and wear of the metallic components and their effects on adjacent bone with physiological weight distribution [135]. Tibial and fibular defects have a variety of solutions ranging from surgically inserted plates and bone grafts to even tissue engineering. However, several drawbacks can appear due to the mechanical stress occurring in the adjacent joints of these bones. Through different tissue engineering solutions made available by 3D bioprinting, faster functional recovery and improved healing were obtained while also decreasing the number of needed revisions [136].

In a retrospective study on 14 patients reporting on the implantation of titanium alloy 3D-printed prostheses, the effectiveness and compatibility for the reconstruction of the tibial diaphyseal critical defects caused by osteomyelitis were assessed [137]. Although numerous methods are reported for the treatment of defects larger than 10 cm, it was concluded that besides four patients that needed a second intervention due to fixation screw failure, this method is optimal for the reconstruction of the tibial bone; it also appears very promising taking into consideration the possible addition of various bioactive substances [137].

In the case of the fibula, the only applications available in the literature regarding 3D printing are fracture plates and additional instruments used for fibular bone fracture. However, in any case of an entire tibial replacement, we need to consider the interaction of the prosthesis with the fibula and identify ways of fixating it in the surrounding muscles and cartilage but also to the fibula. In a reported study about tenogenic differentiation, it was shown that MSCs can differentiate into tendon cells [138]. As previously shown, there are reported studies where MSCs are bioprinted as scaffolds. Therefore, a solution for the fixation of muscles to the fibula is creation of a bioprinted tendon that promotes cell differentiation and could easier attach the muscles to the bone.

In Figure 3, a visualization of the process of 3D printing using metals can be observed. In the application of metal-based prostheses, the possibility that they could pierce the bone or the surrounding tissues needs to be mentioned. Even though these products perform very well and do not easily degrade or break under mechanical stress, this possibility always exists as a potential complication, with increasing chances in case of great efforts or sudden movements [139].

### 2.3.2. Non-Metal-Based 3D-Bioprinted Constructions

PEEK (polyether–ether–ketone) is a biodegradable material that exhibits great physical and mechanical properties, such as low Young's modulus [140]. Its introduction encouraged studies and development of prostheses models and it was rapidly concluded that it could present better results than titanium constructs. Even though it is not yet fully clinically approved, PEEK could represent the next ideal material with medical applications, especially in orthopedics [140].

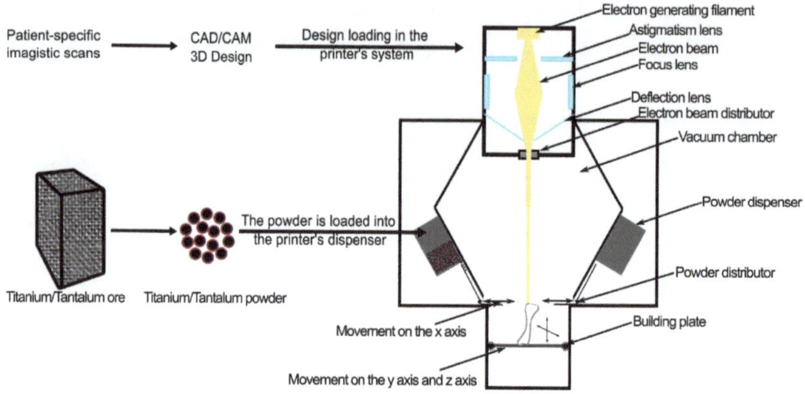


**Figure 3.** Electron Beam Melting (EBM) is the most frequently used technology for 3D printing metals such as titanium or tantalum. After the metal is processed in powder form, a special component distributes the powder as a thin layer at the top of the construction where an electron beam melts it, forming a new layer according to CAD software instructions.

In the case of a 23-year-old patient who presented with chronic right clavicle osteomyelitis, a 3D-printed clavicle was the solution. The part was accurately 3D-printed using CT scans and designed for fixation in the acromial end of the clavicle and the sternal stalk using PEEK. This provided optimal resistance of the prosthesis to the mechanical stress in the scapular girdle by reducing the stress-shielding effect while also ensuring no inflammatory responses and stimulating of osteogenesis [24,141].

It is interesting to note that bones not subjected to high mechanical stress as those in the shoulder girdle are replaced by 3D-printed prostheses made of materials with weaker mechanical results than titanium or PEEK but which present properties closer to the bone as well as enhanced bioactive and osteogenic capacities, such as hydroxyapatite, β-TCP, or PLLA.

PEEK presents numerous qualities and functionality when used in the construction of a prosthesis [24], and in the past few years, research teams are striving to develop and use polymers instead of metals. Scaphoid prostheses were designed and 3D-printed using a PEEK medical filament to demonstrate the effectiveness of the printing from a financial point of view and to showcase the ease with which a construct can be built specifically to the patient's needs [142].

The bioactivity problem of the titanium alloy in tibial defects was addressed in a study using additional bioceramic granules made from β-TCP for osteoinductive activity promotion and enhanced metabolic activity [143]. In these cases, patients aged 13 or younger who presented with an osteosarcoma-induced defect in the tibial bone were subjected to bone replacement with biocompatible and bioactive titanium-bioceramic prostheses, and all the patients healed properly and had no relapse [143]. Compared to cases of critical long bone defects, the authors of this study managed to use an integrated polymer in metal prostheses in a human body; given the young age of the patients, it can be concluded that this method overcame many drawbacks that were considered great challenges for the future of 3D bioprinting in orthopedics.

To demonstrate the effectiveness of polymers, the behavior of these prostheses in joints must be assessed to adequately evaluate the interaction with the surrounding tissues and to eliminate the risks of bone damage or mechanical failure; these complications are less likely to occur in the case of 3D-printed metallic parts.

We present below a compilation of comprehensive information on the technical features of various biomaterials and the devices used in bioprinting along their physical properties (Table 1).

**Table 1.** Characteristics of various bones manufactured with biomaterials using 3D bioprinting.

| Body Part | 3D Printing Technology | Biocompatible Material | Compatible 3D Printer | Properties and Mentions | Reference |
| --- | --- | --- | --- | --- | --- |
| | | | **Bones of the Upper Limb** | | |
| Clavicle | SLA | PEEK | For guiding plate—UP BOX+ 3D printer (Beijing Tiertime Technology Co, Ltd., Beijing, China); | - Low Young's modulus;<br>- Reduced stress-shielding effect;<br>- Biological strength;<br>- Smooth surface; | [141] |
| | EBM | Ti | EBM S12 system (Arcam AB, Mölndal, Sweden) | - High Young's modulus: 110 GPa in comparison with cortical bone: 7–30 GPa;<br>- High stress-shielding effect;<br>- Satisfactory shoulder function and satisfactory ROM: flexion 90°, extension 35°, abduction 80°; | [69] |
| Scapula | EBM | Ti | EBM S12 system (Arcam AB, Mölndal, Sweden) | - High Young's modulus: 110 GPa in comparison with cortical bone: 7–30 GPa;<br>- High stress-shielding effect; | [69] |
| | EBM | Titanium alloy ($TiAl_6V_4$)-Epore | Provided by MUTARS® (Implantcast GmbH, Buxtehude, Germany) | - Porosity: 60%;<br>- Rod thickness: 330–390 μm;<br>- Young's modulus: 3 GPa<br>- Satisfactory shoulder function and ROM; | [79] |
| | FFF | PEEK (polyether-ether-ketone) | Surgeon 200, Jugao-AM, Xi'an, China | - von Mises stress: 22.6 MPa;<br>- Layer thickness: 0.2 mm;<br>- Printing speed: 40 mm/s;<br>- Nozzle temperature: 420 °C;<br>- Density: 1.28–1.32 g/cm$^3$;<br>- Flexural modulus: 3 GPa;<br>- Flexural strength: 110 MPa;<br>- Thermal conductivity: 0.29 W/m/K$^5$. | [140] |
| Humerus | EBM | Titanium alloy with 6% aluminum and 4% vanadium | Not mentioned | Not mentioned | [95] |
| | EBM | Titanium alloy ($TiAl_6V_4$) | Chunli®, Beijing, China | - Pore size: 500 μm;<br>- Porosity rate: 60%. | [96] |
| Ulna/Radius | EBM | Titanium alloy with 6% aluminum and 4% vanadium | Not mentioned | Not mentioned | [95] |
| | EFD-Robocasting | β-Tricalcium Phosphate coated with dipyridamole | EDF Inc., Nordson, Westlake, USA, OH-3D direct-write-micro printer system | - Pore size: 350 μm;<br>- Nozzle diameter: 250 μm;<br>- Dipyramidole coating concentration: 1000 μM; | [40] |

**Table 1.** *Cont.*

| Body Part | 3D Printing Technology | Biocompatible Material | Compatible 3D Printer | Properties and Mentions | Reference |
|---|---|---|---|---|---|
| Ulna/Radius | Bioprinting | PLLA (Resomer L-206, Boehringer Ingelheim Pharma KG, Ingelheim, Germany) | 3D Bioprinter INVIVO 4D2. ROKIT Healthcare, Seoul, Korea | - Compression strength: 80 ± 10 MPa;<br>- PLLA molecular weight: 100,000 g/mol;<br>- Nozzle diameter: 200 μm;<br>- Extrusion temperature: 200 °C;<br>- Ejection pressure: 200–300 kPa;<br>- Pore size: 480 ± 10 μm;<br>- Grid thickness: 187 ± 2 0 μm;<br>- Porosity: 82%;<br>- Compressive strengths: 100 MPa. | [41] |
| Carpals, Metacarpals, Phalanges | EBM | Tantalum | UP BOX, Beijing Tiertime Technology Co., Ltd., Beijing, China | - Grip strength 33.4 ± 2.3 kg;<br>- Pinch strength 8.9 ± 0.7 kg;<br>- Flexion: 54.6° ± 0.8°;<br>- Dorsiflexion: 54.7° ± 1.7°;<br>- Ulnar deviation: 34.6° ± 1.9°;<br>- Radial deviation: 25.9° ± 0.8°;<br>- High porosity: 75%;<br>- Low Young's modulus;<br>- High coefficient of friction;<br>- Thickness: 3.5–4 mm; | [118] |
| | FFF | PEEK (polyether-ether-ketone) | Apium M220 (Apium Additive Technologies GmbH, Karlsruhe, Germany) | - Nozzle diameter: 0.4 mm;<br>- Density: 1.30 g/cm$^3$;<br>- Melting temperature: 340 °C. | [142] |
| | EBM | Titanium alloy ($TiAl_6V_4$) | Shanghai Shenghsi Medical Devices Co., Ltd.; 3D printer—Arcam A1; Arcam, Mölndal, Sweden | Not mentioned | [119] |
| | EBM | Titanium | Not mentioned | Not mentioned | [120] |
| **Bones of the Lower Limb** | | | | | |
| Femur | EBM | Titanium alloy ($TiAl_6V_4$) | Not mentioned | - Pore size: 500 μm;<br>- Porosity: 70%;<br>- Young's modulus—porous titanium alloy: 1500 MPa; solid titanium alloy: 110,000 MPa;<br>- Poisson's ratio: 0.30;<br>- Displacement value in the lateral femoral condyle: varied from 0.01–0.07 mm ≈ 0.01 mm to 0.04 mm. | [134] |

Table 1. *Cont.*

| Body Part | 3D Printing Technology | Biocompatible Material | Compatible 3D Printer | Properties and Mentions | Reference |
|---|---|---|---|---|---|
| Tibia and fibula | SLM | Titanium alloy ($TiAl_6V_4$) | Arcam EBM, Gothenburg, Sweden | - Young's modulus: 1200 ± 48 MPa;<br>- Porosity: 68%;<br>- Pore size: 625 ± 70 μm;<br>- Poisson's ratio: 0.34; | [137] |
| | SLM | Titanium alloy ($TiAl_6V_4$) and β-TCP particles added | Xi'an Bright Laser Technology Co., Ltd. (Xi'an, China) | - Pore diameter bioceramic granules: 500–600 μm;<br>- Diameter of the granules: 1.5–3 mm;<br>- Average operation time: 85–385 min;<br>- Young's modulus: 110 GPa. | [143] |

SLA = Stereo-lithography; EBM = Electron beam melting; FFF = Fused Filament Fabrication; SLM = Selective Laser Melting; EFD = Electric Field Driven; PLLA = Poly-L-lactic acid; PEEK = Polyether–Ether–Ketone; Ti = Titanium; β-TCP = β-Tricalcium Phosphate; ROM = Range of Motion.

### 2.4. Fixation Methods of the Prostheses in the Affected Limb and Future Approaches

One of the greatest challenges in replacing an entire bone with a 3D-printed build, besides biocompatibility and ensuring the desired biological activity, is finding a mechanism to anchor the prosthesis to maintain limb functionality. Thus, in the case of a scapular defect resulting in bone replacement, an electron beam melting 3D-printed titanium scapula was stabilized around the patient's clavicle with a non-absorbable wrap and anchored to the ligaments and bone processes in the small orifices that the prosthesis, as well as the bone, provide [69].

Different parts of the shoulder girdle could be developed using 3D bioprinting as long as a mechanism of fixation is designed, representing a great potential for the replacement of an entire shoulder girdle in the future [144,145]. However, given the complexity of the muscular joint complex of the shoulder girdle, numerous other fixation elements should be added. Current research is centered on the fixation elements of prostheses, with numerous studies proposing holes or anchors where muscles and ligaments can be fixed [146–149]. However, the prostheses are rigid, have surfaces with high friction, and lack softness [150–152]. An optimal fixation needs to extend beyond wire or other materials to just bind the anatomical elements that sustain the bone. Future research should approach different methods to coat the areas of fixation with elastic, resistant, and bioactive materials to ensure an area closer to the biologically active tissue of the body, and this is the case, especially for metal-based prostheses.

One study managed to overcome the technical challenge of the biocompatible materials used (i.e., the high melting point of tantalum: 2996 °C) and managed to build and place a porous tantalum prosthesis designed with peripheral fixation holes as anchor points for the surrounding tendons and muscles, ensuring the comfort of movement and highly efficient biomechanical mobility [118]. Designing numerous holes in the 3D-printed construct might act as a mechanical destabilizer of the construction; however, they are mandatory for the proper implementation of the prosthesis (Figure 4). Nevertheless, a balance between the dimension of the holes and their frequency in the build needs to be identified to ensure the patients with mobility in all the ranges of motion and no rigidity while not interfering with the mechanical properties of the prosthesis [153–155].

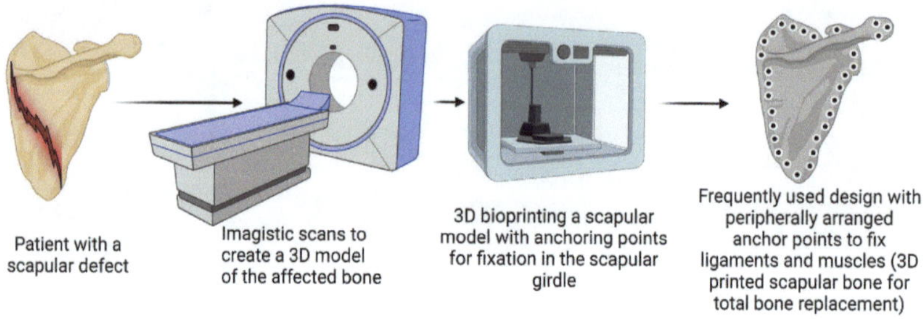


**Figure 4.** Illustration of a design that could be used for creating anchoring points in total bone prostheses. Created in BioRender. Timofticiuc, I. (2024) BioRender.com/q54g477, date of last access—12 October 2024.

For example, the main challenge in saving the functions of the fingers is the fixation of the prostheses at the site of the implantation, and the solution requires the design of anchoring holes and proper positioning to imitate the physiological anchoring points of the tendons and muscles [118,153–155]. Studying the fixation methods in other research, we can observe that many holes are generally designed as anchoring points, but ways to eliminate any risk of complications and to reduce the mechanical frictions of metal–bone tissue interaction need to be identified. Also, no prostheses made entirely from biopolymers are yet reported in humans, a situation that could change in the future.

For total replacement of the clavicle with titanium, the fixation in the scapular girdle is more challenging, therefore ensuring that the titanium model has porosities is essential for the fixation with resorbable wire on the clavicle ligaments [69]. Prosthesis fixation can be satisfactory using muscles and tendons as fixation points; however, the extended manufacturing time and expensive production also need to be considered [95].

Bone prostheses can yield great results in different regions of the body when using adequate materials to meet the specific mechanical properties required, but a few challenges still exist and should be approached by future studies such as designing fixation elements and controlling the tendency of these materials to induce osteogenesis and angiogenesis, which may produce long-term defects at the site of the intervention if overamplified.

## 3. Innovations and Future Directions in 3D Bioprinting for Limb Salvage Surgery

With the input of 3D printing in medical activity, the possibility of creating patient-specific constructs increased exponentially [156]. Once the 3D technologies such as extrusion-based 3D bioprinting, inkjet-based 3D bioprinting, laser-assisted 3D bioprinting, and stereolithographic-based 3D bioprinting developed [133], using viable cells in printed scaffolds has introduced transformative innovations in the surgery field by offering the possibility to fabricate biological active parts that mimic the mechanical and physiological characteristics of the native tissues [157]. For example, it was shown that skin can be either 3D bioprinted at the site of the skin defect or bioprinted separately as a scaffold that can be transplanted after postprocessing in a bioreactor. Given the two possibilities, printing in situ was the optimal, cost-effective solution for different skin injuries due to the controlled evolution of the print in time at the site of the trauma [158].

Innovative for limb salvage surgery is the ability to design parts made of biomaterials with properties that enable osteogenesis and angiogenesis. Furthermore, advances in 3D bioprinting allowed the integration of viable cells in special mixtures called bioinks, thus accelerating the reparative events and integration with the native tissue, which was not possible before the 3D printing input [15]. Besides classical 3D printing of silk fibroin, there are mentions of silk also used as a bioink for 3D bioprinting, also known as "silk-inks" [159]. In a study where silk ink was mixed with different enzymes, gold nanoparticles, or various antibiotics, and printed directly in a Petri dish, it was shown that the scaffold is capable of mineralization while protecting itself from bacteria, thus explaining how silk can be a great candidate for use in a human body, but especially for osteogenesis [160].

Although the results are promising, many challenges persist. The incorporation of viable cells is limited within the scaffolds, and many of the cells used are still in experimental stages [161]. Additionally, the biological activity of the constructs is limited to the number of cells included in the scaffold build [162]. Using excessive viable cells in different limb parts can lead to defective mechanical behavior, especially for weight-bearing applications [163].

Current applications of 3D printing in limb salvage surgery are titanium- and polymer-based prostheses [164,165]. Although there are no reported studies where viable cells are directly incorporated in the titanium build, the bioactive properties of a titanium construct were enhanced by coating it with 3D-bioprinted cell-laden hydrogels [166]. Without affecting the surface of the titanium construct, an enhanced interaction with cells and proteins that promotes differentiation and mineralization was established [166]. While the constructs do not include viable cells, they serve as a precursor to bioprinting applications, with the condition of finding the optimal viable cell composition to not interfere with the mechanical structure of the limb parts printed. This highlights the fact that 3D printing usually addresses structural and mechanical needs, with less focus on bioactive needs, while 3D bioprinting mainly addresses the need for biofunctionality in the parts that are created. Combining these approaches could be the bridge to the next era of medical activity, especially in this category of patients [133]. Future directions include refining bioprinting technologies, enhancing the mechanical aspects of fully bioprinted constructs, and also optimizing the design to better support angiogenesis and nerve regeneration, but also to address the costs that these techniques include [133,167,168]. The roadmap to achieving these goals, in our view, is by making hybrid parts that combine the mechanical stability of simple 3D-printed parts with the biological activity of other softer materials such as polymers used also in classical 3D printing and the biological activity of 3D-bioprinted scaffolds. By adapting these technologies, bioprinting can evolve into a comprehensive tool for limb salvage surgery.

## 4. Conclusions

The literature on 3D bioprinting in limb salvage surgery on the lower limb is scarce compared to studies on the upper limb. This might be due to already perfected solutions of prefabricated prostheses for the lower limb; however, upper limb injuries do not benefit from similar solutions. Partial restorative surgeries or bone replacements can be managed with fewer complications compared to the previous decade, leaving room for further development of material characteristics and properties while improving 3D printing techniques and devices.

Many studies show the possibility of creating bioprinted compounds with various viable human cells. Additionally, many studies report various in vitro studies of how these different cells interact with human-like scaffolds. In our view, the innovation and also the solution for the still rapid development of the merged field of 3D printing and medicine is by creating hybrid constructs that can ensure mechanical properties, functional and biofunctional characteristics, and also builds that promote optimal integration with less to no side effects in patients.

Bioprinting overlaps in many ways with classical orthopedic approaches but has the opportunity to provide additional benefits, advantages, and functionality to the builds, showing tremendous potential for the future of limb salvage surgery. The perspective of building constructs besides bioactive bone prostheses that mimic muscles, nerves, and other tissues is one of the reasons for the extensive research conducted in this promising field that holds the potential for identifying the optimal balance for building full-functionality limb prostheses, the ultimate goal of limb salvage surgeries—the possibility of replacing an entire limb, regardless of the disease or trauma that the patients suffer from.

**Author Contributions:** Conceptualization, I.-A.T., A.C., C.C. and C.S.; methodology, S.D., A.-E.S., N.D.G. and C.S.; resources, I.-A.T., I.A.B. and A.C.D.; writing—original draft preparation, I.-A.T., S.D., A.C., A.-E.S., I.A.B., N.D.G., A.C.D., C.C. and C.S.; writing—review and editing, I.A.B., A.C.D., C.C. and C.S.; visualization, I.-A.T.; supervision, A.C.D., C.C. and C.S. All authors have read and agreed to the published version of the manuscript.

**Funding:** This research received no external funding.

**Data Availability Statement:** No new data were created or analyzed in this study. Data sharing is not applicable to this article.

**Conflicts of Interest:** The authors declare no conflicts of interest.

## References

1. Lääperi, T.; Pohjolainen, T.; Alaranta, H.; Kärkkäinen, M. Lower-limb amputations. *Ann. Chir. Gynaecol.* **1993**, *82*, 183–187. [PubMed]
2. Nosalski, R.; Guzik, T.J. Perivascular adipose tissue inflammation in vascular disease. *Br. J. Pharmacol.* **2017**, *174*, 3496–3513. [CrossRef]
3. Kirilova, M.; Klein, A.; Lindner, L.H.; Nachbichler, S.; Knösel, T.; Birkenmaier, C.; Baur-Melnyk, A.; Dürr, H.R. Amputation for extremity sarcoma: Indications and outcomes. *Cancers* **2021**, *13*, 5125. [CrossRef] [PubMed]
4. Pezzin, L.E.; Dillingham, T.R.; MacKenzie, E.J. Rehabilitation and the long-term outcomes of persons with trauma-related amputations. *Arch. Phys. Med. Rehabil.* **2000**, *81*, 292–300. [CrossRef] [PubMed]
5. Kadam, D. Limb salvage surgery. *Indian J. Plast. Surg. Off. Publ. Assoc. Plast. Surg. India* **2013**, *46*, 265. [CrossRef]
6. Fortington, L.V.; Geertzen, J.H.; van Netten, J.J.; Postema, K.; Rommers, G.M.; Dijkstra, P.U. Short and long term mortality rates after a lower limb amputation. *Eur. J. Vasc. Endovasc. Surg.* **2013**, *46*, 124–131. [CrossRef]
7. Mohamed, J.; Reetz, D.; van de Meent, H.; Schreuder, H.; Frölke, J.P.; Leijendekkers, R. What Are the Risk Factors for Mechanical Failure and Loosening of a Transfemoral Osseointegrated Implant System in Patients with a Lower-limb Amputation? *Clin. Orthop. Relat. Res.* **2022**, *480*, 722–731. [CrossRef] [PubMed]
8. Bäcker, H.C.; Wu, C.H.; Kienzle, A.; Perka, C.; Gwinner, C. Mechanical failure of total hip arthroplasties and associated risk factors. *Arch. Orthop. Trauma Surg.* **2023**, *143*, 1061–1069. [CrossRef] [PubMed]
9. Toh, R.X.; Yeo, Z.N.; Liow, M.H.L.; Yeo, S.J.; Lo, N.N.; Chen, J.Y. Debridement, Antibiotics, and Implant Retention in Periprosthetic Joint Infection: What Predicts Success or Failure? *J. Arthroplast.* **2021**, *36*, 3562–3569. [CrossRef] [PubMed]
10. Feng, Y.; Zhu, S.; Mei, D.; Li, J.; Zhang, J.; Yang, S.; Guan, S. Application of 3D Printing Technology in Bone Tissue Engineering: A Review. *Curr. Drug Deliv.* **2021**, *18*, 847–861. [CrossRef]
11. Fleischhacker, E.; Sprecher, C.M.; Milz, S.; Saller, M.M.; Gleich, J.; Siebenbürger, G.; Helfen, T.; Böcker, W.; Ockert, B. Functional outcomes before and after implant removal in patients with posttraumatic shoulder stiffness and healed proximal humerus fractures: Does implant material (PEEK vs. titanium) have an impact?—A pilot study. *BMC Musculoskelet. Disord.* **2022**, *23*, 95. [CrossRef]
12. Choi, J.; Lee, E.J.; Jang, W.B.; Kwon, S.-M. Development of Biocompatible 3D-Printed Artificial Blood Vessels through Multidimensional Approaches. *J. Funct. Biomater.* **2023**, *14*, 497. [CrossRef] [PubMed]
13. Kong, Z.; Wang, X. Bioprinting technologies and bioinks for vascular model establishment. *Int. J. Mol. Sci.* **2023**, *24*, 891. [CrossRef] [PubMed]
14. Tharakan, S.; Khondkar, S.; Ilyas, A. Bioprinting of stem cells in multimaterial scaffolds and their applications in bone tissue engineering. *Sensors* **2021**, *21*, 7477. [CrossRef] [PubMed]
15. Gungor-Ozkerim, P.S.; Inci, I.; Zhang, Y.S.; Khademhosseini, A.; Dokmeci, M.R. Bioinks for 3D bioprinting: An overview. *Biomater. Sci.* **2018**, *6*, 915–946. [CrossRef]
16. Fang, Y.; Guo, Y.; Liu, T.; Xu, R.; Mao, S.; Mo, X.; Zhang, T.; Ouyang, L.; Xiong, Z.; Sun, W. Advances in 3D bioprinting. *Chin. J. Mech. Eng. Addit. Manuf. Front.* **2022**, *1*, 100011. [CrossRef]
17. Dey, M.; Ozbolat, I.T. 3D bioprinting of cells, tissues and organs. *Sci. Rep.* **2020**, *10*, 14023. [CrossRef] [PubMed]
18. Sun, W.; Starly, B.; Daly, A.C.; Burdick, J.A.; Groll, J.; Skeldon, G.; Shu, W.; Sakai, Y.; Shinohara, M.; Nishikawa, M. The bioprinting roadmap. *Biofabrication* **2020**, *12*, 022002. [CrossRef] [PubMed]
19. Lemons, J.; Lucas, L. Properties of biomaterials. *J. Arthroplast.* **1986**, *1*, 143–147. [CrossRef]
20. Mei, J.; Zhu, X.-Z.; Wang, Z.-Y.; Cai, X.-S. Functional outcomes and quality of life in patients with osteosarcoma treated with amputation versus limb-salvage surgery: A systematic review and meta-analysis. *Arch. Orthop. Trauma Surg.* **2014**, *134*, 1507–1516. [CrossRef] [PubMed]
21. Chen, G.; Yin, Y.; Chen, C. Limb-salvage surgery using personalized 3D-printed porous tantalum prosthesis for distal radial osteosarcoma: A case report. *Medicine* **2021**, *100*, e27899. [CrossRef] [PubMed]
22. Park, J.W.; Jung, S.H.; Yang, J.H.; Kim, J.H.; Oh, S.E.; Kang, H.G. Whole blood titanium concentration after limb salvage surgery with three-dimensional-printed Ti6Al4V implants. *Clin. Orthop. Surg.* **2023**, *15*, 864. [CrossRef] [PubMed]

23. Rezvani Ghomi, E.; Nourbakhsh, N.; Akbari Kenari, M.; Zare, M.; Ramakrishna, S. Collagen-based biomaterials for biomedical applications. *J. Biomed. Mater. Res. Part B Appl. Biomater.* **2021**, *109*, 1986–1999. [CrossRef]
24. Timofticiuc, I.-A.; Călinescu, O.; Iftime, A.; Dragosloveanu, S.; Caruntu, A.; Scheau, A.-E.; Badarau, I.A.; Didilescu, A.C.; Caruntu, C.; Scheau, C. Biomaterials adapted to VAT photopolymerization in 3D printing: Characteristics and medical applications. *J. Funct. Biomater.* **2023**, *15*, 7. [CrossRef]
25. Estrada, S.A.M.; Armendáriz, I.O.; García, A.T.; Paz, J.F.H.; González, C.A.R. Evaluation of in vitro bioactivity of 45S5 bioactive glass/poly lactic acid scaffolds produced by 3D printing. *Int. J. Compos. Mater.* **2017**, *7*, 144–149.
26. Nasiri, G.; Ahmadi, S.; Shahbazi, M.-A.; Nosrati-Siahmazgi, V.; Fatahi, Y.; Dinarvand, R.; Rabiee, M.; Haftlang, F.; Kim, H.S.; Rabiee, N. 3D printing of bioactive materials for drug delivery applications. *Expert Opin. Drug Deliv.* **2022**, *19*, 1061–1080. [CrossRef] [PubMed]
27. Jin, W.; Chu, P.K. Orthopedic implants. *Encycl. Biomed. Eng.* **2019**, *1*, 425–439.
28. Wu, C.A.; Zhu, Y.; Woo, Y.J. Advances in 3D bioprinting: Techniques, applications, and future directions for cardiac tissue engineering. *Bioengineering* **2023**, *10*, 842. [CrossRef]
29. Du, X.; Wei, D.; Huang, L.; Zhu, M.; Zhang, Y.; Zhu, Y. 3D printing of mesoporous bioactive glass/silk fibroin composite scaffolds for bone tissue engineering. *Mater. Sci. Eng. C* **2019**, *103*, 109731. [CrossRef]
30. Wei, L.; Wu, S.; Kuss, M.; Jiang, X.; Sun, R.; Reid, P.; Qin, X.; Duan, B. 3D printing of silk fibroin-based hybrid scaffold treated with platelet rich plasma for bone tissue engineering. *Bioact. Mater.* **2019**, *4*, 256–260. [CrossRef] [PubMed]
31. Sun, W.; Gregory, D.A.; Tomeh, M.A.; Zhao, X. Silk fibroin as a functional biomaterial for tissue engineering. *Int. J. Mol. Sci.* **2021**, *22*, 1499. [CrossRef] [PubMed]
32. Wang, Q.; Han, G.; Yan, S.; Zhang, Q. 3D printing of silk fibroin for biomedical applications. *Materials* **2019**, *12*, 504. [CrossRef]
33. Lin, D.; Li, M.; Wang, L.; Cheng, J.; Yang, Y.; Wang, H.; Ye, J.; Liu, Y. Multifunctional hydrogel based on silk fibroin promotes tissue repair and regeneration. *Adv. Funct. Mater.* **2024**, *34*, 2405255. [CrossRef]
34. Rastogi, P.; Kandasubramanian, B. Review of alginate-based hydrogel bioprinting for application in tissue engineering. *Biofabrication* **2019**, *11*, 042001. [CrossRef]
35. Gonzalez-Fernandez, T.; Tenorio, A.J.; Campbell, K.T.; Silva, E.A.; Leach, J.K. Alginate-based bioinks for 3D bioprinting and fabrication of anatomically accurate bone grafts. *Tissue Eng. Part A* **2021**, *27*, 1168–1181. [CrossRef]
36. Moncal, K.K.; Ozbolat, V.; Datta, P.; Heo, D.N.; Ozbolat, I.T. Thermally-controlled extrusion-based bioprinting of collagen. *J. Mater. Sci. Mater. Med.* **2019**, *30*, 55. [CrossRef]
37. Liu, G.; Chen, J.; Wang, X.; Liu, Y.; Ma, Y.; Tu, X. Functionalized 3D-printed ST2/gelatin methacryloyl/polcaprolactone scaffolds for enhancing bone regeneration with vascularization. *Int. J. Mol. Sci.* **2022**, *23*, 8347. [CrossRef]
38. Amenorfe, L.P.; Agorku, E.S.; Sarpong, F.; Voegborlo, R.B. Innovative exploration of additive incorporated biopolymer-based composites. *Sci. Afr.* **2022**, *17*, e01359. [CrossRef]
39. Barré-Sinoussi, F.; Montagutelli, X. Animal models are essential to biological research: Issues and perspectives. *Future Sci. OA* **2015**, *1*, FSO63. [CrossRef]
40. Witek, L.; Alifarag, A.M.; Tovar, N.; Lopez, C.D.; Cronstein, B.N.; Rodriguez, E.D.; Coelho, P.G. Repair of critical-sized long bone defects using dipyridamole-augmented 3D-printed bioactive ceramic scaffolds. *J. Orthop. Res.* **2019**, *37*, 2499–2507. [CrossRef]
41. Hong, Y.R.; Kim, T.-H.; Lee, K.; Lim, J.O.; Oh, C.-W. Bioactive bone substitute in a rabbit ulna model: Preclinical study. *Tissue Eng. Regen. Med.* **2023**, *20*, 1205–1217. [CrossRef] [PubMed]
42. Zhao, H.; Shen, S.; Zhao, L.; Xu, Y.; Li, Y.; Zhuo, N. 3D printing of dual-cell delivery titanium alloy scaffolds for improving osseointegration through enhancing angiogenesis and osteogenesis. *BMC Musculoskelet. Disord.* **2021**, *22*, 734. [CrossRef]
43. Rajendran, S.; Palani, G.; Kanakaraj, A.; Shanmugam, V.; Veerasimman, A.; Gądek, S.; Korniejenko, K.; Marimuthu, U. Metal and polymer based composites manufactured using additive manufacturing—A brief review. *Polymers* **2023**, *15*, 2564. [CrossRef] [PubMed]
44. Lauer, A.; Wolf, P.; Mehler, D.; Götz, H.; Rüzgar, M.; Baranowski, A.; Henrich, D.; Rommens, P.M.; Ritz, U. Biofabrication of SDF-1 functionalized 3D-printed cell-free scaffolds for bone tissue regeneration. *Int. J. Mol. Sci.* **2020**, *21*, 2175. [CrossRef]
45. Yang, Y.; Chu, L.; Yang, S.; Zhang, H.; Qin, L.; Guillaume, O.; Eglin, D.; Richards, R.G.; Tang, T. Dual-functional 3D-printed composite scaffold for inhibiting bacterial infection and promoting bone regeneration in infected bone defect models. *Acta Biomater.* **2018**, *79*, 265–275. [CrossRef] [PubMed]
46. Ma, L.; Cheng, S.; Ji, X.; Zhou, Y.; Zhang, Y.; Li, Q.; Tan, C.; Peng, F.; Zhang, Y.; Huang, W. Immobilizing magnesium ions on 3D printed porous tantalum scaffolds with polydopamine for improved vascularization and osteogenesis. *Mater. Sci. Eng. C* **2020**, *117*, 111303. [CrossRef] [PubMed]
47. Wang, W.; Liu, P.; Zhang, B.; Gui, X.; Pei, X.; Song, P.; Yu, X.; Zhang, Z.; Zhou, C. Fused Deposition Modeling Printed PLA/Nano β-TCP Composite Bone Tissue Engineering Scaffolds for Promoting Osteogenic Induction Function. *Int. J. Nanomed.* **2023**, *18*, 5815–5830. [CrossRef]
48. Zheng, P.; Yao, Q.; Mao, F.; Liu, N.; Xu, Y.; Wei, B.; Wang, L. Adhesion, proliferation and osteogenic differentiation of mesenchymal stem cells in 3D printed poly-ε-caprolactone/hydroxyapatite scaffolds combined with bone marrow clots. *Mol. Med. Rep.* **2017**, *16*, 5078–5084. [CrossRef]
49. Wafi, A.; Kolli, V.; Azhar, B.; Poole, G.; Budge, J.; Moxey, P.; Loftus, I.; Holt, P. Amputation of the Unsalvageable Leg in Vascular Patients with Cancer. *Vasc. Endovasc. Surg.* **2023**, *57*, 697–705. [CrossRef]

50. Bradley, J.A.; Bellon, J.R. Quality of Life and Limb: Reducing Lymphedema Risk After Breast Cancer Therapy. *Int. J. Radiat. Oncol. Biol. Phys.* **2020**, *106*, 225–229. [CrossRef] [PubMed]
51. Tampa, M.; Georgescu, S.R.; Mitran, C.I.; Mitran, M.I.; Matei, C.; Scheau, C.; Constantin, C.; Neagu, M. Recent Advances in Signaling Pathways Comprehension as Carcinogenesis Triggers in Basal Cell Carcinoma. *J. Clin. Med.* **2020**, *9*, 3010. [CrossRef] [PubMed]
52. Bryce, Y.; Emmanuel, A., Jr.; Agrusa, C.; Ziv, E.; Harnain, C.; Huq, S.; Martin, E.S. Acute limb ischemia in a cancer patient has high morbidity, high mortality, and atypical presentation: A tertiary cancer center's retrospective study. *BMC Cancer* **2021**, *21*, 916. [CrossRef]
53. Oh, G.-W.; Nguyen, V.-T.; Heo, S.-Y.; Ko, S.-C.; Kim, C.S.; Park, W.S.; Choi, I.-W.; Jung, W.-K. 3D PCL/fish collagen composite scaffolds incorporating osteogenic abalone protein hydrolysates for bone regeneration application: In vitro and in vivo studies. *J. Biomater. Sci. Polym. Ed.* **2021**, *32*, 355–371. [CrossRef] [PubMed]
54. Bodnárová, S.; Gromošová, S.; Hudák, R.; Rosocha, J.; Živčák, J.; Plšíková, J.; Vojtko, M.; Tóth, T.; Harvanová, D.; Ižariková, G. 3D printed Polylactid Acid based porous scaffold for bone tissue engineering: An in vitro study. *Acta Bioeng. Biomech.* **2019**, *21*, 101–110. [CrossRef] [PubMed]
55. Liu, H.; Li, W.; Liu, C.; Tan, J.; Wang, H.; Hai, B.; Cai, H.; Leng, H.-J.; Liu, Z.-J.; Song, C.-L. Incorporating simvastatin/poloxamer 407 hydrogel into 3D-printed porous Ti6Al4V scaffolds for the promotion of angiogenesis, osseointegration and bone ingrowth. *Biofabrication* **2016**, *8*, 045012. [CrossRef]
56. Jamalpour, M.R.; Yadegari, A.; Vahdatinia, F.; Amirabad, L.M.; Jamshidi, S.; Shojaei, S.; Shokri, A.; Moeinifard, E.; Omidi, M.; Tayebi, L. 3D-printed bi-layered polymer/hydrogel construct for interfacial tissue regeneration in a canine model. *Dent. Mater.* **2022**, *38*, 1316–1329. [CrossRef] [PubMed]
57. El-Habashy, S.E.; El-Kamel, A.H.; Essawy, M.M.; Abdelfattah, E.-Z.A.; Eltaher, H.M. Engineering 3D-printed core–shell hydrogel scaffolds reinforced with hybrid hydroxyapatite/polycaprolactone nanoparticles for in vivo bone regeneration. *Biomater. Sci.* **2021**, *9*, 4019–4039. [CrossRef]
58. Teotia, A.K.; Dienel, K.; Qayoom, I.; van Bochove, B.; Gupta, S.; Partanen, J.; Seppälä, J.; Kumar, A. Improved bone regeneration in rabbit bone defects using 3D printed composite scaffolds functionalized with osteoinductive factors. *ACS Appl. Mater. Interfaces* **2020**, *12*, 48340–48356. [CrossRef] [PubMed]
59. Zhang, M.; Zhai, X.; Ma, T.; Huang, Y.; Jin, M.; Yang, H.; Fu, H.; Zhang, S.; Sun, T.; Jin, X. Sequential therapy for bone regeneration by cerium oxide-reinforced 3D-printed bioactive glass scaffolds. *ACS Nano* **2023**, *17*, 4433–4444. [CrossRef] [PubMed]
60. Gerdes, S.; Ramesh, S.; Mostafavi, A.; Tamayol, A.; Rivero, I.V.; Rao, P. Extrusion-based 3D (bio) printed tissue engineering scaffolds: Process–structure–quality relationships. *ACS Biomater. Sci. Eng.* **2021**, *7*, 4694–4717. [CrossRef] [PubMed]
61. Dragosloveanu, S.; Petre, M.A.; Gherghe, M.E.; Nedelea, D.G.; Scheau, C.; Cergan, R. Overall Accuracy of Radiological Digital Planning for Total Hip Arthroplasty in a Specialized Orthopaedics Hospital. *J. Clin. Med.* **2023**, *12*, 4503. [CrossRef] [PubMed]
62. Nordqvist, A.; PETERSSON, C. The incidence of fractures of the clavicle. *Clin. Orthop. Relat. Res. (1976–2007)* **1994**, *300*, 127–132. [CrossRef]
63. Robinson, C.M. Fractures of the clavicle in the adult: Epidemiology and classification. *J. Bone Jt. Surg. Br. Vol.* **1998**, *80*, 476–484. [CrossRef]
64. Marsh, J.; Slongo, T.; Agel, J. Tarsal-metatarsal dislocation (80-C5). Fracture and dislocation classification compendium–2007: Orthopaedic Trauma Association classification, database and outcomes committee. *J. Orthop. Trauma* **2007**, *21*, 126–127.
65. Canadian Orthopaedic Trauma Society. Nonoperative treatment compared with plate fixation of displaced midshaft clavicular fractures. A multicenter, randomized clinical trial. *J. Bone Jt. Surg. Am.* **2007**, *89*, 1–10. [CrossRef]
66. Van der Meijden, O.A.; Gaskill, T.R.; Millett, P.J. Treatment of clavicle fractures: Current concepts review. *J. Shoulder Elb. Surg.* **2012**, *21*, 423–429. [CrossRef]
67. Kim, H.N.; Liu, X.N.; Noh, K.C. Use of a real-size 3D-printed model as a preoperative and intraoperative tool for minimally invasive plating of comminuted midshaft clavicle fractures. *J. Orthop. Surg. Res.* **2015**, *10*, 91. [CrossRef]
68. van Doremalen, R.F.; van der Linde, R.A.; Kootstra, J.J.; van Helden, S.H.; Hekman, E.E. Can 3D-printing avoid discomfort-related implant removal in midshaft clavicle fractures? A four-year follow-up. *Arch. Orthop. Trauma Surg.* **2021**, *141*, 1899–1907. [CrossRef]
69. Fan, H.; Fu, J.; Li, X.; Pei, Y.; Li, X.; Pei, G.; Guo, Z. Implantation of customized 3-D printed titanium prosthesis in limb salvage surgery: A case series and review of the literature. *World J. Surg. Oncol.* **2015**, *13*, 308. [CrossRef]
70. Chen, W.; Xu, K.; Tao, B.; Dai, L.; Yu, Y.; Mu, C.; Shen, X.; Hu, Y.; He, Y.; Cai, K. Multilayered coating of titanium implants promotes coupled osteogenesis and angiogenesis in vitro and in vivo. *Acta Biomater.* **2018**, *74*, 489–504. [CrossRef] [PubMed]
71. Shen, X.; Shukla, P. A Review of Titanium Based Orthopaedic Implants (Part-I): Physical Characteristics, Problems and the need for Surface Modification. *Int. J. Peen. Sci. Technol.* **2020**, *1*, 301–332.
72. Cole, P.A.; Freeman, G.; Dubin, J.R. Scapula fractures. *Curr. Rev. Musculoskelet. Med.* **2013**, *6*, 79–87. [CrossRef]
73. Puchner, S.E.; Panotopoulos, J.; Puchner, R.; Schuh, R.; Windhager, R.; Funovics, P.T. Primary malignant tumours of the scapula—A review of 29 cases. *Int. Orthop.* **2014**, *38*, 2155–2162. [CrossRef]
74. Houdek, M.T.; Wilke, B.K.; Barlow, J.D. Management of scapular tumors. *Orthop. Clin.* **2023**, *54*, 101–108. [CrossRef]
75. Guo, Q.; Li, X.; Tang, Y.; Huang, Y.; Luo, L. Augmented reality and three-dimensional plate library-assisted posterior minimally invasive surgery for scapula fracture. *Int. Orthop.* **2022**, *46*, 875–882. [CrossRef] [PubMed]

76. Luo, G.; Zhang, Y.; Wang, X.; Chen, S.; Li, D.; Yu, M. Individualized 3D printing-assisted repair and reconstruction of neoplastic bone defects at irregular bone sites: Exploration and practice in the treatment of scapular aneurysmal bone cysts. *BMC Musculoskelet. Disord.* **2021**, *22*, 984. [CrossRef]
77. Yung, C.S.-Y.; Fang, C.; Fang, E.; Siu, Y.-C.; Yee, D.K.H.; Wong, K.K.-H.; Poon, K.-C.; Leung, M.M.F.; Wan, J.; Lau, T.-W. Surgeon-designed patient-specific instrumentation improves glenoid component screw placement for reverse total shoulder arthroplasty in a population with small glenoid dimensions. *Int. Orthop.* **2023**, *47*, 1267–1275. [CrossRef] [PubMed]
78. Huang, D.; Wang, J.; Ye, Z.; Chen, F.; Liu, H.; Huang, J. Biomechanical study of 3D-printed titanium alloy pad for repairing glenoid bone defect. *J. Orthop. Surg.* **2024**, *32*, 10225536241257169. [CrossRef]
79. Trikoupis, I.G.; Mavrodontis, I.I.; Papadopoulos, D.V.; Goumenos, S.D.; Georgoulis, D.A.; Gavriil, P.; Melissaridou, D.; Savvidou, O.D.; Kontogeorgakos, V.A.; Papagelopoulos, P.J. 3D-printed glenoid implant reconstruction, after partial scapulectomy for malignant tumors: A case series. *Eur. J. Orthop. Surg. Traumatol.* **2024**, *34*, 1557–1562. [CrossRef]
80. Kargozar, S.; Mollazadeh, S.; Kermani, F.; Webster, T.J.; Nazarnezhad, S.; Hamzehlou, S.; Baino, F. Hydroxyapatite Nanoparticles for Improved Cancer Theranostics. *J. Funct. Biomater.* **2022**, *13*, 100. [CrossRef] [PubMed]
81. Scheau, C.; Draghici, C.; Ilie, M.A.; Lupu, M.; Solomon, I.; Tampa, M.; Georgescu, S.R.; Caruntu, A.; Constantin, C.; Neagu, M.; et al. Neuroendocrine Factors in Melanoma Pathogenesis. *Cancers* **2021**, *13*, 2277. [CrossRef] [PubMed]
82. Fornetti, J.; Welm, A.L.; Stewart, S.A. Understanding the Bone in Cancer Metastasis. *J. Bone Miner. Res.* **2018**, *33*, 2099–2113. [CrossRef] [PubMed]
83. Han, W.; El Botty, R.; Montaudon, E.; Malaquin, L.; Deschaseaux, F.; Espagnolle, N.; Marangoni, E.; Cottu, P.; Zalcman, G.; Parrini, M.C.; et al. In vitro bone metastasis dwelling in a 3D bioengineered niche. *Biomaterials* **2021**, *269*, 120624. [CrossRef]
84. Liu, D.; Liang, J.; Yang, H. Combining robotics and 3D printing facilitates closed reduction of humeral shaft fractures using a minimally invasive plate as a reduction template: A proof-of-concept study. *Int. J. Med. Robot. Comput. Assist. Surg.* **2024**, *20*, e2656. [CrossRef] [PubMed]
85. Tilton, M.; Armstrong, A.; Sanville, J.; Chin, M.; Hast, M.W.; Lewis, G.S.; Manogharan, G.P. Biomechanical testing of additive manufactured proximal humerus fracture fixation plates. *Ann. Biomed. Eng.* **2020**, *48*, 463–476. [CrossRef]
86. Hu, C.; Qiu, B.; Cen, C.; Luo, Q.; Cao, Y. 3D printing assisted MIPO for treatment of complex middle-proximal humeral shaft fractures. *BMC Musculoskelet. Disord.* **2024**, *25*, 93. [CrossRef] [PubMed]
87. Li, Z.; Lu, M.; Zhang, Y.; Gong, T.; Wang, J.; Luo, Y.; Zhou, Y.; Min, L.; Tu, C. Computer-aided Design and 3D-printed Personalized Stem-plate Composite for Precision Revision of the Proximal Humerus Endoprosthetic Replacement: A Technique Note. *Orthop. Surg.* **2023**, *15*, 3000–3005. [CrossRef]
88. Ke, S.; Zhang, B.; He, Y.; Zhou, Y.; Hu, X.; Fan, Y.; Wang, M.; Zhang, Y.; Wang, C. Reconstruction Strategy for Upper Extremity Defects After Bone Tumor Resection Based on 3D Customized Bone Cement Mold. *Surg. Innov.* **2024**, *31*, 307–317. [CrossRef]
89. Thomrungpiyathan, T.; Luenam, S.; Lohwongwatana, B.; Sirichativapee, W.; Nabudda, K.; Puncreobutr, C. A custom-made distal humerus plate fabricated by selective laser melting. *Comput. Methods Biomech. Biomed. Eng.* **2021**, *24*, 585–596. [CrossRef] [PubMed]
90. Kim, H.; Chung, Y.-G.; Jang, J.S.; Kim, Y.; Park, S.B.; Song, H.S. Why locking plates for the proximal humerus do not fit well. *Arch. Orthop. Trauma Surg.* **2022**, *142*, 219–226. [CrossRef] [PubMed]
91. Chen, J.; Zhang, W.; Chen, P. Three-dimensional printed bone cement prostheses can be used to treat bone defects in the distal humerus. *JSES Rev. Rep. Tech.* **2022**, *2*, 584–591. [CrossRef]
92. Wang, Q.; Hu, J.; Guan, J.; Chen, Y.; Wang, L. Proximal third humeral shaft fractures fixed with long helical PHILOS plates in elderly patients: Benefit of pre-contouring plates on a 3D-printed model—A retrospective study. *J. Orthop. Surg. Res.* **2018**, *13*, 203. [CrossRef] [PubMed]
93. Shuang, F.; Hu, W.; Shao, Y.; Li, H.; Zou, H. Treatment of intercondylar humeral fractures with 3D-printed osteosynthesis plates. *Medicine* **2016**, *95*, e2461. [CrossRef] [PubMed]
94. Periferakis, A.; Periferakis, A.-T.; Troumpata, L.; Dragosloveanu, S.; Timofticiuc, I.-A.; Georgatos-Garcia, S.; Scheau, A.-E.; Periferakis, K.; Caruntu, A.; Badarau, I.A.; et al. Use of Biomaterials in 3D Printing as a Solution to Microbial Infections in Arthroplasty and Osseous Reconstruction. *Biomimetics* **2024**, *9*, 154. [CrossRef] [PubMed]
95. Ackmann, T.; Klingebiel, S.; Gosheger, G.; Rachbauer, A.; Theil, C.; Andreou, D. Reconstruction of Total Bone Defects following Resection of Malignant Tumors of the Upper Extremity with 3D Printed Prostheses: Presentation of Two Patients with a Follow-Up of Three Years. *Case Rep. Orthop.* **2020**, *2020*, 8822466. [CrossRef]
96. Liang, H.; Guo, W.; Yang, Y.; Li, D.; Yang, R.; Tang, X.; Yan, T. Efficacy and safety of a 3D-printed arthrodesis prosthesis for reconstruction after resection of the proximal humerus: Preliminary outcomes with a minimum 2-year follow-up. *BMC Musculoskelet. Disord.* **2022**, *23*, 635. [CrossRef]
97. Dragosloveanu, S.; Petre, M.A.; Cretu, B.; Mihailescu, A.A.; Cergan, R.; Scheau, C. Etiology of Total Knee Arthroplasty Revisions: A Two-Decade Institutional Perspective. *Cureus* **2024**, *16*, e55263. [CrossRef] [PubMed]
98. Wu, N.; Li, S.; Liu, Y.; Zhang, A.; Chen, B.; Han, Q.; Wang, J. Novel exploration of 3D printed personalized total elbow arthroplasty to solve the severe bone defect after internal fixation failure of comminuted distal humerus fracture: A case report. *Medicine* **2020**, *99*, e21481. [CrossRef] [PubMed]
99. Dragosloveanu, S.; Petre, M.-A.; Gherghe, M.E.; Baz, R.O.; Cergan, R.; Scheau, C. Elbow Reconstruction with Megaprosthesis: An Effective Strategy for Salvage Surgery in Trauma Patients. *Diagnostics* **2024**, *14*, 724. [CrossRef] [PubMed]

100. Hamiti, Y.; Yalikun, A.; Lu, C.; Yusufu, A.; Yushan, M. Ilizarov technique in the treatment of bone defects of the radius and ulna: A systematic review and meta-analysis. *J. Orthop. Surg. Res.* **2023**, *18*, 642. [CrossRef]
101. Sharma, A.; Desando, G.; Petretta, M.; Chawla, S.; Bartolotti, I.; Manferdini, C.; Paolella, F.; Gabusi, E.; Trucco, D.; Ghosh, S. Investigating the role of sustained calcium release in silk-gelatin-based three-dimensional bioprinted constructs for enhancing the osteogenic differentiation of human bone marrow derived mesenchymal stromal cells. *ACS Biomater. Sci. Eng.* **2019**, *5*, 1518–1533. [CrossRef]
102. Axpe, E.; Oyen, M.L. Applications of alginate-based bioinks in 3D bioprinting. *Int. J. Mol. Sci.* **2016**, *17*, 1976. [CrossRef] [PubMed]
103. Theus, A.S.; Ning, L.; Kabboul, G.; Hwang, B.; Tomov, M.L.; LaRock, C.N.; Bauser-Heaton, H.; Mahmoudi, M.; Serpooshan, V. 3D bioprinting of nanoparticle-laden hydrogel scaffolds with enhanced antibacterial and imaging properties. *Iscience* **2022**, *25*, 104947. [CrossRef] [PubMed]
104. Duncan, S.F.; Saracevic, C.E.; Kakinoki, R. Biomechanics of the hand. *Hand Clin.* **2013**, *29*, 483–492. [CrossRef] [PubMed]
105. Wan, S.-x.; Meng, F.-b.; Zhang, J.; Chen, Z.; Yu, L.-b.; Wen, J.-j. Experimental study and preliminary clinical application of mini-invasive percutaneous internal screw fixation for scaphoid fracture under the guidance of a 3D-printed guide plate. *Curr. Med. Sci.* **2019**, *39*, 990–996. [CrossRef] [PubMed]
106. Rong, C.; Zhu, S.; Zhang, Q.; Xu, H.; Zhang, L.; Han, Q. Minimally Invasive Percutaneous Screw Guided by 3-Dimensional–Printed Guide for the Treatment of Scaphoid Fractures. *J. Hand Surg.* **2023**, *48*, 1279.e1–1279.e7. [CrossRef]
107. Chiu, Y.-C.; Ho, T.-Y.; Hsu, C.-E.; Yeh, C.-W.; Ting, Y.-N.; Tsai, M.-T.; Hsu, J.-T. Biomechanical analysis of plate versus K-wire fixation for metacarpal shaft fractures with wedge-shaped bone defects. *BMC Musculoskelet. Disord.* **2024**, *25*, 350. [CrossRef]
108. Chiu, Y.-C.; Hsu, C.-E.; Ho, T.-Y.; Ting, Y.-N.; Wei, B.-H.; Tsai, M.-T.; Hsu, J.-T. Comparison of the fixation ability of headless compression screws and locking plate for metacarpal shaft transverse fracture. *Medicine* **2021**, *100*, e27375. [CrossRef]
109. Chiu, Y.-C.; Ho, T.-Y.; Ting, Y.-N.; Tsai, M.-T.; Huang, H.-L.; Hsu, C.-E.; Hsu, J.-T. Effect of oblique headless compression screw fixation for metacarpal shaft fracture: A biomechanical in vitro study. *BMC Musculoskelet. Disord.* **2021**, *22*, 146. [CrossRef]
110. Chiu, Y.-C.; Hsu, C.-E.; Ho, T.-Y.; Ting, Y.-N.; Tsai, M.-T.; Hsu, J.-T. Bone plate fixation ability on the dorsal and lateral sides of a metacarpal shaft transverse fracture. *J. Orthop. Surg. Res.* **2021**, *16*, 441. [CrossRef] [PubMed]
111. Ho, T.-Y.; Hsu, C.-E.; Wang, W.-C.; Ting, Y.-N.; Tsai, M.-T.; Chiu, Y.-C.; Hsu, J.-T. Biomechanical study of the fixation ability of the dorsal and volar locking plate for transverse metacarpal neck fractures. *Medicine* **2023**, *102*, e34981. [CrossRef]
112. Chiu, Y.-C.; Ho, T.-Y.; Hsu, C.-E.; Ting, Y.-N.; Tsai, M.-T.; Hsu, J.-T. Comparison of the fixation ability between lag screw and bone plate for oblique metacarpal shaft fracture. *J. Orthop. Surg. Res.* **2022**, *17*, 72. [CrossRef]
113. Chiu, Y.-C.; Hsu, C.-E.; Ho, T.-Y.; Ting, Y.-N.; Tsai, M.-T.; Hsu, J.-T. Biomechanical study on fixation methods for horizontal oblique metacarpal shaft fractures. *J. Orthop. Surg. Res.* **2022**, *17*, 374. [CrossRef]
114. Diao, E.; Moy, O.J. Common tumors. *Orthop. Clin. N. Am.* **1992**, *23*, 187–196. [CrossRef]
115. Averill, R.M.; Smith, R.J.; Campbell, C.J. Giant-cell tumors of the bones of the hand. *J. Hand Surg.* **1980**, *5*, 39–50. [CrossRef] [PubMed]
116. Cioffi, A.; Rovere, G.; Bosco, F.; Sinno, E.; Stramazzo, L.; Liuzza, F.; Ziranu, A.; Romeo, M.; Vigni, G.E.; Galvano, N. Treatment of Scaphoid Non-Unions with Custom-Made 3D-Printed Titanium Partial and Total Scaphoid Prostheses and Scaphoid Interosseous Ligament Reconstruction. *Healthcare* **2023**, *11*, 3123. [CrossRef]
117. Rossello, M.I. A case of total scaphoid titanium custom-made 3D-printed prostheses with one-year follow-up. *Case Rep. Plast. Surg. Hand Surg.* **2020**, *7*, 7–12. [CrossRef] [PubMed]
118. Zhang, C.; Chen, H.; Fan, H.; Xiong, R.; He, R.; Huang, C.; Peng, Y.; Yang, P.; Chen, G.; Wang, F. Carpal bone replacement using personalized 3D printed tantalum prosthesis. *Front. Bioeng. Biotechnol.* **2023**, *11*, 1234052. [CrossRef] [PubMed]
119. Xu, L.; Qin, H.; Cheng, Z.; Jiang, W.-B.; Tan, J.; Luo, X.; Huang, W. 3D-printed personalised prostheses for bone defect repair and reconstruction following resection of metacarpal giant cell tumours. *Ann. Transl. Med.* **2021**, *9*, 1421. [CrossRef] [PubMed]
120. Beltrami, G. Custom 3D-printed finger proximal phalanx as salvage of limb function after aggressive recurrence of giant cell tumour. *Case Rep.* **2018**, *2018*, bcr-2018-226007. [CrossRef]
121. Daia, C.; Scheau, C.; Neagu, G.; Andone, I.; Spanu, A.; Popescu, C.; Stoica, S.I.; Verenca, M.C.; Onose, G. Nerve conduction study and electromyography findings in patients recovering from COVID-19—Case report. *Int. J. Infect. Dis.* **2021**, *103*, 420–422. [CrossRef] [PubMed]
122. Hussain, S.A.; Walters, S.; Ahluwalia, A.K.; Trompeter, A. Fracture-related infections. *Br. J. Hosp. Med.* **2023**, *84*, 1–10. [CrossRef] [PubMed]
123. Legrand, M.; Jourdan, M.L.; de Pinieux, G. Histopathogenesis of bone- and soft-tissue tumor spectrum with USP6 gene rearrangement: Multiple partners involved in the tissue repair process. *Histol. Histopathol.* **2023**, *38*, 247–260. [CrossRef]
124. Wang, C.; Ma, Z.; Yuan, K.; Ji, T. Using scaffolds as drug delivery systems to treat bone tumor. *Nanotechnology* **2022**, *33*, 212002. [CrossRef]
125. Shaikh, A.; Bhardwaj, S.; Vashista, V. Learning complex upper-limb movements through practicing movement elements. *Hum. Mov. Sci.* **2023**, *90*, 103121. [CrossRef]
126. Barbosa, G.M.; Calixtre, L.B.; Fonseca Fialho, H.R.; Locks, F.; Kamonseki, D.H. Measurement properties of upper extremity physical performance tests in athletes: A systematic review. *Braz. J. Phys. Ther.* **2024**, *28*, 100575. [CrossRef] [PubMed]
127. Dragosloveanu, S.; Popov, V.M.; Cotor, D.-C.; Dragosloveanu, C.; Stoica, C.I. Percutaneous Chevron Osteotomy: A Prospective Randomized Controlled Trial. *Medicina* **2022**, *58*, 359. [CrossRef] [PubMed]

128. Gupta, T.; Ghosh, S.B.; Bandyopadhyay-Ghosh, S.; Sain, M. Is it possible to 3D bioprint load-bearing bone implants? A critical review. *Biofabrication* **2023**, *15*, 042003. [CrossRef] [PubMed]
129. Dragosloveanu, S.; Dragosloveanu, C.D.M.; Cotor, D.C.; Stoica, C.I. Short vs. long intramedullary nail systems in trochanteric fractures: A randomized prospective single center study. *Exp. Ther. Med.* **2022**, *23*, 106. [CrossRef]
130. Jeyapalina, S.; Beck, J.P.; Bachus, K.N.; Bloebaum, R.D. Cortical bone response to the presence of load-bearing percutaneous osseointegrated prostheses. *Anat. Rec.* **2012**, *295*, 1437–1445. [CrossRef]
131. Schajowicz, F.; Schajowicz, F. Giant-cell tumor (osteoclastoma). In *Tumors and Tumorlike Lesions of Bone and Joints*; Springer: New York, NY, USA, 1981; pp. 205–242.
132. Kyriakos, M. Intracortical osteosarcoma. *Cancer* **1980**, *46*, 2525–2533. [CrossRef] [PubMed]
133. Agarwal, S.; Saha, S.; Balla, V.K.; Pal, A.; Barui, A.; Bodhak, S. Current developments in 3D bioprinting for tissue and organ regeneration—A review. *Front. Mech. Eng.* **2020**, *6*, 589171. [CrossRef]
134. Hu, X.; Lu, M.; Zhang, Y.; Wang, Y.; Min, L.; Tu, C. A biomechanical comparison between cement packing combined with extra fixation and three-dimensional printed strut-type prosthetic reconstruction for giant cell tumor of bone in distal femur. *J. Orthop. Surg. Res.* **2022**, *17*, 151. [CrossRef] [PubMed]
135. Dragosloveanu, S.; Capitanu, B.-S.; Josanu, R.; Vulpe, D.; Cergan, R.; Scheau, C. Radiological Assessment of Coronal Plane Alignment of the Knee Phenotypes in the Romanian Population. *J. Clin. Med.* **2024**, *13*, 4223. [CrossRef] [PubMed]
136. Henkel, J.; Savi, F.M.; Berner, A.; Fountain, S.; Saifzadeh, S.; Steck, R.; Epari, D.R.; Woodruff, M.A.; Knackstedt, M.; Schuetz, M.A. Scaffold-guided bone regeneration in large volume tibial segmental defects. *Bone* **2021**, *153*, 116163. [CrossRef] [PubMed]
137. Liu, B.; Wang, L.; Li, X.; Chen, Z.; Hou, G.; Zhou, F.; Wang, C.; Tian, Y. Applying 3D-printed prostheses to reconstruct critical-sized bone defects of tibial diaphysis (> 10 cm) caused by osteomyelitis and aseptic non-union. *J. Orthop. Surg. Res.* **2024**, *19*, 418. [CrossRef] [PubMed]
138. Lui, P.; Rui, Y.; Ni, M.; Chan, K. Tenogenic differentiation of stem cells for tendon repair—What is the current evidence? *J. Tissue Eng. Regen. Med.* **2011**, *5*, e144–e163. [CrossRef]
139. Pisanu, F.; Andreozzi, M.; Fiori, E.; Altamore, F.; Bartoli, M.; Caggiari, G.; Ortu, S.; Rios, M.; Manunta, A.F.; Doria, C. Surgical management of hip prosthetic failure in metallosis: A case series and literature review. *J. Orthop.* **2021**, *28*, 10–20. [CrossRef] [PubMed]
140. Sun, C.; Kang, J.; Yang, C.; Zheng, J.; Su, Y.; Dong, E.; Liu, Y.; Yao, S.; Shi, C.; Pang, H. Additive manufactured polyether-ether-ketone implants for orthopaedic applications: A narrative review. *Biomater. Transl.* **2022**, *3*, 116.
141. Chen, C.; Yin, Y.; Xu, H.; Li, Z.; Wang, F.; Chen, G. Personalized three-dimensional printed polyether-ether-ketone prosthesis for reconstruction after subtotal removal of chronic clavicle osteomyelitis: A case report. *Medicine* **2021**, *100*, e25703. [CrossRef] [PubMed]
142. Honigmann, P.; Sharma, N.; Schumacher, R.; Rueegg, J.; Haefeli, M.; Thieringer, F. In-Hospital 3D Printed Scaphoid Prosthesis Using Medical-Grade Polyetheretherketone (PEEK) Biomaterial. *BioMed Res. Int.* **2021**, *2021*, 1301028. [CrossRef] [PubMed]
143. Lu, Y.; Chen, G.; Long, Z.; Li, M.; Ji, C.; Wang, F.; Li, H.; Lu, J.; Wang, Z.; Li, J. Novel 3D-printed prosthetic composite for reconstruction of massive bone defects in lower extremities after malignant tumor resection. *J. Bone Oncol.* **2019**, *16*, 100220. [CrossRef]
144. Alkaissy, R.T.S. *Development of a Biphasic Scaffold in the Context of Rotator Cuff Repairs*; University of Oxford: Oxford, UK, 2022.
145. Amirouche, F.; Koh, J. Biomechanics of Human Joints. In *Orthopaedic Biomechanics in Sports Medicine*; Springer: Cham, Switzerland, 2021; pp. 3–13.
146. Ock, J.; Seo, J.; Koh, K.H.; Kim, N. Comparing the biomechanical properties of conventional suture and all-suture anchors using patient-specific and realistic osteoporotic and non-osteoporotic phantom using 3D printing. *Sci. Rep.* **2023**, *13*, 20976. [CrossRef] [PubMed]
147. Hsieh, Y.-Y.; Wu, L.-C.; Tsuang, F.-Y.; Chen, C.-H.; Chiang, C.-J. Pull-Out capability of a 3D printed threadless suture anchor with rectangular cross-section: A biomechanical study. *Appl. Sci.* **2021**, *11*, 12128. [CrossRef]
148. Chen, C.-H.; Chang, W.-J.; Chen, Y.-S.; Chen, K.H.; Huang, S.-F.; Hsueh, H.-R.; Li, C.-B.; Lin, C.-L. Development of a novel hybrid suture anchor for osteoporosis by integrating titanium 3D printing and traditional machining. *Int. J. Bioprint.* **2022**, *8*, 608. [CrossRef]
149. Burdis, R.; Chariyev-Prinz, F.; Kelly, D.J. Bioprinting of biomimetic self-organised cartilage with a supporting joint fixation device. *Biofabrication* **2021**, *14*, 015008. [CrossRef]
150. Allen, Q.; Raeymaekers, B. Surface texturing of prosthetic hip implant bearing surfaces: A review. *J. Tribol.* **2021**, *143*, 040801. [CrossRef]
151. Hall, R.; Unsworth, A. Friction in hip prostheses. *Biomaterials* **1997**, *18*, 1017–1026. [CrossRef] [PubMed]
152. Shah, R.; Gashi, B.; Hoque, S.; Marian, M.; Rosenkranz, A. Enhancing mechanical and biomedical properties of protheses-surface and material design. *Surf. Interfaces* **2021**, *27*, 101498. [CrossRef]
153. Arnold, C.; Monsees, D.; Hey, J.; Schweyen, R. Surface quality of 3D-printed models as a function of various printing parameters. *Materials* **2019**, *12*, 1970. [CrossRef]
154. Wang, H.; Lim, J.Y. Metal-ceramic bond strength of a cobalt chromium alloy for dental prosthetic restorations with a porous structure using metal 3D printing. *Comput. Biol. Med.* **2019**, *112*, 103364. [CrossRef] [PubMed]

155. Górski, F.; Wichniarek, R.; Kuczko, W.; Żukowska, M. Study on properties of automatically designed 3d-printed customized prosthetic sockets. *Materials* **2021**, *14*, 5240. [CrossRef] [PubMed]
156. Pathak, K.; Saikia, R.; Das, A.; Das, D.; Islam, M.A.; Pramanik, P.; Parasar, A.; Borthakur, P.P.; Sarmah, P.; Saikia, M. 3D printing in biomedicine: Advancing personalized care through additive manufacturing. *Explor. Med.* **2023**, *4*, 1135–1167. [CrossRef]
157. Dalgarno, K. *The Impact and Potential for 3D Printing and Bioprinting in the Medical Devices Industry*; Newcastle University: London, UK, 2020.
158. Ozbolat, I.T. Bioprinting scale-up tissue and organ constructs for transplantation. *Trends Biotechnol.* **2015**, *33*, 395–400. [CrossRef] [PubMed]
159. Agostinacchio, F.; Mu, X.; Dirè, S.; Motta, A.; Kaplan, D.L. In situ 3D printing: Opportunities with silk inks. *Trends Biotechnol.* **2021**, *39*, 719–730. [CrossRef]
160. Tao, H.; Marelli, B.; Yang, M.; An, B.; Onses, M.S.; Rogers, J.A.; Kaplan, D.L.; Omenetto, F.G. Inkjet printing of regenerated silk fibroin: From printable forms to printable functions. *Adv. Mater.* **2015**, *27*, 4273–4279. [CrossRef]
161. Zhang, J.; Wehrle, E.; Rubert, M.; Müller, R. 3D bioprinting of human tissues: Biofabrication, bioinks, and bioreactors. *Int. J. Mol. Sci.* **2021**, *22*, 3971. [CrossRef] [PubMed]
162. Liu, N.; Zhang, X.; Guo, Q.; Wu, T.; Wang, Y. 3D bioprinted scaffolds for tissue repair and regeneration. *Front. Mater.* **2022**, *9*, 925321. [CrossRef]
163. Klak, M.; Kowalska, P.; Dobrzański, T.; Tymicki, G.; Cywoniuk, P.; Gomółka, M.; Kosowska, K.; Bryniarski, T.; Berman, A.; Dobrzyń, A. Bionic organs: Shear forces reduce pancreatic islet and mammalian cell viability during the process of 3D bioprinting. *Micromachines* **2021**, *12*, 304. [CrossRef]
164. Zhu, X.; Hu, J.; Lin, J.; Song, G.; Xu, H.; Lu, J.; Tang, Q.; Wang, J. 3D-printed modular prostheses for reconstruction of intercalary bone defects after joint-sparing limb salvage surgery for femoral diaphyseal tumours. *Bone Jt. Open* **2024**, *5*, 317. [CrossRef] [PubMed]
165. Vitiello, R.; Matrangolo, M.R.; El Motassime, A.; Perna, A.; Cianni, L.; Maccauro, G.; Ziranu, A. Three-dimension-printed custom-made prosthetic reconstructions in bone tumors: A single center experience. *Curr. Oncol.* **2022**, *29*, 4566–4577. [CrossRef] [PubMed]
166. Kotlarz, M.; Ferreira, A.M.; Gentile, P.; Dalgarno, K. Bioprinting of cell-laden hydrogels onto titanium alloy surfaces to produce a bioactive Interface. *Macromol. Biosci.* **2022**, *22*, 2200071. [CrossRef]
167. Kim, D.Y.; Liu, Y.; Kim, G.; An, S.B.; Han, I. Innovative Strategies in 3D Bioprinting for Spinal Cord Injury Repair. *Int. J. Mol. Sci.* **2024**, *25*, 9592. [CrossRef] [PubMed]
168. Islam, A.; Vakitbilir, N.; Almeida, N.; França, R. Advances in 3D Bioprinting for Neuroregeneration: A Literature Review of Methods, Bioinks, and Applications. *MICRO* **2024**, *4*, 490–508. [CrossRef]

Journal of
Functional Biomaterials

MDPI

*Article*

# Development of Prevascularized Synthetic Block Graft for Maxillofacial Reconstruction

**Borvornwut Buranawat [1,†], Abeer Shaalan [2,†], Devy F. Garna [2] and Lucy Di Silvio [2,*]**

1 Center for Implant Dentistry and Periodontics, Faculty of Dentistry and Research Unit in Innovations in Periodontics, Oral Surgery and Advanced Technology in Implant Dentistry, Thammasat University, Bangkok 10200, Thailand; borvornw@staff.tu.ac.th

2 Center for Oral, Clinical and Translational Sciences, Faculty of Dentistry, Oral & Craniofacial Sciences, King's College London, London SE1 9RT, UK; shaalan.abeer@kcl.ac.uk (A.S.); devy.garna@kcl.ac.uk (D.F.G.)

* Correspondence: lucy.di_silvio@kcl.ac.uk

† These authors contributed equally to this work.

**Abstract:** Cranio-maxillofacial bone reconstruction, especially for large defects, remains challenging. Synthetic biomimetic materials are emerging as alternatives to autogenous grafts. Tissue engineering aims to create natural tissue-mimicking materials, with calcium phosphate-based scaffolds showing promise for bone regeneration applications. This study developed a porous calcium metaphosphate (CMP) scaffold with physicochemical properties mimicking natural bone, aiming to create a prevascularized synthetic bone graft. The scaffold, fabricated using sintered monocalcium phosphate with poly (vinyl alcohol) as a porogen, exhibited pore sizes ranging from 0 to 400 µm, with the highest frequency between 80 and 100 µm. The co-culture of endothelial cells (ECs) with human alveolar osteoblasts (aHOBs) on the scaffold led to the formation of tube-like structures and intrinsic VEGF release, reaching 10,455.6 pg/mL This level approached the optimal dose for vascular formation. Conversely, the co-culture with mesenchymal stem cells did not yield similar results. Combining ECs and aHOBs in the CMP scaffold offers a promising approach to developing prevascularized grafts for cranio-maxillofacial reconstruction. This innovative strategy can potentially enhance vascularization in large tissue-engineered constructs, addressing a critical limitation in current bone regeneration techniques. The prevascularized synthetic bone graft developed in this study could significantly improve the success rate of maxillofacial reconstructions, offering a viable alternative to autogenous grafts.

**Keywords:** prevascularization; porous calcium phosphate block graft; bone tissue engineering; growth factors

## 1. Introduction

Cranio-maxillofacial bone defects, whether resulting from congenital deformities, trauma, disease, or cancer, pose significant clinical challenges, impacting not only physical function but also esthetics and psychological well-being. Approximately 2 million bone grafting procedures are performed globally each year, with 6% of these aimed at repairing cranio-maxillofacial defects [1]. Bone is a dynamic, highly vascularized tissue with regenerative and healing potential that is reliant on the close spatial and temporal connection of blood vessels and bone cells. Current treatments for bone repair typically involve autografts and allografts, which, despite being the gold standard, face challenges such as limited tissue availability, donor site morbidity, disease transmission risks, and potential immunogenic rejection [2,3]. The limitations of traditional transplanted grafts have sparked increased attention towards developing advanced synthetic bone graft materials over the past century, aiming to restore organ and tissue function [4,5].

Tissue engineering has evolved as an emerging therapy with the potential to replace or regenerate tissues or organs. This usually necessitates a scaffold to provide the structural architecture and act as a vehicle for incorporated factors to enhance the recruitment of stem cells. The importance of scaffolds has been highlighted by the current advances that are occurring in novel biomaterial design with bioactive potential, able to influence cell behaviour directly. However, large bone defects present a major hurdle: insufficient vascularization in the early stages post implantation, which limits nutrient and oxygen supply to the scaffold, leading to poor cell survival and integration. In vivo, blood vessels provide essential support to bone tissue, ensuring its regeneration and healing potential [6–8], but the supply of oxygen and nutrients is often limited to cells in a proximity of 100–200 μm from the next capillary [9]. In the case of large tissue-engineered constructs, the survival of cells in the centre cannot solely rely on nutrient supply by diffusion. Growth, function, and survival post implantation are entirely dependent on the ingrowth of blood vessels from the host [10]. Therefore, additional strategies that serve to enhance vascularization are essential for the survival of large tissue-engineered grafts.

An optimal scaffold for bone tissue engineering should exceed simple osteoconductive properties. It must actively stimulate osteoinduction while concurrently promoting angiogenesis and vascularization, thereby tackling the combined challenges of bone regeneration and adequate blood supply. An ideal scaffold for bone tissue engineering should mimic bone's chemistry and structure, featuring high porosity (>40–60%) and interconnected pores. This design facilitates cell migration, nutrient exchange, and fluid transport, all crucial for cell survival and vascularization [11].

In vivo prevascularization, an early strategy to enhance vascularization, involves implanting the scaffold in a primary site for weeks to develop a microvascular network before reimplantation at the defect site. This method provides immediate vascularization through microsurgical attachment to local vasculature.

In vitro, prevascularization has emerged as a promising strategy to enhance scaffold performance and survival. This approach requires only one surgical procedure and reduces the time the scaffold remains in the body. Creating a pre-existing vascular network accelerates overall construct vascularization, as host vessels need only connect to the outer regions, potentially leading to faster graft integration [9,12]. This approach also involves the co-culture of endothelial cells with other cell types, such as osteoblasts, and aims to create capillary-like structures before implantation. In conditions simulating the physiological niche, especially in a three-dimensional environment, endothelial cells naturally organize into tubular networks [13,14].

Prevascular structures formed in vitro can rapidly connect to host vasculature upon implantation, accelerating graft vascularization and survival. This is crucial in bone tissue engineering, where the interplay between bone cells and blood vessels is essential [8,15–17]. For effective prevascularization, endothelial cells are typically combined with other cell types. The challenge lies in optimizing culture conditions that support both vascular network formation and tissue development, ensuring the creation of a functional prevascularized construct.

Calcium metaphosphates (CMPs) are a distinct type of bioactive ceramic with a polymeric structure [$Ca(PO_3)_2$] [18]. They have gained significant attention as potential bone substitute materials due to their close resemblance to the calcium phosphate found in bone, despite having a slightly different chemical structure compared to hydroxyapatite (HA). CMP is known to elicit specific biological responses at the material–tissue interface, promoting the formation of a strong bond between the material and surrounding tissue [19].

This study aims to develop a novel 3D porous calcium metaphosphate (CMP) scaffold that supports osteoconduction and vascularization for cranio-maxillofacial reconstruction. By establishing a co-culture model of endothelial cells and osteoblasts, we sought to create a prevascular network within the scaffold, focusing on its fundamental biological interactions and vascularization potential as critical first steps toward developing an effective bone graft material for large, complex bone defects.

## 2. Materials and Methods

### 2.1. Scaffold Fabrication

Porous scaffolds of CMP were produced by mixing commercial monocalcium bisphosphate monohydrate (Ca $(H_2PO_4)_2{\cdot}H_2O$) (Fluka) and commercial polyvinyl alcohol (PVA) in a 4:1 weight ratio, 0.7 g of the powder mixture was placed in a 12 mm diameter stainless steel mould, and the mixture was pressed at 10 MPa (INSTRON) for 2 min to yield a solid disc before being heated to 900 °C at 10 °C/min and remaining at 900 °C for 6 h before being furnace-cooled to room temperature. Pores were created in the scaffolds by the burning of PVA, the pore-forming agent [20].

### 2.2. Scaffold Characterization

The phase purity of CMP scaffolds was determined by X-ray diffractometry (XRD, JEOL JDX 3530) and Fourier Transform Infrared spectroscopy (FTIR, Perken-Elmer Spectrum one). For morphology studies, the scaffolds were fixed on carbon-coated stubs and then gold-coated before being viewed under an FEI Quanta (Field Emission Gun SEM). Energy-dispersive X-ray analysis (EDX) was also employed to provide information on the chemical composition and respective proportions (At%) of the scaffold. Porosity was determined using both X-ray micro-computed tomography (μ-CT) (Skyscan 1172, Skyscan, Belgium) and mercury intrusion porosimetry.

Water uptake and solubility are key factors influencing the degradation rate of porous CMP materials. To determine the dry weight, HA and CMP samples were dried overnight at 110 °C in a drying oven. After weighing, samples ($n$ = 4) were immersed in 3 mL of distilled water and stored at 37 °C for 56 days. At specific intervals, samples were removed, blotted with filter paper to remove surface water, and weighed using a digital balance. The percentage of weight change was calculated using

$$\%\ \text{Hydration} = (\text{Final weight} - \text{Initial weight})/\text{Initial weight} \times 100$$

After each measurement, the water volume was replenished to 3 mL. This process was repeated throughout this study to monitor changes over time.

### 2.3. Cells and Growth Conditions

#### 2.3.1. Human Alveolar Osteoblast Cells (aHOBs)

The primary aHOBs were isolated (ethics and patient consent approved, 05/Q1803/85) and characterized as previously described [21,22]. Cells were incubated in a humidified atmosphere with 5% $CO_2$ at 37 °C. The growth medium used was Dulbecco's Modified Eagle's Medium (DMEM; D6046), containing 10% fetal calf serum (FCS), 5% of HEPES, 1% minimal essential medium (MEM), 20 mM L-glutamines, 100 units/mL of penicillin, 0.1 mg/mL of streptomycin, and 15% ascorbate powder (all from Sigma, Leeds, UK). Only cells from passages 6–8 were used in this study.

#### 2.3.2. Human Umbilical Vein Endothelial Cells (HUVECs)

Primary human endothelial cells isolated from the umbilical vein (HUVECs) were purchased from Cascade Biologics® (Life Technologies, Scotland, UK). Cells were resuscitated and cultured in a humidified atmosphere (37 °C, 5% $CO_2$) in Medium 200 with the addition of serum growth supplements bFGF (20 ng/mL), EFG (10 ng/mL), and human plasma fibronectin (10 μg/mL) (all from Invitrogen, Morecambe, UK). Only HUVECs from passages 5–8 were used in the experiments.

#### 2.3.3. Human Bone Marrow Mesenchymal Stem Cells (hBMSCs)

Undifferentiated human bone marrow mesenchymal stem cells (hBMSCs) were exploited for their potential role in stimulating endothelial tubular formation in the co-culture system. Briefly, primary human hBMSCs were obtained from fresh bone marrow from human iliac crest aspiration (ethics and patient consent approved, KCH REC REF 08/H0808/10) as described previously [23]. Cells were cultured in Dulbecco's Modified Eagle's Medium (DMEM; Special D6429), containing 20% fetal calf serum (FCS), 100 units/mL of penicillin, and 0.1 mg/mL of streptomycin (all from Sigma, Leeds, UK), and 10 ng/mL of fibroblast growth factor (FGF) (Prepotech, London, UK) was also added. Only cells from passages 6–8 were used in this study.

### *2.4. Optimization of VEGF Concentration*

The response of HUVEC to different concentrations of VEGF was investigated. The VEGF was loaded at concentrations of 5, 10, 20, 30, 50, and 100 ng/mL. Results were obtained on days 1, 4, and 7 by cell counting and methyl thiazolyl tetrazolium (MTT) cell viability assay. To minimize the serum confounding effect, a medium with a 1% low serum supplement was selected for this study to ensure that the sole effect of VEGF on HUVEC could be observed.

### *2.5. Optimization of Co-Culture Media*

To determine the optimal media for co-culture, different ratios of HUVEC to MSC and HOB media were investigated. Equal numbers of cells were seeded in direct contact in a 24-well plate. After 24 h, the media were changed; six different media ratios were tested (Table 1).

**Table 1.** Different ratios of culture media used in co-culture proliferation assay.

| HOB or hBMSC Medium (%) | HUVEC Medium (%) |
|---|---|
| 100 | 0 |
| 70 | 30 |
| 60 | 40 |
| 50 | 50 |
| 40 | 60 |
| 0 | 100 |

The co-culture of HUVEC and aHOB or hBMSC was allowed to proliferate for 21 days. The Alamar Blue assay was conducted on days 2, 5, 7, 14, and 21 to determine cell activity and viability in each of the media ratios. To assess whether each cell type proliferated equally within the co-culture system using the optimum ratio of media, determined previously, cells were labelled with cell trackers to allow the identification of specific cell types for cell counting. The immunofluorescent staining of HUVEC, aHOB, and hBMSC cells was carried out using CellTrackers (Invitrogen, Morecambe, UK). Red (C34552) was used for both aHOB and hBMSC and green (C7025) was used for the HUVECs.

### 2.6. VEGF Release from Co-Culture

To determine the amount of VEGF released in the co-culture system, supernatants of co-culture cells in optimized media were collected on days 4, 7, 14, and 21; particulates were removed by centrifugation; and the supernatant was stored at −80 °C for later analysis. VEGF release from the co-culture was measured using the Quantikine® Human VEGF Immunoassay (R&D systems, Oxfordshire, UK). Optical density was determined using a DYNEX Opsys technologies reader (test wavelength: 450 nm; reference wavelength: 570 nm).

### 2.7. Angiogenesis Assay (Endothelial Tube Formation)

A collagen gel sandwich culture was utilized to visualize tubule formation. The gel was prepared by mixing 0.7 mL of 10× Eagle's DMEM solution with 6 mL of rat-tail type I collagen, which was dissolved in 0.1 M acetic acid at a protein concentration of 2.035 mg/mL. This mixture was then neutralized using 5 M and 1 M sodium hydroxide. Following the preparation of the gel, 300 µL of the collagen solution was added to each well of a 24-well plate and incubated for 30 min to allow it to set. A 250 µL cell suspension was prepared for three conditions: (A) HUVEC, (B) HUVEC with HOB, and (C) HUVEC with hBMSC. Each suspension ($1 \times 10^5$ cells/well) was added on top of the set collagen and incubated for 60 min for cell adhesion. Then, 300 µL of collagen was layered over the cells to form a "sandwich" and incubated until set. Following this, 1 mL of medium was added to the wells: HUVEC-specific media for group (A) and optimized co-culture media for groups (B) and (C).

Cultures were allowed to grow for 14 days with microscopic observations every 12 h. The media were changed on day 7 without disturbing the collagen construct using low-power vacuum suction. Endothelial tube morphogenesis was examined by phase contrast microscopy (Olympus IX51, Nagano, Japan) and images were captured using a Colorview II digital camera (Olympus, Nagano, Japan). At the end of the assay, both semi-quantitative CD31 ELISA and tubule area were assessed using a CD31 ELISA & Histology Staining Kit (TCS cell works, Buckingham, UK). Optical density was determined using a DYNEX Opsys technologies reader (test wavelength: 405 nm; reference wavelength: 570 nm). For image analysis, four randomly selected fields of view were photographed in each quadruplicate well per condition. Images were captured using low magnification (×40) and converted to binary format using LCS Leica confocal software (version 2.5, Leica GmbH, Germany). The binary threshold function was adjusted to obtain the best contrast of tubules with the background. Tubule area was calculated as the total number of pixels in threshold-adjusted images and then converted to µm$^2$.

### 2.8. Phenotypic Characterization of HUVEC and aHOB

To evaluate the stability of EC and osteoblast phenotype within the co-culture, and to further establish the optimum seeding conditions for tubular formation in the 3D βCMP scaffold, semi-quantitative PCR was performed to verify both EC and osteoblast-specific markers (Table 2). RNA was isolated from a monolayer of aHOB, and the HUVEC co-culture from day 14 was extracted. Reverse transcription was performed using a Thermal Cycler Veriti (Applied Biosystems, UK). The PCR product was loaded onto 1.2% *w*/*v* agarose gel (Bioline, Germany), the gel was viewed by a PC-linked UV transilluminator, and amplified DNA fragments were determined using the DNA ladders.

**Table 2.** Primer's nucleotide sequences and expected PCR product sizes.

| Target Gene | Sequence (5′→3′) | Product Size |
|---|---|---|
| GAPDH | | |
| Forward | ACC ACA GTC CAT GCC ATC AC | 452 bp |
| Reverse | TCC ACC ACC CTG TTG CTG TA | |
| VEGFR-2 | | |
| Forward | GTG ACC AAC ATG GAG TCG TG | 660 bp |
| Reverse | CCA GAG ATT CCA TGC CAC TT | |
| Angiopoietin 1 | | |
| Forward | AGA GGC ACG GAA GGA GTG TG | 410 bp |
| Reverse | CTA TCT CCA GCA TGG TAG CCG | |
| Tie 2 | | |
| Forward | CGA GTT CGA GGA GAG GCA ATC | 148 bp |
| Reverse | TCA GGT ACT TCA TGC CGG G | |
| ALP | | |
| Forward | CCA CGT CTT CAC ATT TGG TG | 196 bp |
| Reverse | AGA CTG CGC CTG GTA GTT GT | |
| Runx2 | | |
| Forward | CAG ACC AGC AGC ACT CCA TA | 178 bp |
| Reverse | CAG CGT CAA CAC CAT CAT TC | |
| Col1 | | |
| Forward | CCA AAT CTG TCT CCC CAG A | 213 bp |
| Reverse | TCA AAA ACG AAG GGG AGA T | |

### 2.9. Three-Dimensional Co-Cultures of HUVEC and aHOB on βCMP Scaffold

Following sterilization of the βCMP scaffolds, cells were seeded at $5 \times 10^5$ per scaffold with an equal proportion of HUVEC to aHOB cells. After incubation for 60 min, 400 μL of collagen type I (as described above) was added to each well. Once the collagen was set, 1 mL of co-culture media (40% HOB: 60% HUVEC) with an additional 10 ng/mL of VEGF was added. The medium was changed after 7 days. All incubations were carried out in a humidified atmosphere (37 °C, 5% $CO_2$) for 14 days.

### 2.10. Scanning Electron Microscopy for Cell Morphology

On day 14, samples were fixed and processed, and SEM was used to examine the morphology of cells and tubular structures.

### 2.11. Immunocytochemistry

The expression pattern of the endothelial cell adhesion molecules (PECAM-1 or CD31, von Willebrand factor) and structural protein vimentin was examined by the immunofluorescent staining of cellular constructs using a Leica multi-photon 2 confocal microscope (Leica GmbH, Germany) with an acoustic–optical beam-splitter spectral scan head (AOBS) to visualize the tubular networks inside the βCMP scaffold. The dilution factor of each primary and secondary antibody is summarized in Table 3. The tubular formation inside of the porous βCMP scaffold was confirmed by real-time recording for different depths of βCMP, using the 3D time-lapse function of LCS Leica software. The scaffolds were also stained immunohistochemically by both CD31 and vWF to identify the microtubule formation (TCS Cell works, Buckingham, UK).

**Table 3.** Dilutions of fluorescent stains for primary and secondary antibodies.

| Antibodies | Dilution Used | |
|---|---|---|
| | Primary | Secondary |
| PECAM-1, CD31 | 1:50 | 1:1000 |
| Von Willebrand (vWF) | 1:8000 | 1:1000 |
| Phalloidin (direct staining) | 1:100 | |
| Vimentin | 1:100 | 1:1000 |

### 2.12. Statistical Analysis

All cellular experiments were performed in quadruplicates and repeated at least three times, demonstrating reliable reproducibility. Data are expressed as mean ± standard deviation (SD). Potential outliers were examined using the interquartile range (IQR) method, with any identified outliers reported in the results section. Statistical analyses were performed using STATA® statistical software version 17. The significance level was predetermined at $p < 0.05$ for all tests.

The Shapiro–Wilk test was conducted to assess the normality of data distribution. For normally distributed data, one-way analysis of variance (ANOVA) was used to compare means among groups, followed by Tukey's post hoc test for multiple comparisons. For data not following a normal distribution, the non-parametric Kruskal–Wallis's test was employed, with the subsequent Dunn's procedure for pairwise comparisons.

## 3. Results

### 3.1. Characterization of CMP Scaffold

#### 3.1.1. X-Ray Diffraction

The XRD diffraction pattern of the CMP showed sharp diffraction-characteristic peaks that appeared at around 25.28°, 28.50°, and 31.76° (Figure 1). This corresponds to the characteristic peaks of crystalline β-meta calcium phosphate as published earlier [24,25] and by the Joint Committee on Powder Diffraction Standards (JCPDS no. 11-0039).

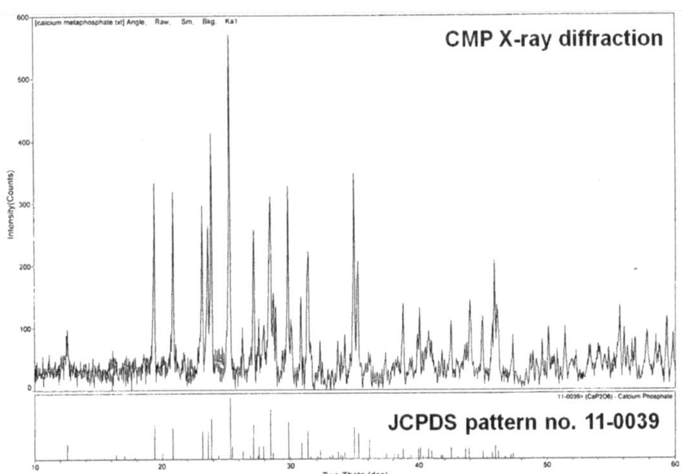


**Figure 1.** X-ray diffraction patterns for the CMP scaffold showing sharp, high peaks at 25.28°, 28.50°, and 31.75°. The peaks observed correspond to predominant phases of crystalline β-meta calcium phosphate (JCPDS 110039).

### 3.1.2. Infrared Spectroscopy

The infrared spectra of the CMP showed strong characteristic absorption peaks at 1241 $cm^{-1}$, 1114 $cm^{-1}$, 1055 $cm^{-1}$, 935 $cm^{-1}$, and 788 $cm^{-1}$ (Figure 2). These results for the P–O bond and also the $PO_3$ group correspond to those reported by Briche et al. [26]. No characteristic peaks of PVA and organic residues were observed in the βCMP scaffold, confirming that they had been obliterated following the sintering process.

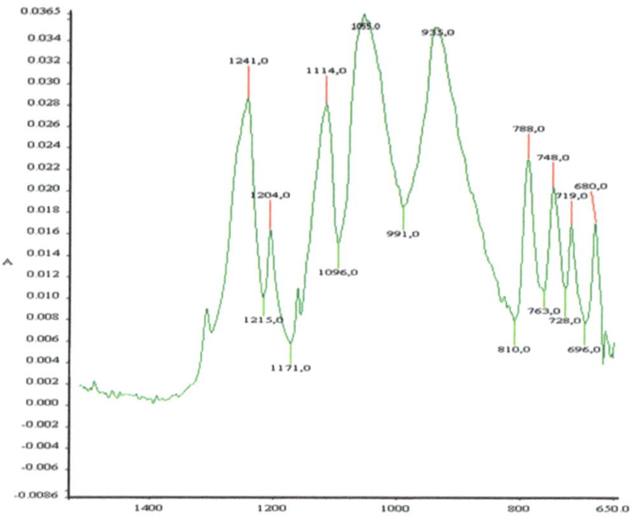


**Figure 2.** FTIR spectrum of calcium metaphosphate scaffold shows expansion of the fingerprint region.

### 3.1.3. Morphology and Pore Structure of CMP Scaffold

The topography of the CMP was observed by SEM (Figure 3A,B) to possess a predominant porosity over a wide range of pore sizes from 80 to 100 μm. In addition, microporosity pores (>400 μm) were also observed across the surface of the scaffold. EDX microanalysis results showed porous CMP with a Ca/P ratio of 0.48 ± 0.046 ($n$ = 4) (Figure 4).

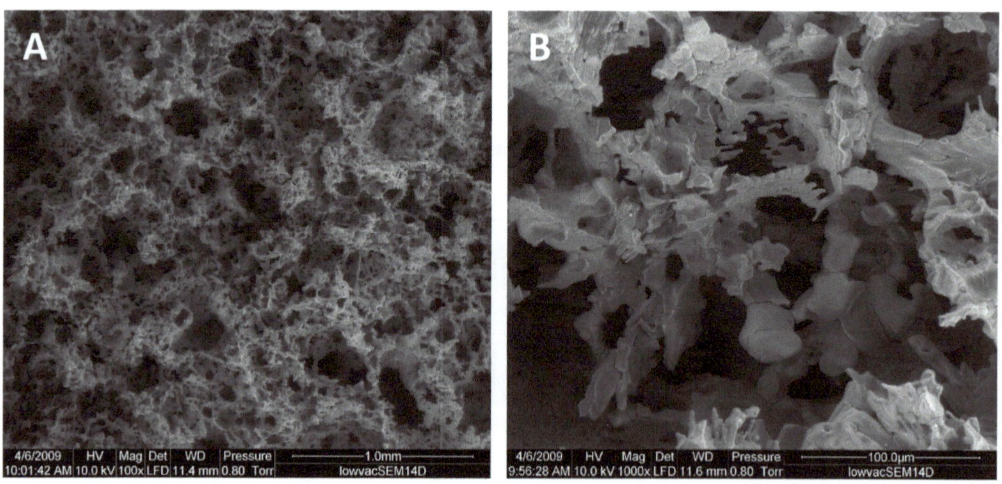


**Figure 3.** SEM micrographs of porous CMP scaffold: (**A**) ×100 and (**B**) ×1000 viewed under low vacuum at 10.0 kV.

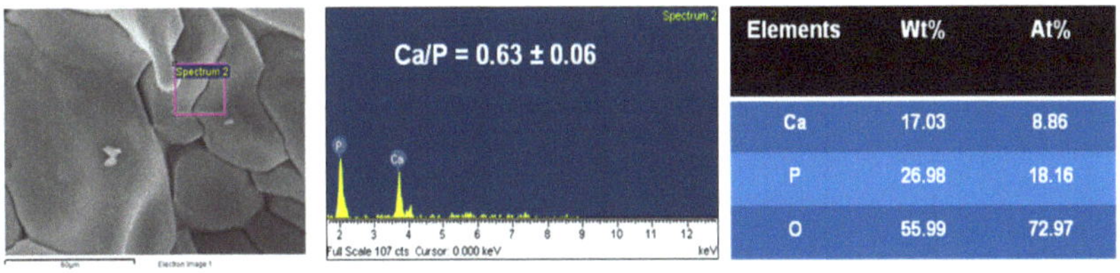


**Figure 4.** EDS microanalysis of the chemical composition of CMP scaffold and tabulated data on Ca, P, and O elemental proportions by weight (Wt%) and by number of atoms (At%).

The proportion of the number of atoms corresponded to the chemical composition of β-calcium metaphosphate ($CaP_2O_6$). The pore diameter frequency distribution and % porosity data were collected via MIP. Pores were within the 0–217 μm range studied, and 100 μm pores were the most frequent within the structure of CMP (Figure 5), although smaller and larger pores were also detected.

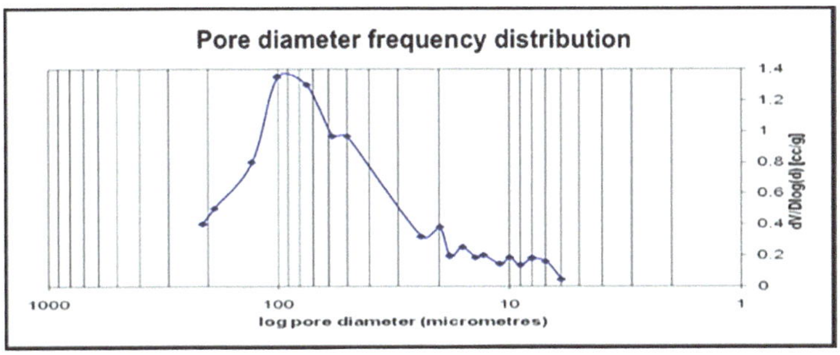


**Figure 5.** Pore size distribution of CMP obtained from mercury intrusion porosimetry.

In addition, with the same method, 71% of total porosity was also observed in the CMP scaffold. The actual pore structure of CMP was determined by μ-CT. Rendered 3D scans of the CMP scaffold revealed good interconnectivity from the top to bottom of the construct with an approximate porosity of 68.6%. μCT structural analysis values are shown in Table 4.

**Table 4.** Micro-CT analysis of porous CMP scaffold.

| Description | Abbreviation | Value | Unit |
|---|---|---|---|
| Structure thickness | St.Th | 0.0353 | Mm |
| Structure separation | St.Sp | 0.072 | Mm |
| Number of objects | Obj.N | 4675 | |
| Number of closed pores | Po.N(cl) | 336 | |
| Volume of closed pores | Po.V(cl) | 0.000256 | $mm^3$ |
| Surface of closed pores | Po.S(cl) | 0.14 | $mm^2$ |
| Closed porosity | Po(cl) | 0.00769 | % |
| Open porosity | PO(op) | 68.93 | % |
| Total volume of pore space | Po.V(tot) | 7.28 | $mm^3$ |
| Total porosity | Po(tot) | 68.6 | % |
| Connectivity | Conn | 42748 | |
| Connectivity density | Conn.Dn | 4030 | $1/mm^3$ |

The interconnectivity of the porous CMP scaffold was confirmed by using the "flight recorder" function of CTvox software, which allows observation of the internal structures throughout the CMP scaffold.

### 3.1.4. Water Uptake

After immersion in distilled water, the weights of HA and CMP were recorded over 56 days (Figure 6). CMP exhibited higher water uptake during the first 2 h compared to HA, which swelled more slowly at the start. Over time, HA showed a gradual increase in water uptake, while CMP displayed a decreasing trend, reaching a final swelling of 30.65% of its initial dry weight after 56 days. Weight fluctuations were observed in both materials throughout this study.

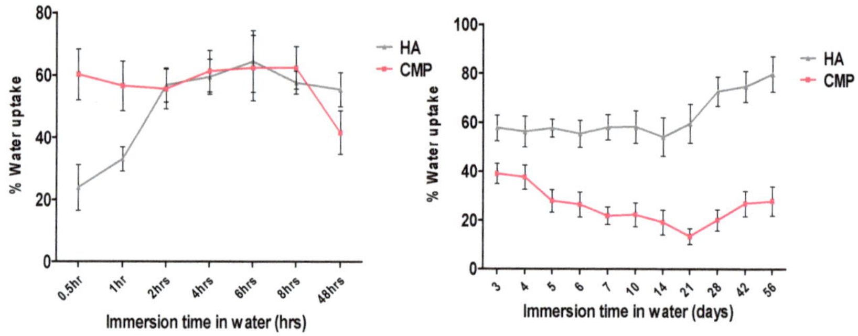


**Figure 6.** Graph showing % water uptake of HA and CMP at 37 °C cover period of 56 days (time(x) axis not to scale, error bar = SD).

### *3.2. Optimization of VEGF Concentrations*

Results were obtained using cell counts and the MTT assay (Figure 7).

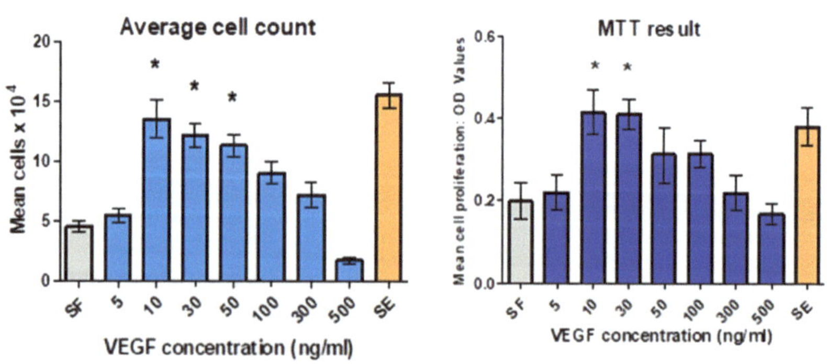


**Figure 7.** The dose-dependent effect of varying VEGF concentrations on HUVEC proliferation; grey columns represent EC media supplement-free (SF) and brown columns represent EC media with supplements (SE). Data presented as mean ± standard deviation (SD) from quadruplicates and three independent experiments. One-way analysis of variance (ANOVA) was used to compare the means among groups; * $p < 0.05$ was considered statistically significant.

The average cell number obtained for days 1, 4, and 7 indicated that high doses of VEGF (500 ng/mL) downregulated HUVEC proliferation, with the optimum stimulatory dose found to be between 10 and 30 ng/mL. Statistical analysis revealed a significant difference between optimum doses and serum-free ($p < 0.05$). In addition, it was evident from both the cell counts and MTT assay that 5 ng/mL of VEGF was found to not affect cell proliferation.

### 3.3. Optimization of Co-Culture Media

To determine the ideal medium for the maximum proliferation of cells within the co-culture system, different ratios were investigated. Over 21 days, an increasing trend was observed universally. The ratio of 60% HUVEC: 40% HOB media was optimum for HUVEC/HOB co-culture and 30% HUVEC: 70% MSC for HUVEC/hBMSC co-culture (Figure 8).

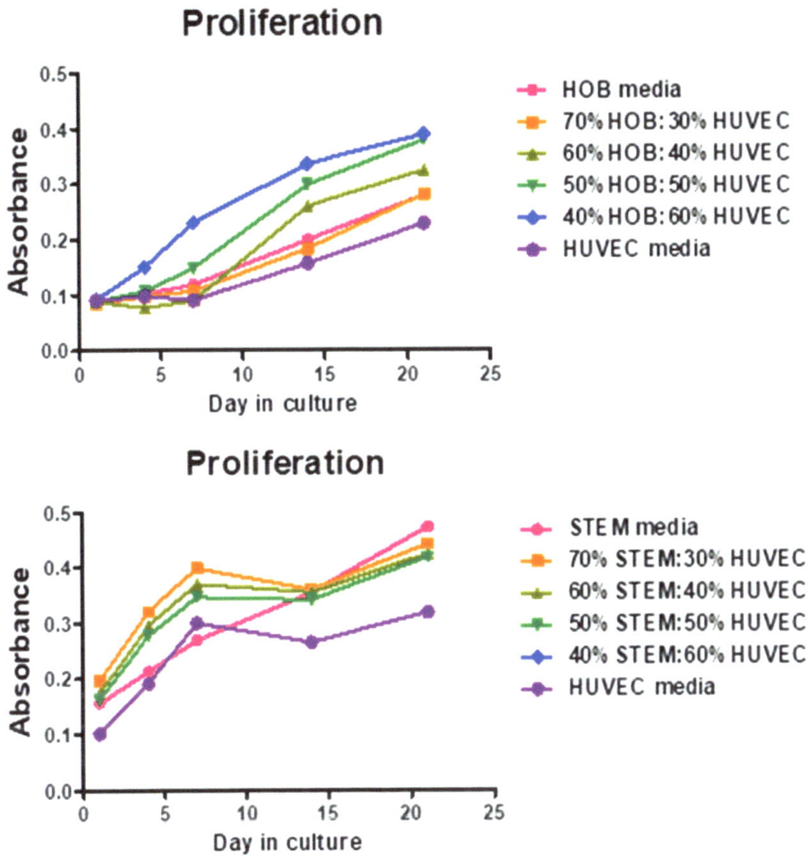


**Figure 8.** AlamarBlue cell proliferation assay over 21 days with various ratios of co-culture media of aHOB and HUVEC. The highest cell growth was found in the 60%HUVEC:40%HOB ratio. Statistical analysis revealed a significant difference between optimum doses and serum-free ($p < 0.05$).

In addition, the growth of each cell type was also confirmed using immunofluorescent tracking and cell counts were confirmed using fluorescent microscopy (Figure 9A,B).

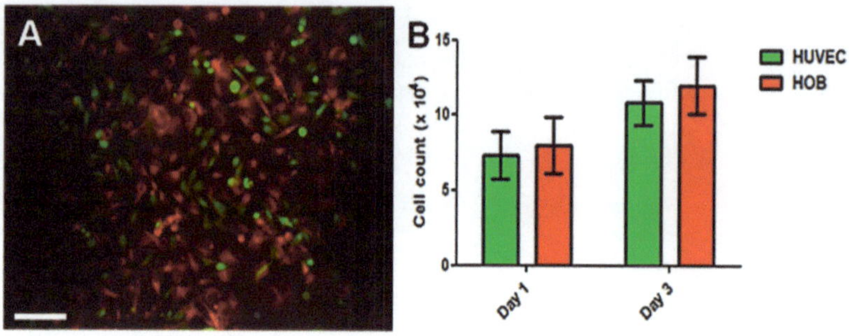


**Figure 9.** (**A**) Fluorescent micrographs showing co-cultures of alveolar osteoblast cells (aHOBs) in red and umbilical vein endothelial cells (HUVECs) in green, stained with CellTracker™ (scale bar = 150 µm); (**B**) no significant difference was observed between the numbers of each cell type on either day 1 or day 3, with $p$-values of $p = 0.79$ and $p = 0.64$ for days 1 and 3, respectively. Results are expressed as the mean value ± standard deviation (SD), derived from four replicate samples across three separate experimental runs.

### 3.4. VEGF Release from Co-Culture

Before adding the exogenous VEGF to the cells in co-culture to examine the effect on tubular formation, the amount of intrinsic VEGF released from each cell type and in the co-cultured cells was investigated. Figure 10 shows that VEGF release increased with time.

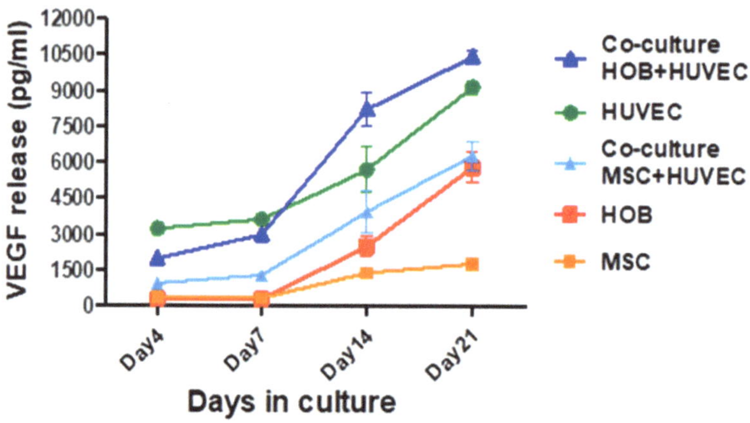


**Figure 10.** The amounts of VEGF released in co-culture (aHOB/HUVEC and hBMSC/HUVEC) and in monoculture for HUVEC, aHOB, and hBMSC. The data are presented as the average ± standard deviation (SD), calculated from quadruplicate samples obtained from three independent experimental iterations. The ratio of 60% HUVEC: 40% HOB media was optimum for HUVEC/HOB co-culture ($p < 0.001$) and 30% HUVEC: 70% MSC for HUVEC/hBMSC co-culture ($p < 0.05$). Data were analyzed using Stata™ statistical software. One-way analysis of variance (ANOVA) was used to compare the means among groups, and non-parametric Kruskal–Wallis analysis was used where the data were not normally distributed.

The highest VEGF release was observed in the co-culture of aHOB/HUVEC up to 10,455.6 pg/mL on day 21 followed by HUVEC monoculture. In contrast, very low levels of VEGF were released by hBMSC in monoculture. Both the co-culture of aHOB/HUVEC and hBMSC/HUVEC released more VEGF than the monoculture of aHOB or hBMSC alone (Figure 10).

### 3.5. Angiogenesis Assay

HUVECs in all culture conditions, except for the co-culture with hBMSC (with and without VEGF), appeared more elongated and organized to form aggregates. By day 10, a more organized tubular-like network formation was evident. Interestingly, co-cultures of HUVEC and aHOB with VEGF formed tubule networks that contained more total junctions and longer tubules (Figure 11A,B). In contrast, for the co-culture of HUVEC and hBMSC, no concomitant cell aggregates or lumenization of the nascent capillary-like structure was observed (Figure 11C).

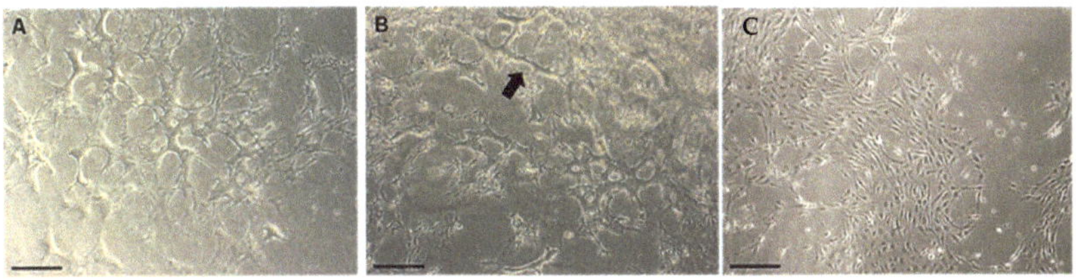


**Figure 11.** (**A**) Phase contrast micrographs showing a greater number of networks of branching and anastomosing cords of cells at day 10; (**B**) a longer tube length (arrow) was observed in the co-culture of HUVEC/HOB with VEGF; (**C**) Co-culture of HUVEC/hBMSC (Scale bar = 200 µm).

At the end of the experiment, quantification of angiogenesis was measured using CD31/PECAM-1 ELISA and image analysis. The emergent tubular structures were visualized with CD31 staining. The area occupied by aggregates of HUVEC was reconstructed using image software (Figure 12A,B).

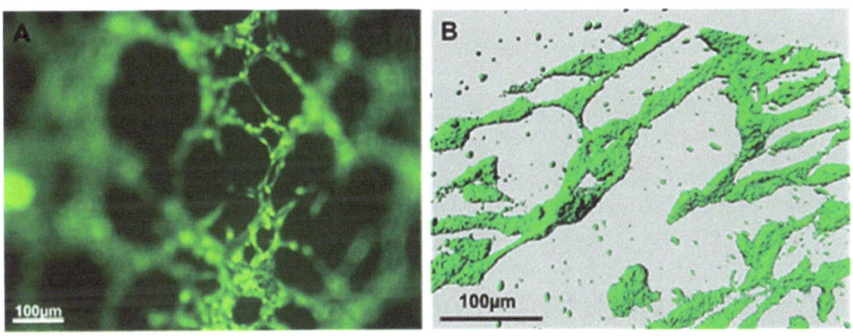


**Figure 12.** (**A**) Fluorescent micrograph of tubular structures of HUVEC stained with CD31 antibody. (**B**) Reconstructed image of HUVEC using LCS Leica confocal software (version 2.5).

The results obtained from CD31 ELISA confirmed a degree of tubule development in the wells. These showed that tubular formation in collagen gel was greatly enhanced by the co-culture of HUVEC and aHOB in the presence of VEGF (Figure 13A). An additional role of VEGF was observed; the results showed a greater effect in co-culture than monoculture when VEGF was added to the respective culture media. Furthermore, the total area of tubules (Figure 13B) was similar to the ELISA results, with statistical significance ($p < 0.001$) in co-cultures of HUVEC/aHOB + VEGF when compared to HUVEC/hBMSCs.

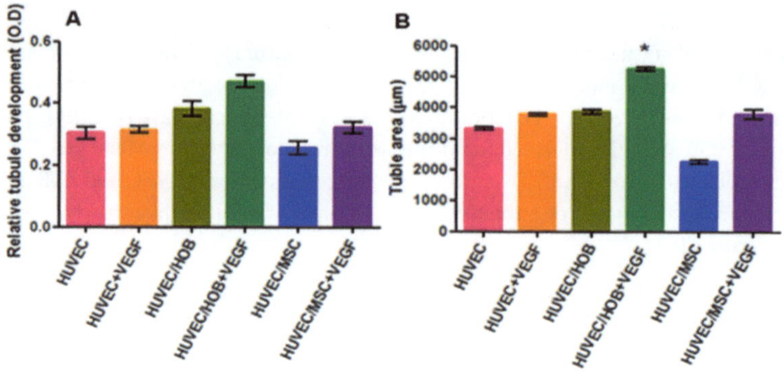


**Figure 13.** Comparison of the relative amount of tubular formation in different culture systems using (**A**) CD31 ELISA and (**B**) image analysis software. Data presented as mean ± standard deviation (SD) from quadruplicates obtained from triple-repeated experiments. One-way analysis of variance (ANOVA) indicated a significant difference among the culture groups ($p < 0.01$). Tukey's post hoc test showed that the mean values of the co-cultures of HUVEC/aHOB + VEGF were statistically significantly higher than co-cultures of HUVEC/hBMSCs (* $p < 0.01$).

### 3.6. Phenotypic Characteristics of Co-Culture of HUVEC and aHOB

The co-culture of HUVEC and aHOB in the presence of 10 ng/mL of VEGF demonstrated ideal conditions for initiating in vitro prevascularization of the CMP scaffold. The ability of the cells to retain phenotypic characteristics in the experimental conditions was confirmed by RT-PCR. The results for PCR showed both EC (VEGFR-2, Angiopoietin1, and Tie-2) and osteoblast (ALP, Runx2, and Col1) mRNA to be present in co-culture cell lysates (Figure 14). Although these results were only qualitative, they confirmed the expression of endothelial and osteoblast cell phenotypic markers for up to 14 days in co-culture.

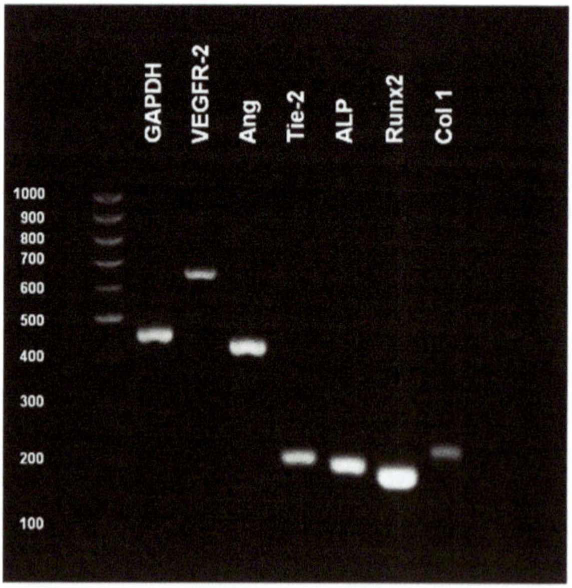


**Figure 14.** Reverse-transcriptase polymerase chain reaction (RT-PCR) for endothelial and osteoblast marker expression from selected co-culture conditions (HUVEC/aHOB+VEGF) after 14 days. Endothelial cell markers (VEGFR-2, Angiopoietin-1, Tie-2) and osteoblast markers (ALP, Runx2, col1) observed in cell lysates of co-culture confirmed the phenotypic expression of endothelial cells.

### 3.7. Prevascularization of 3D βCMP Scaffold

After 14 days of an ideal co-culture system, the outgrowth of co-culture cells adhering to the surface and also inside of the porous CMP scaffold was evident. SEM revealed tube-like structures across the surface (Figure 15A) and inside of the CMP scaffold (Figure 15B).

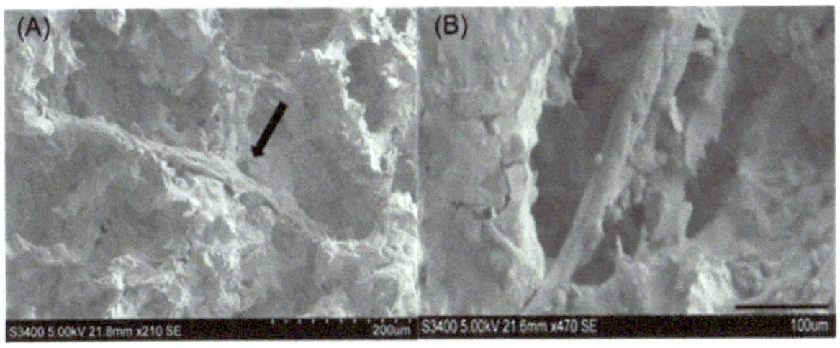


**Figure 15.** (**A**) The SEM image shows the tube-like structure across the surface of CMP (arrow). (**B**) A tubular structure inside the calcium metaphosphate (CMP) scaffold.

Immunofluorescent staining of EC with CD31 (Figure 16A,B), vWF (Figure 16C,D), and actin and vimentin (Figure 16E,F) demonstrated the organization of cells forming capillary-like structures inside the porous CMP scaffold.

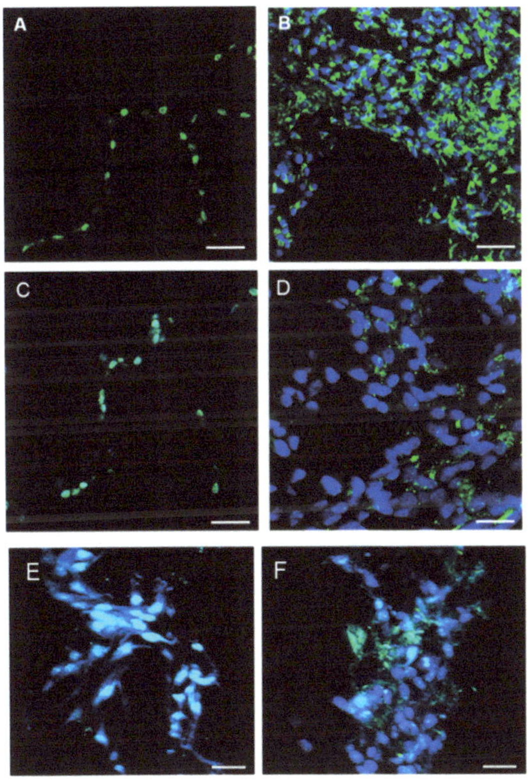


**Figure 16.** (**A**) Immunofluorescence staining of CD31, EC marker, inside the pore structure of CMP, and (**B**) image from the outside looking in through half of the fractured CMP (scale bar = 100 μm). (**C**) Immunofluorescent staining for vWF, EC marker, inside the pore structure of CMP, and (**D**) image from the outside looking in through the fractured CMP (scale bar = 100 μm). Immunofluorescent staining for (**E**) actin and (**F**) vimentin filaments inside the 3D scaffold (scale bar = 100 μm).

Each EC marker showed the organization of cells forming capillary-like structures inside the porous CMP. This was further confirmed by capturing images at different depths of the scaffold (Supplementary Materials). This animation confirmed that cells were able to infiltrate the interconnecting pores of the scaffold and arrange themselves in an orderly manner to form tubule-like structures.

The qualitative immunohistochemistry of EC markers in co-culture showed that cells were evenly distributed throughout the porous surface of the CMP scaffold (Figure 17A). Distinct differences in $CD31^+$ cells were observed between the monolayer (Figure 17B) and in 3D CMP, which were organized into capillary-like networks (Figure 17C). In addition, tubular-like structures with branches were confirmed by vWF staining as viewed by non-inverted microscopy (Figure 17D).

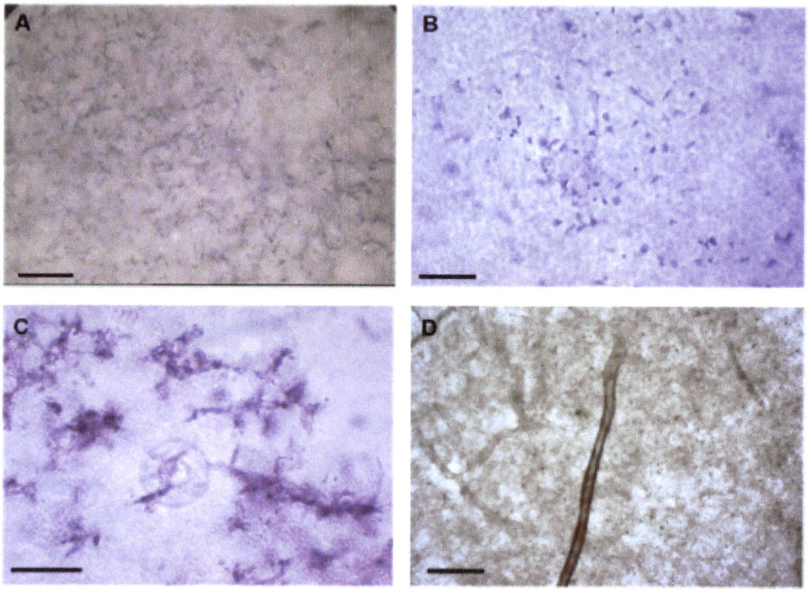


**Figure 17.** Immunohistochemical staining of (**A**) CD31 on CMP (10× magnifications), (**B**,**C**) CD31-positive ECs, and (**D**) VWF staining of a tubular structure in porous CMP (40× magnifications) (scale bar = 100 μm).

## 4. Discussion

Our study aimed to develop a cell-seeded scaffold for a prevascularized bone graft to address insufficient vascularization in large bone defects. While composite materials like polycaprolactone (SPLC) [27] or silk fibroin (SF) [28] have been used, calcium phosphate-based materials are preferred due to their similarity to natural bone, non-toxicity, biocompatibility, and osteoconductive properties [19]. Various synthesis methods for calcium phosphate bioceramics include co-precipitation and sintering. The sintering process, including heating rate, temperature, and duration, is crucial for achieving the desired properties. βCMP was formed by heating MCP to 900 °C to form the crystalline. PVA acted as a pore-forming agent during sintering, creating a highly porous microstructure through the release of water and carbon dioxide [20].

The FTIR, XRD, and EDX data confirmed that the chemical composition of both scaffolds was crystalline β-calcium metaphosphate (β-Ca $(PO_3)_2$). Low-vacuum SEM revealed a porous βCMP topography with mixed pore sizes. MIP and μCT analysis confirmed a wide range of pore sizes from macro- (>400 μm) to micro (<80 μm)-porosity, aligning with the optimal range for bone tissue engineering (100–500 μm) [11], while the optimal pore size for bone ingrowth was claimed to be 100–400 μm [29]. Larger pores facilitate cellular migration and proliferation, while micropores support nutrient, gas, and ion exchange. Three-dimensional modelling using CTvol software (skyscan, Kontich, Belgium) demonstrated good pore interconnectivity, promoting cell infiltration and colonization. The scaffold's pore structure, with the highest frequency between 80 and 100 μm, effectively balances mechanical strength with biological requirements for cell infiltration and vascularization, making it suitable for bone tissue engineering applications.

The total porosity of βCMP, measured by MIP (71%) and μCT analysis (68.3%), falls within the appropriate range for bone tissue engineering application as the natural bone porosity ranges from 50 to 90% [11]. While increasing porosity typically reduces the mechanical properties, this study prioritizes creating a material that allows nutrient ingress and cell migration. The focus was on maintaining an average porosity of 71%, with emphasis on pore size and interconnectivity.

Calcium metaphosphate (CMP) scaffolds exhibit a higher water uptake compared to hydroxyapatite (HA), indicating a more porous structure and faster degradation rate. This characteristic suggests that CMP may have compromised mechanical properties, making it less suitable for load-bearing applications. However, the increased porosity and degradation rate of CMP can be advantageous in non-load-bearing scenarios where gradual material resorption is desired, as it facilitates tissue integration and remodelling.

MTT assay and cell counts showed that the optimal VEGF dose for HUVEC was 10–30 ng/mL, with 5 ng/mL being ineffective. Therefore, 10 ng/mL was selected as the lowest effective dose, aligning with several studies [30–32]. In contrast, Silva and Mooney (2010) found 30 ng/mL optimal for human microvascular dermal endothelial cells (HDMECs), highlighting cell-specific responses. In vivo, GF levels are tightly regulated, as excess VEGF can cause abnormal vessel formation [33]. Determining the minimum effective concentration is crucial to achieve optimal results without side-effects like receptor downregulation.

Various studies have explored co-culture conditions for endothelial cells (ECs) and bone cells. This study found optimal media ratios of 60% HUVEC to 40% HOB media, and 30% HUVEC to 70% MSC media for maximal cell proliferation. Cell trackers confirmed equal growth and survival of both cell types. Achieving similar proliferation rates and maintaining phenotypes of both cell types are crucial for successful co-culture systems. The ideal cell ratio for vasculogenesis in vitro is debated. Unger et al. suggested a ratio of 5:1 of the endothelial cells to osteoblasts [34], while another study found that lower percentages of HUVECs stimulated prevascular network formation [9]. Our study demonstrated equal growth of HUVECs and aHOBs in co-culture. RT-PCR analysis of osteoblasts (ALP, RUNX2, Col1) and EC (VEGFR-2, Ang, Tie2) markers confirmed the maintenance of phenotypic expression in co-culture.

Collagen matrices allowed direct observation of cell organization and microcapillary-like tube formation, resembling the natural ECM for vessel formation [35]. The vasculogenic process was influenced by cell type and exogenous VEGF. HUVEC-hBMSC co-cultures in collagen gel proliferated but did not form networks without VEGF after 14 days. However, HUVEC-aHOB co-cultures and the HUVEC monoculture with VEGF formed tubule-like structures, consistent with Donovan D's findings [36]. The EC–osteoblast relationship enhanced network formation without exogenous VEGF through crosstalk and support. VEGF release experiments showed that HUVEC-aHOB co-cultures produced intrinsic VEGF up to 10,455.6 pg/m, near the optimal dose of VEGF (10 ng/mL).

The collagen scaffold provides a more physiological environment for cells, mimicking the natural ECM [37,38]. Collagen promotes cell migration, including EC, and EC binding to the ECM via integrins is crucial for VEGF-induced angiogenesis [39]. Unlike other biomaterials, βCMP demonstrated HUVEC adhesion, orientation, and microcapillary-like tube formation without surface modification in both monoculture and co-culture. This contrasts with studies requiring fibronectin coating for HUVEC adhesion, proliferation, and survival [34]. βCMP's success may be due to its properties and culture conditions. Unlike polymeric scaffolds, βCMP promotes cellular interaction with adsorbed proteins (including fibronectin) and media-supplied nutrients and growth factors.

Our study has several limitations that should be acknowledged. Primarily, the study predominantly utilizes human umbilical vein endothelial cells (HUVECs) for the endothelial component of the co-culture. Although HUVECs are a common model for endothelial cells, they may not accurately reflect the behaviour of endothelial cells found in bone tissue. Employing bone-specific endothelial cells could yield more relevant insights for bone tissue engineering applications. Furthermore, this study does not evaluate the long-term performance of the prevascularized scaffold or its degradation profile in physiological conditions, both of which are critical for understanding its behaviour in vivo. It is also important to note that our study does not cover the mechanical properties of the scaffold, which are crucial for bone tissue engineering applications. These limitations highlight the need for further research, which will focus on refining this approach to maximize its clinical applications, aiming to bridge the gap between scaffold implantation and successful vascular integration in complex bone defects.

## 5. Conclusions

This study demonstrates that the calcium metaphosphate (CMP) scaffold exhibits promising structural and biological properties for bone tissue engineering, particularly in cranio-maxillofacial reconstruction. By co-culturing osteoblasts and endothelial cells, we successfully established a prevascularized network within the scaffold, addressing the critical challenge of insufficient vascularization in large bone defects. The scaffold's porosity, interconnectivity, and ability to promote cell infiltration and capillary-like structure formation make it a strong candidate for further investigation. Future research will focus on refining this approach to enhance clinical applications by bridging the gap between scaffold implantation and successful vascular integration in complex bone defects. Additionally, future studies will include mechanical testing, such as compressive strength and fatigue resistance, to ensure the scaffold's suitability for load-bearing applications. Together, these efforts aim to improve the efficacy of synthetic bone grafts, leading to faster healing and better functional outcomes, particularly in maxillofacial and large bone reconstructions.

**Supplementary Materials:** The following supporting information can be downloaded at: https://www.mdpi.com/article/10.3390/jfb16010018/s1, Figure S1. The process of CMP fabrication. (A) The commercial powders of MCP and PVA were used in a 4:1 ratio by weight, and (B) mixed and homogenized by using a porcelain pestle and mortar. (C) The mixture was divided into 0.8 g samples and put into a stainless steel mould before being pressed at 10 MPa. (D) The solid discs were obtained after pressing in an Instron machine. (E) The sintering temperature was 8 °C/minute until 900 °C was reached, and then kept at 900 °C for 6 h, before allowing to cool down. (F) The sintered CMP discs were polished and soaked with PBS for 24 h before sterilization with gamma radiation. Figure S2. Overview of in vitro prevascularization model. aHOB or hBMSCs were co-cultured with HUVEC in specially conditioned media and culture conditions. Tubular formation in the presence of VEGF was assessed using collagen gel. The optimum condition was then applied to the cell-seeded scaffolds to allow a vascularized network formation inside of the CMP construct. Table S1. Plate layout tubular formation assay with or without GF supplements.

**Author Contributions:** Conceptualization, methodology, B.B. and L.D.S.; validation, formal analysis, investigation, B.B.; writing—original draft preparation, B.B. and A.S.; writing—review and editing, D.F.G. and L.D.S.; supervision, L.D.S.; funding acquisition, B.B. All authors have read and agreed to the published version of the manuscript.

**Funding:** This research was supported by the Thammasat University research fund, Contract No. TUFT 93/64.

**Institutional Review Board Statement:** The study was conducted in accordance with the Declaration of Helsinki, and approved by the Ethics Committee of Kings College Hospital REC (protocol code 08/H0808/104 and date of approval 21 May 2008).

**Informed Consent Statement:** Informed consent was obtained from all subjects involved in the study.

**Data Availability Statement:** The original contributions presented in the study are included in the article/Supplementary Materials. Further inquiries can be directed to the corresponding author.

**Acknowledgments:** The authors are highly grateful to Phil Salmon for supporting this research with micro-CT analysis at Skyscan, Belgium.

**Conflicts of Interest:** The authors declare no conflicts of interest.

## References

1. Zhang, X.; Xie, C.; Lin, A.S.; Ito, H.; Awad, H.; Lieberman, J.R.; Rubery, P.T.; Schwarz, E.M.; O'Keefe, R.J.; Guldberg, R.E. Periosteal progenitor cell fate in segmental cortical bone graft transplantations: Implications for functional tissue engineering. *J. Bone Miner. Res.* **2005**, *20*, 2124–2137. [CrossRef] [PubMed]
2. Lambert, F.; Lecloux, G.; Léonard, A.; Sourice, S.; Layrolle, P.; Rompen, E. Bone regeneration using porous titanium particles versus bovine hydroxyapatite: A sinus lift study in rabbits. *Clin. Implant Dent. Relat. Res.* **2013**, *15*, 412–426. [CrossRef] [PubMed]
3. White, A.A.; Best, S.M.; Kinloch, I.A. Hydroxyapatite–carbon nanotube composites for biomedical applications: A review. *Int. J. Appl. Ceram. Technol.* **2007**, *4*, 1–13. [CrossRef]
4. Board, P. *PDQ Cancer Information Summaries [Internet]*; National Cancer Institute (US): Bethesda, MD, USA, 2019.
5. Agarwal, R.; García, A.J. Biomaterial strategies for engineering implants for enhanced osseointegration and bone repair. *Adv. Drug Deliv. Rev.* **2015**, *94*, 53–62. [CrossRef] [PubMed]
6. Tan, H.; Yang, B.; Duan, X.; Wang, F.; Zhang, Y.; Jin, X.; Dai, G.; Yang, L. The promotion of the vascularization of decalcified bone matrix in vivo by rabbit bone marrow mononuclear cell-derived endothelial cells. *Biomaterials* **2009**, *30*, 3560–3566. [CrossRef]
7. Rady, A.A.; Hamdy, S.M.; Abdel-Hamid, M.A.; Hegazy, M.G.; Fathy, S.A.; Mostafa, A.A. The role of VEGF and BMP-2 in stimulation of bone healing with using hybrid bio-composite scaffolds coated implants in animal model. *Bull. Natl. Res. Cent.* **2020**, *44*, 1–9. [CrossRef]
8. Jang, H.-J.; Yoon, J.-K. The Role of Vasculature and Angiogenic Strategies in Bone Regeneration. *Biomimetics* **2024**, *9*, 75. [CrossRef] [PubMed]
9. Rouwkema, J.; Rivron, N.C.; van Blitterswijk, C.A. Vascularization in tissue engineering. *Trends Biotechnol.* **2008**, *26*, 434–441. [CrossRef] [PubMed]

10. Parfitt, A.M. The mechanism of coupling: A role for the vasculature. *Bone* **2000**, *26*, 319–323. [CrossRef]
11. Karageorgiou, V.; Kaplan, D. Porosity of 3D biomaterial scaffolds and osteogenesis. *Biomaterials* **2005**, *26*, 5474–5491. [CrossRef]
12. Asakawa, N.; Shimizu, T.; Tsuda, Y.; Sekiya, S.; Sasagawa, T.; Yamato, M.; Fukai, F.; Okano, T. Pre-vascularization of in vitro three-dimensional tissues created by cell sheet engineering. *Biomaterials* **2010**, *31*, 3903–3909. [CrossRef] [PubMed]
13. Madri, J.A.; Pratt, B.M.; Tucker, A.M. Phenotypic modulation of endothelial cells by transforming growth factor-beta depends upon the composition and organization of the extracellular matrix. *J. Cell Biol.* **1988**, *106*, 1375–1384. [CrossRef]
14. Padmanaban, A.M.; Ganesan, K.; Ramkumar, K.M. A Co-Culture System for Studying Cellular Interactions in Vascular Disease. *Bioengineering* **2024**, *11*, 1090. [CrossRef] [PubMed]
15. Black, A.F.; Berthod, F.; L'heureux, N.; Germain, L.; Auger, F.A. In vitro reconstruction of a human capillary-like network in a tissue-engineered skin equivalent. *FASEB J.* **1998**, *12*, 1331–1340. [CrossRef] [PubMed]
16. Tremblay, P.-L.; Hudon, V.; Berthod, F.; Germain, L.; Auger, F.A. Inosculation of Tissue-Engineered Capillaries with the Host's Vasculature in a Reconstructed Skin Transplanted on Mice. *Am. J. Transplant.* **2005**, *5*, 1002–1010. [CrossRef]
17. Huang, J.; Liao, C.; Yang, J.; Zhang, L. The role of vascular and lymphatic networks in bone and joint homeostasis and pathology. *Front. Endocrinol.* **2024**, *15*, 1465816. [CrossRef]
18. Liao, L.; Chen, L.; Chen, A.-Z.; Pu, X.-M.; Kang, Y.-Q.; Yao, Y.-D.; Liao, X.-M.; Huang, Z.-b.; Yin, G.-F. Preparation and characteristics of novel poly-L-lactide/β-calcium metaphosphate fracture fixation composite rods. *J. Mater. Res.* **2007**, *22*, 3324–3329. [CrossRef]
19. Jung, Y.; Kim, S.-S.; Kim, Y.H.; Kim, S.-H.; Kim, B.-S.; Kim, S.; Choi, C.Y.; Kim, S.H. A poly(lactic acid)/calcium metaphosphate composite for bone tissue engineering. *Biomaterials* **2005**, *26*, 6314–6322. [CrossRef]
20. Gauthier, O.; Bouler, J.-M.; Aguado, E.; Pilet, P.; Daculsi, G. Macroporous biphasic calcium phosphate ceramics: Influence of macropore diameter and macroporosity percentage on bone ingrowth. *Biomaterials* **1998**, *19*, 133–139. [CrossRef] [PubMed]
21. Di Silvio, L. Osteoblasts in bone tissue engineering. *Proc. Inst. Mech. Eng. Part H J. Eng. Med.* **2010**, *224*, 1415–1440.
22. Di-Silvo, L. *A Novel Application of Two Biomaterials for the Delivery of Growth Hormone and Its Effect on Osteoblasts*; University of London: London, UK, 1995.
23. Tsiridis, E.; Ali, Z.; Bhalla, A.; Heliotis, M.; Gurav, N.; Deb, S.; DiSilvio, L. In vitro and in vivo optimization of impaction allografting by demineralization and addition of rh-OP-1. *J. Orthop. Res.* **2007**, *25*, 1425–1437. [CrossRef] [PubMed]
24. Jaw, K. The effects on the devitrification mechanism for a certain composition of $CaO/P_2O_5$ glasswith additives of HAp, TCP and $\beta$-$CaP_2O_6$ whisker. *J. Therm. Anal. Calorim.* **2006**, *83*, 151–156. [CrossRef]
25. McIntosh, A.O.; Jablonski, W.L. X-Ray Diffraction Powder Patterns of Calcium Phosphates. *Anal. Chem.* **1956**, *28*, 1424–1427. [CrossRef]
26. Briche, S.; Zambon, D.; Boyer, D.; Chadeyron, G.; Mahiou, R. Sol–gel derived Y(PO3)3 polyphosphate: Synthesis and characterization. *Opt. Mater.* **2006**, *28*, 615–620. [CrossRef]
27. Fuchs, S.; Ghanaati, S.; Orth, C.; Barbeck, M.; Kolbe, M.; Hofmann, A.; Eblenkamp, M.; Gomes, M.; Reis, R.L.; Kirkpatrick, C.J. Contribution of outgrowth endothelial cells from human peripheral blood on in vivo vascularization of bone tissue engineered constructs based on starch polycaprolactone scaffolds. *Biomaterials* **2009**, *30*, 526–534. [CrossRef]
28. Ghanaati, S.; Unger, R.E.; Webber, M.J.; Barbeck, M.; Orth, C.; Kirkpatrick, J.A.; Booms, P.; Motta, A.; Migliaresi, C.; Sader, R.A.; et al. Scaffold vascularization in vivo driven by primary human osteoblasts in concert with host inflammatory cells. *Biomaterials* **2011**, *32*, 8150–8160. [CrossRef] [PubMed]
29. Dorozhkin, S.V.; Epple, M. Biological and Medical Significance of Calcium Phosphates. *Angew. Chem. Int. Ed.* **2002**, *41*, 3130–3146. [CrossRef]
30. Asahara, T.; Takahashi, T.; Masuda, H.; Kalka, C.; Chen, D.; Iwaguro, H.; Inai, Y.; Silver, M.; Isner, J.M. VEGF contributes to postnatal neovascularization by mobilizing bone marrow-derived endothelial progenitor cells. *EMBO J* **1999**, *18*, 3964–3972. [CrossRef]
31. Zambarakji, H.J.; Nakazawa, T.; Connolly, E.; Lane, A.M.; Mallemadugula, S.; Kaplan, M.; Michaud, N.; Hafezi-Moghadam, A.; Gragoudas, E.S.; Miller, J.W. Dose-Dependent Effect of Pitavastatin on VEGF and Angiogenesis in a Mouse Model of Choroidal Neovascularization. *Investig. Ophthalmol. Vis. Sci.* **2006**, *47*, 2623–2631. [CrossRef]
32. Sarkanen, J.-R.; Mannerstrom, M.; Vuorenpaa, H.; Uotila, J.; Ylikomi, T.; Heinonen, T. Intra-laboratory pre-validation of a human cell based in vitro angiogenesis assay for testing angiogenesis modulators. *Front. Pharmacol.* **2011**, *1*, 147. [CrossRef] [PubMed]
33. Kaigler, D.; Cirelli, J.A.; Giannobile, W.V. Growth factor delivery for oral and periodontal tissue engineering. *Expert Opin. Drug Deliv.* **2006**, *3*, 647–662. [CrossRef]
34. Unger, R.E.; Sartoris, A.; Peters, K.; Motta, A.; Migliaresi, C.; Kunkel, M.; Bulnheim, U.; Rychly, J.; James Kirkpatrick, C. Tissue-like self-assembly in cocultures of endothelial cells and osteoblasts and the formation of microcapillary-like structures on three-dimensional porous biomaterials. *Biomaterials* **2007**, *28*, 3965–3976. [CrossRef]

35. Gauvin, R.; Guillemette, M.; Dokmeci, M.; Khademhosseini, A. Application of microtechnologies for the vascularization of engineered tissues. *Vasc. Cell* **2011**, *3*, 24. [CrossRef] [PubMed]
36. Donovan, D.; Brown, N.J.; Bishop, E.T.; Lewis, C.E. Comparison of three in vitro human 'angiogenesis' assays with capillaries formed in vivo. *Angiogenesis* **2001**, *4*, 113–121. [CrossRef]
37. Montesano, R.; Orci, L.; Vassalli, P. In vitro rapid organization of endothelial cells into capillary-like networks is promoted by collagen matrices. *J. Cell Biol.* **1983**, *97*, 1648–1652. [CrossRef]
38. Glowacki, J.; Mizuno, S. Collagen scaffolds for tissue engineering. *Biopolymers* **2008**, *89*, 338–344. [CrossRef] [PubMed]
39. Schultz, G.S.; Wysocki, A. Interactions between extracellular matrix and growth factors in wound healing. *Wound Repair Regen.* **2009**, *17*, 153–162. [CrossRef]

Journal of
*Functional Biomaterials*

*Review*

# Exploring Mechanical Features of 3D Head and Neck Cancer Models

**Aleksandra Evangelista [1], Franca Scocozza [2,*], Michele Conti [2,3], Ferdinando Auricchio [2], Bice Conti [4], Rossella Dorati [4], Ida Genta [4], Marco Benazzo [1] and Silvia Pisani [4]**

1 Department of Otorhinolaryngology, Fondazione IRCCS Policlinico San Matteo, Via Golgi 19, 27100 Pavia, Italy; a.evangelista@smatteo.pv.it (A.E.); m.benazzo@smatteo.pv.it (M.B.)
2 Department of Civil Engineering and Architecture, University of Pavia, Via Ferrata 3, 27100 Pavia, Italy; michele.conti@unipv.it (M.C.); ferdinando.auricchio@unipv.it (F.A.)
3 3D and Computer Simulation Laboratory, IRCCS Policlinico San Donato, Piazza Edmondo Malan 2, San Donato Milanese, 20097 Milano, Italy
4 Department of Drug Sciences, University of Pavia, Via Taramelli 12, 27100 Pavia, Italy; bice.conti@unipv.it (B.C.); rossella.dorati@unipv.it (R.D.); ida.genta@unipv.it (I.G.); silvia.pisani@unipv.it (S.P.)
* Correspondence: franca.scocozza@unipv.it

**Abstract:** Head and neck squamous cell carcinoma (HNSCC) presents significant challenges in oncology due to its complex biology and poor prognosis. Traditional two-dimensional (2D) cell culture models cannot replicate the intricate tumor microenvironment, limiting their usefulness in studying disease mechanisms and testing therapies. In contrast, three-dimensional (3D) in vitro models provide more realistic platforms that better mimic the architecture, mechanical features, and cellular interactions of HNSCC. This review explores the mechanical properties of 3D in vitro models developed for HNSCC research. It highlights key 3D culture techniques, such as spheroids, organoids, and bioprinted tissues, emphasizing their ability to simulate critical tumor characteristics like hypoxia, drug resistance, and metastasis. Particular attention is given to stiffness, elasticity, and dynamic behavior, highlighting how these models emulate native tumor tissues. By enhancing the physiological relevance of in vitro studies, 3D models offer significant potential to revolutionize HNSCC research and facilitate the development of effective, personalized therapeutic strategies. This review bridges the gap between preclinical and clinical applications by summarizing the mechanical properties of 3D models and providing guidance for developing systems that replicate both biological and mechanical characteristics of tumor tissues, advancing innovation in cancer research and therapy.

**Keywords:** HNSCC; 3D models; mechanical properties; 3D bioprinting; cancer models

## 1. Introduction

Head and neck squamous cell carcinoma (HNSCC) ranks as the sixth most prevalent cancer worldwide. Primarily located in the oral cavity, larynx, and pharynx, it arises from the mucosal epithelium; these areas are adjacent to numerous critical structures, complicating the possibility of extensive surgical removal. This tumor is often diagnosed at a late stage, exhibits rapid progression, and shows resistance to antitumor treatment strategies [1]. Developing reliable preclinical models is crucial for gaining a deeper understanding of the molecular mechanisms underlying HNSCC treatment resistance and progression. These models are also crucial for identifying more effective therapeutic strategies.

Drug screening in monolayer cell cultures (2D in vitro model) remains the primary approach for discovering new therapeutic agents. Immortalized cell lines obtained from

 https://doi.org/10.3390/jfb16030074

HNSCC tumors serve as an important tool for assessing the efficacy of antitumor treatments, exploring mechanisms of resistance, and enhancing early diagnostic and screening methods. The advantages of cell lines as the simplest in vitro tumor model are evident: they are easy to use, allow for precise control of external factors, are economically accessible, and have a wide range of applications [2]. However, three-dimensional (3D) in vitro models, which more accurately mimic the architecture and cellular environment of tumor tissue, may be superior in predicting drug efficacy and tumor progression. Studies using 3D cell cultures have demonstrated significant variations in radiation and drug sensitivity, akin to those observed in in vivo tumors [3]. The main advantages of 3D models compared to the traditional 2D are their ability to better mimic the complexity and behavior of primary tumors while 2D models fall short in replicating the physiological environment of living tissues. In contrast, 3D models, particularly those using cell lines or primary cells, provide a more accurate representation of the tumor microenvironment by promoting cell–cell and cell–extracellular matrix (ECM) interactions. This leads to enhanced cell proliferation, differentiation, and morphology that closely resemble in vivo conditions. However, 3D models come with challenges such as increased costs, more time-consuming examination processes, and technical difficulties in handling [4]. While the cost and technical demands of 3D models are acknowledged, they offer significant advantages in terms of predictive accuracy for tumor progression and therapeutic response. These benefits, particularly in drug screening and the reduction of animal testing, provide a strong justification for their adoption despite the higher initial investment. A comparative cost–benefit analysis would help to further demonstrate how these models could ultimately lead to more effective and personalized treatments, potentially offsetting costs in the long term [5].

Thus, robust preclinical models are necessary to investigate the mechanisms of treatment resistance and progression in HNSCC, which will help to refine and improve therapeutic strategies. In recent years, the development of patient-specific 3D cell models represents a significant advancement in HNSCC research, offering a tailored approach to testing chemotherapeutic drugs with greater specificity, enhancing our ability to combat treatment resistance and advance personalized therapeutic strategies for patients. These advancements help rationalize the use of animals in research, aligning with the principles of "the 3Rs" (reduction, replacement, and refinement) in animal experimentation [1,6,7].

This review aims to provide a comprehensive summary of the latest and most innovative 3D in vitro models developed for head and neck squamous cell carcinoma (HNSCC) research, with a particular focus on their mechanical properties (Figure 1). The development of 3D models still faces challenges, including standardizing mechanical properties across systems, reproducing the complexity of the native extracellular matrix, and scaling models for high-throughput screening. While research efforts have been initiated to address some of these challenges, such as refining mechanical tunability and enhancing matrix composition, others—such as the dynamic simulation of vascularization or immune interactions—remain largely unexplored. Highlighting these gaps more explicitly is essential to map the trajectory of future research. Addressing these limitations is essential to fully realize the potential of 3D in vitro models as transformative tools in cancer research [8].

Understanding and replicating in vitro the mechanical characteristics of the tumor microenvironment is crucial for enhancing the physiological relevance of these 3D models. These capabilities bridge the gap between conventional in vitro methods and in vivo studies, enhancing the predictive power of drug testing and accelerating the development of effective therapies for HNSCC. This review also explores how mechanical properties influence tumor growth, metastasis, and treatment response, providing direct clinical applications. By closely replicating the structural and biomechanical characteristics of head and neck cancers (HNCs), 3D models enable the development of more effective therapies, support personalized treatment testing, and offer insights to refine surgical strategies. Ultimately, this approach contributes to advancing therapeutic strategies and improving clinical outcomes for patients with HNCs [9].

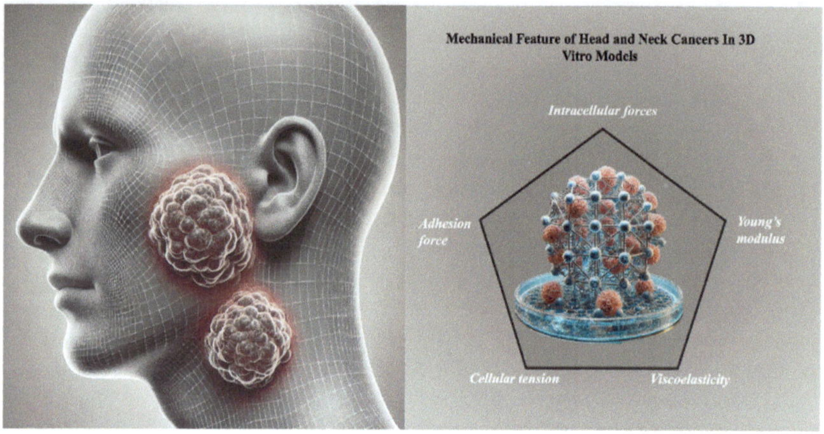


**Figure 1.** This review explores the mechanical features of head and neck cancers (HNCs) in 3D in vitro models aiming to enhance our understanding of tumor biomechanics with direct clinical applications. This approach facilitates the development of more effective therapies, enables testing of personalized treatments, and offers insights to improve surgical strategies.

## 2. Mechanical Properties of HNSCC Models

Cancer is a complex, multi-phase condition marked by abnormal regulation and uncontrolled cell growth, leading to the development of solid tumors. Mechanical abnormalities present within the tumor microenvironment (TME), including compressive forces and matrix stiffness, affect cancer cells at the molecular, cellular, and tissue level to fuel tumor growth and metastasis [10]. Studies show that examining the mechanical characteristics of cells and tissues in a developing tumor is essential for understanding how cancers maintain their molecular structure and organization. Various mechanical properties are altered in cancer cells, such as cell tension, hydrostatic pressure, adhesion strength, elasticity (Young's modulus E), and viscosity ($\eta$) [11].

Among the many mechanical properties analyzed in mechanobiological studies, stiffness is one of the most frequently assessed metrics. It is typically measured using Young's modulus, which represents the ratio of stress ($\sigma$), or the applied force per unit area, to strain ($\varepsilon$), which quantifies the relative change in length compared to the material's original length [12]. However, only stiffness does not fully capture the true mechanical behavior of biological materials due to the highly heterogeneous nature of both cells and tissues, and these structures typically display a time-dependent response rather than linear-elastic deformation when subjected to an external force.

A related concept used in certain measurement systems is compliance ($\delta$), which is the inverse of stiffness and represents the flexibility of a material.

Cancerous cells undergo significant changes in their cytoskeleton and plasma membrane, which profoundly affect the physical properties of the surrounding tissue. Research has consistently shown that these alterations lead to a general decrease in cellular tension, a phenomenon closely linked to malignant progression. One notable consequence of these structural changes is the reduced shear modulus observed in cancerous cells compared to healthy ones. By analyzing the mechanical properties of cancer cells and tissues (Table 1), scientists can gain valuable insights into how the modulation of specific biomolecules or pharmacological treatments might influence cancer cell aggressiveness—either by enhancing or suppressing it [11,13]. Furthermore, understanding these mechanical alterations plays a crucial role in the development of increasingly realistic and predictive 3D models.

**Table 1.** Mechanical properties of distinct human cancer cell types reported in the literature.

| Cancer | Normal | Malignant | Ref. |
|---|---|---|---|
| Esophageal | EPC2:<br>E[(1)] = 4.72 kPa (modal) | CP-A:<br>E = 3.08 kPa (modal)<br>CP-D:<br>E = 2.64 kPa (modal) | [14] |
| Melanoma | Human epidermal melanocytes, adult<br>(HEMa):<br>E = 14.3 ± 0.8 kPa | VGP (primary tumor):<br>E = 9.91 ± 0.55 kPa<br>Skin metastasis<br>(WM239):<br>E = 7.8 ± 0.61 kPa<br>Lung metastasis<br>(A375P):<br>E = 5.7 ± 0.61 kPa | [15] |
| Oral squamous cell | OKF-4:<br>$\delta^{(2)} = 0.69 \pm 0.46 \times 10^{-2}$ Pa$^{-1}$<br>OKF-6:<br>$\delta = 0.75 \pm 0.49 \times 10^{-2}$ Pa$^{-1}$ | CAL-33:<br>$\delta = 1.99 \pm 1.63 \times 10^{-2}$ Pa$^{-1}$<br>CAL-27:<br>$\delta = 1.59 \pm 0.75 \times 10^{-2}$ Pa$^{-1}$<br>BHY (OSCC):<br>$\delta = 1.86 \pm 0.76 \times 10^{-2}$ Pa$^{-1}$<br>HNCs:<br>$\delta = 1.75 \pm 0.76 \times 10^{-2}$ Pa$^{-1}$ | [16] |
| Squamous cell carcinoma | Human mammary fibroblasts:<br>E ~1 kPa | SCC38:<br>E ~0.75 kPa | [17] |
| Thyroid | S748:<br>E ~2211–6879 Pa | S277:<br>E ~1189–1365 Pa | [18] |

(1) Young's modulus (E); (2) Compliance (δ).

The tumor microenvironment (TME) is a dynamic and complex system where both cellular and extracellular components interact to influence tumor growth, progression, and response to therapy. Among the factors shaping the TME, mechanical properties play a pivotal role, directly impacting processes such as cell migration, invasion, and drug resistance. These mechanical characteristics are not solely determined by the tumor cells but are also profoundly influenced by components of the TME, including integrins and stromal elements. Integrins, for instance, are significant therapeutic targets in squamous cell carcinoma (SCC). Among these, cilengitide, a specific integrin inhibitor, has been clinically evaluated in combination with 5-fluorouracil (5-FU), cisplatin, and cetuximab, an epidermal growth factor receptor (EGFR) inhibitor, in studies aimed at improving therapeutic efficacy [19].

However, the role of additional TME factors in HNSCC progression remains incompletely understood. The immune system, for example, plays a dual role in HNSCC, both promoting tumor elimination and, in some cases, facilitating immune evasion through immunosuppressive elements such as regulatory T cells (Tregs), tumor-associated macrophages (TAMs), and myeloid-derived suppressor cells (MDSCs). Additionally, stromal components, including cancer-associated fibroblasts (CAFs), actively contribute to tumor progression by remodeling the extracellular matrix (ECM), promoting angiogenesis, and modulating immune responses. Vascularization is another critical aspect, as abnormal tumor vasculature can create hypoxic regions that drive treatment resistance and tumor aggressiveness. These factors collectively shape the TME and influence therapeutic response, highlighting the need for further research to develop more effective combination therapies targeting both cellular and mechanical components of the TME [20].

Targeting the mechanical properties of the tumor microenvironment (TME) represents an emerging strategy in cancer therapy, particularly in head and neck squamous cell carcinoma (HNSCC) and other solid tumors. Table 2 highlights several clinical trials investigating agents that modulate integrins, stromal components, and extracellular matrix (ECM) stiffness to enhance treatment efficacy. Translating therapies that target the mechanical properties of the TME into clinical practice remains a challenge due to the complex and dynamic nature of tumor–stroma interactions. While preclinical studies have demonstrated the potential of targeting integrins and stromal components to improve therapeutic efficacy, clinical outcomes have often been disappointing, emphasizing the need for refined approaches.

**Table 2.** Clinical trials investigating agents targeting the mechanical properties of the Tumor Microenvironment (TME).

| Target | Agent | Cancer Type | Combined with | Clinicaltrial.gov ID |
|---|---|---|---|---|
| Integrin | Cilengitide | Squamous cell carcinoma | 5-FU + cisplatin + cetuximab (EGFR inhibitor) (PFE) | NCT00705016 |
| Stromal components | PEGPH20 (HA) (discontinued) | Esophageal | Leucovorin, cisplatin, paclitaxel, oxaliplatin, fluorouracil, atezolizumab, cobimetinib, ramucirumab, BL-8040, linagliptin, tiragolumab | NCT03281369 |
| Stromal components | Saridegib (GPCR inhibitor) | Head and neck squamous cell carcinoma (HNSCC) | Cetuximab | NCT01255800 |

One of the most studied integrin inhibitors, cilengitide, which targets $\alpha v\beta 3$ and $\alpha v\beta 5$, was evaluated in squamous cell carcinoma in combination with 5-FU, cisplatin, and cetuximab (NCT00705016). Although preclinical studies suggested that integrin inhibition could enhance chemotherapy sensitivity, clinical trials failed to show significant survival benefits. This outcome underscores the complexity of integrin signaling and suggests that successful integration of these therapies may require better patient stratification and combination with immune-modulating agents. PEGPH20, a hyaluronidase enzyme designed to degrade hyaluronic acid (HA) and reduce ECM stiffness, was investigated in esophageal cancer (NCT03281369). Despite the initial promise, the drug was discontinued due to a lack of efficacy and potential toxicities, highlighting the challenge of targeting ECM components effectively. Similarly, saridegib, a GPCR inhibitor targeting the Hedgehog signaling pathway, was tested in HNSCC in combination with cetuximab (NCT01255800). While the Hedgehog pathway is known to play a role in ECM remodeling and stromal cell activation, clinical translation of GPCR inhibitors remains difficult due to an incomplete understanding of their effects on tumor–stromal interactions. These challenges suggest that future efforts in targeting the mechanical properties of the TME will require biomarker-driven patient selection and optimized combination strategies to improve therapeutic outcomes [21].

### 2.1. Types of 3D Models for Head and Neck Cancer

Three-dimensional cultivation involves the following techniques: growing cellular spheroids and organoids, utilizing bioink, sowing on scaffolds, and decellularized tissues, microfluidics, "organs-on-a-chip", and 3D bioprinting (Figure 2).

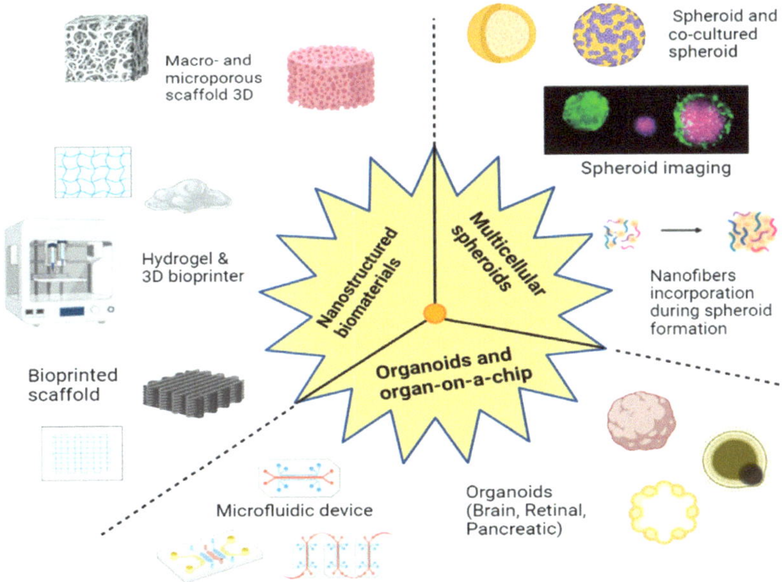


**Figure 2.** Schematic representation of the most promising technologies and tools for the engineering of 3D in vitro models. Figure created with BioRender (https://www.biorender.com/ (accessed on 16 February 2025) Shiz Aoki, Toronto, Canada).

Choosing one of these approaches depends on many factors, including the aim, experimental time frame, and material contents. At present, three-dimensional cell systems are most developed using technologies based on cell spheroids, scaffolds, and hydrogels. These methods are favored due to their affordability, simplicity, scalability, and suitability for high-throughput analysis, making them particularly valuable for drug testing [22].

#### 2.1.1. Spheroid Models

Multi-cellular spheroids derived from tumor cells are among the simplest and most reproducible in vitro tumor models that can accurately reflect how tumor tissue responds to therapy. Spheroids exhibit cellular zoning, which becomes more pronounced as their size increases. When spheroids reach a diameter of around 500 μm, they develop a hypoxic zone and areas of necrosis. Histological examination of large spheroids reveals several distinct layers: an external layer of rapidly proliferating cells, a central layer of senescent or quiescent cells, and an inner layer of necrotic cells. These diverse layers arise due to the restricted diffusion of oxygen and nutrients across the multi-cellular structure [1,23].

Spheroid formation occurs naturally when cell–cell interactions outweigh interactions between cells and the culture surface. As a result, all primary techniques for spheroid formation are designed to foster these conditions. These methods involve hanging drop technique, growing cells on ultra-low-adhesion surfaces in dishes or vials, and using rotational systems or magnetic fields. In each of these methods (Figure 3), the key objective is to minimize contact between cells and the culture substrate. Primary cultures are inherently heterogeneous and thus provide more relevant models for personalized medicine. To better replicate the different compositions of tumor tissue, heterospheroids (also known as heterotypic or co-culture spheroids) are used, consisting of tumor cells associated with other cells found in vivo, such as immune cells, fibroblasts, or endothelial cells [1,24].

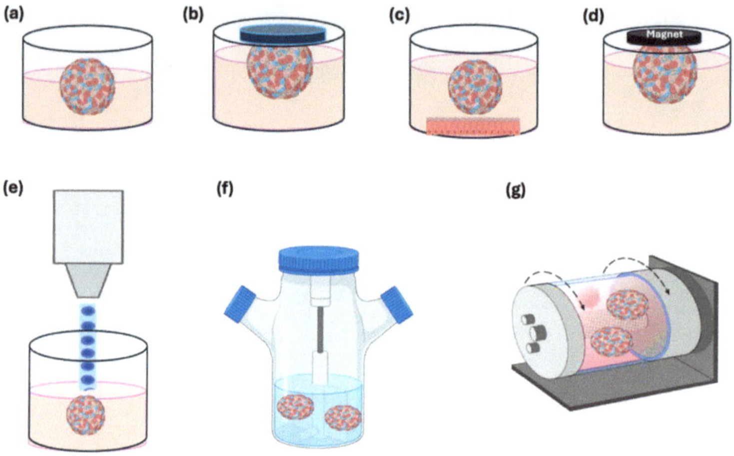


**Figure 3.** Different methods of cell spheroid method. (**a**) the use of a low-adhesive curved surface, (**b**) the hanging drop method, (**c**) the use of microstructured substrates, (**d**) magnetic levitation using magnetic culture, (**e**) bioprinting, (**f**) cultivation of suspension culture in stirred bioreactors, and (**g**) in spinner flasks.

In many respects, spheroids closely resemble tumor tissue, making them a relevant preclinical model for assessing the efficacy and toxicity of a wide range of anticancer drugs. However, they often fail to properly include intratumoral heterogeneity and the biomechanical and biochemical cues provided by surrounding tissues due to the lack of other supporting cell types and the extracellular matrix that contribute to the tumor microenvironment [22].

Kadlets et al. have developed stable protocols for HNSCC spheroid formation and highlighted their distinct characteristics in comparison to traditional 2D cell culture techniques using FaDu, CAL27, and SCC25 head and neck squamous cell carcinoma cells [25]. The research analyzed the expression of key HNSCC proteins in spheroids and compared the findings with a 2D cell model. Although derived from the same cell line, the spheroids and monolayer cultures exhibited variations in protein expression intensity and staining patterns. Also, Melissaridou et al., in their research, confirmed how the 3D cell cultures (five HNSCC cell lines, namely LK0858B, LK0902, LK0917, LK1108, and LK1122 were used) imitate the in vivo behavior of neoplastic cells within the tumor, suggesting that a 3D culture model is superior to 2D monolayers in the search for new therapeutic targets [26].

To recreate a tumor microenvironment (TME) closer to real conditions, Francois et al. developed a 3D human heterotypic model consisting of head and neck squamous cell carcinoma (HNSCC) cells and different subtypes of macrophages to replicate the interactions between immune cells and cancer cells [27]. The goal is to develop a model for screening immunomodulatory nanomedicines designed to target tumor-associated macrophages (TAMs) in solid head and neck tumors, either as standalone treatments or in combination with standard therapies. A summary of studies comparing 2D and 3D spheroid models is provided in Table 3A.

#### 2.1.2. Organoid Models

The development of organoid technology, which merges the benefits of spheroids (cell self-organization in 3D) and tissue engineering models (presence of extracellular matrix), has significantly advanced research into the interactions between tumor cells and ECM (Figure 4). As a result, organoids exhibit high genetic and phenotypic similarity to native tissues, preserving the original intratumoral heterogeneity. Organoids used for modeling HNSCC are typically derived from the resected tumor tissue of patients. In recent years, organoids have also been successfully generated from normal and tumor tissues of various organs, including the brain, lungs, esophagus, stomach, intestines, liver, pancreas, kidneys, and salivary glands, among others [1,28].

The number of studies successfully producing HNSCC organoids is limited due to logistical challenges (minimizing the time from tumor tissue resection to delivery to the laboratory), often insufficient volume of biologic material, and stringent requirements for both the qualitative and quantitative composition of the culture medium. Moreover, the efficiency of generating organoids from head and neck tumor tissue rarely exceeds 60–70%, even in well-established laboratories. The primary factor affecting this efficiency is believed to be the quality of the initial biological material, as necrotic tumor tissue has a low organoid-forming capacity [1,29].

Creating organoids requires significant material and time investments, specialized expertise, and close collaboration between clinicians and cell biology researchers. The result is a tumor model that can be maintained in vitro for extended periods, preserving genetic stability while closely resembling the original tissue's morphology. Organoids are considered valuable in vitro tumor models because they retain a unique set of biomarkers from the donor tissue. Growing evidence indicates that organoids can predict the treatment response of the tumors from which they are derived. Numerous studies highlight the prognostic potential of organoids in predicting how solid tumors will respond to radiotherapy and its combination with other treatments. Furthermore, organoids can be cultured and cryopreserved, facilitating the creation of organoid biobanks containing various cancer subtypes from multiple patients, making them an essential resource for preclinical research [1,30].

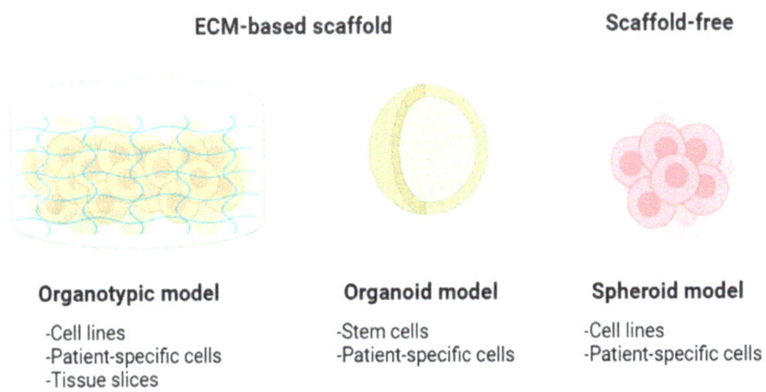


**Figure 4.** An illustration of organotypic culture models. Organotypic models offer cell–cell and ECM interactions within a 3D culture system. These models involve embedding disaggregated cells or tissues in ECM-based scaffolds. Specifically, organoids are a subtype of organotypic models derived from stem cells or patient-specific cells. In contrast, spheroids can be formed using either single or multiple standard cell lines or patient-derived cells, with or without the inclusion of ECM-based scaffolds. Figure created with BioRender (https://www.biorender.com/, 2025, Shiz Aoki, Toronto, Canada) and adapted from Moya-Garcia et al. [31].

Some studies comparing 2D and 3D organoid models are summarized in Table 3B.

#### 2.1.3. Scaffold-Based Models

To enhance the relevance of in vitro tumor models, tissue engineering approaches, such as cell culture on 3D scaffolds, have been utilized. The first HNSCC model utilizing a synthetic scaffold was introduced in 2007. This model involved culturing oral squamous cell carcinoma (OSCC-3) cells within a highly porous poly(lactide-co-glycolide) (PLG) scaffold.

Scaffolds are three-dimensional structures derived from various sources, characterized by parameters such as porosity, mechanical properties, and surface chemistry. They are engineered to replicate the extracellular matrix, offering structural support to cells while encouraging adhesion, proliferation, and differentiation. Natural materials like alginic acid, chitosan, collagen, fibronectin, and hyaluronic acid are preferred over synthetic ones due to their closer resemblance to the human body. In contrast, synthetic polymers (e.g., poly-ε-caprolactone (PCL), polyvinyl alcohol (PVA)) are used in the manufacture of scaffolds to provide better mechanical strength, processability, and more controlled degradation rates. Scaffolds of natural and synthetic origin are often used to create biomimetic tumors and subsequently used in anticancer drug trials. Thus, the use of polylactide scaffolds may help mimic the tumor microenvironment [22,32].

Furthermore, in the field of scaffolds, developments are underway to realize hybrid scaffolds that study the correlation between mechanical and surface chemical properties on the one hand and cellular responses on the other. Understanding these interactions will help to achieve maximum biocompatibility, high cell proliferation, and differentiation when implanting materials at the site of injury. Further advancement and optimization of scaffold-based HNSCC models, considering essential factors such as material cytotoxicity, carcinogenicity, and others, could be beneficial for studying various cancer-related processes. Additionally, these models could help identify similar materials suitable for use as grafts in severe cancer lesions [22,33].

HNSCC has been studied with models using various scaffolds including sandwich-like collagen scaffolds [34], microtiter plates [35], decellularized tongue extracellular matrix [36], poly(L-lactide-co-ε-caprolactone) (PLCL) scaffolds [37], and 3D-printed scaffolds based on β-tricalcium phosphate [38]. Thus, scaffold-based models provide for co-culture with various cell types, considering the physicochemical properties of the extracellular matrix (as in hydrogel-based models) and the influence of microstructure/topography/curvature on tumor 3D growth. For example, these models could focus on testing diagnostic agents to detect cancer markers related to cell adhesion or chemotherapeutic agents targeting the cytoskeleton [22,39].

#### 2.1.4. Bioprinted and Hydrogel-Based Models

In recent years, 3D tissue printing has advanced significantly. This technique involves building three-dimensional structures by precisely layering bioink, which contains cells, cytokines, and extracellular matrix components. Bioink typically consists of a biocompatible hydrogel embedded with single cells or cell spheroids [22,40]. These techniques differ considerably in various factors, such as equipment and material costs, printing speed, resolution, limitations on the maximum size of the printed object, and the types of hydrogels that can be used. At present, there are only a few studies detailing the successful application of bioprinting methods for modeling HNSCC. Kort-Mascort et al. showed that their 3D bioprinted model of HNSCC effectively serves as an advanced tissue-engineered model. In this approach, a hydrogel scaffold is employed, and the printing method allows precise control over tissue architecture, surpassing traditional gel layering techniques. However, to date, bioprinted HNSCC models have been developed primarily using immortalized cell lines, primarily due to the high cell density required for achieving the desired outcomes [41].

A key goal for researchers is to create 3D models using patient-derived HNSCC cells to better replicate biological features and potentially advance personalized medicine applications. A promising strategy involves utilizing synthetic extracellular matrices that replicate the characteristics of natural extracellular matrices found in vivo. These synthetic matrices can be composed of natural polymers, such as alginate, chitosan, and pectin, or chemically synthesized polymers like PEG and PVA. The primary requirements for these hydrogels include biocompatibility and suitable physicochemical properties. Additionally, their characteristics—particularly mechanical properties such as density, stiffness, viscoelasticity, and plasticity—can be precisely adjusted and regulated through chemical or biotechnological synthesis. Compared to natural matrices, synthetic matrices offer greater control over the simulation of the tumor cell microenvironment, enabling more accurate modeling of in vivo conditions. The mechanical properties of hydrogels affect tumor cell proliferation, migration, and cell function formation through cell surface adhesion proteins, linker proteins, and cytoskeletal networks, and stimulate signaling for spheroid and organoid development [42].

Thus, the ability to modulate properties allows for the specific setting and selection of specific types of tumor cultures with different morphology and cellular behavior concerning HNSCC. As a result, hydrogel-based models can be used to test anticancer drugs in terms of penetration into tumor cells via the extracellular matrix.

#### 2.1.5. Tumor Explants and Histocultures

Another 3D cell model is the patient-derived tumor explant (PDE) culture, where a tissue fragment is maintained alive under ex vivo conditions. This model involves minimal manipulation: the tissue is mechanically fragmented into pieces approximately 1–3 $mm^3$ and then placed in a culture medium. This approach maintains the different cellular and extracellular components of the original tumor, including both the extracellular matrix and associated tumor cells. Despite its advantages in maintaining tumor tissue architecture and ease of production, the use of a PDE as an in vitro model is limited by its fragility. Typically, PDEs are employed for rapid evaluation of drug efficacy and/or toxicity within 5–7 days post-isolation [1,43]. It has been observed that the viability of HNSCC explants declines from 90% to 30% within a week of cultivation.

An alternative approach for this type of 3D model is histoculture. In histoculture, tumor tissue is mechanically processed not with surgical instruments but using a vibratome, which produces thick, unfixed tissue sections. Similar to explants, these sections preserve the tumor cells within their native microenvironment, including the extracellular matrix, immune cells, and stromal components. As a result, explants and histocultures of HNSCC are relatively simple to obtain and efficient for quickly evaluating tumor tissue responses to drug treatments, demonstrating their potential for use in personalized medicine applications [44].

#### 2.1.6. Microfluidics-Based Models (Tumor-on-a-Chip)

Tumor-on-a-chip is a technique that has seen significant development in the past decade, allowing for precise manipulation of small liquid volumes and control over nutrient concentrations in both space and time. This is achieved through microchannels (ranging from 1–1000 μm in cross-section) where the liquid flow remains laminar. In addition, microfluidics has the advantage of being able to handle small amounts of experimental samples and reagents. Microfluidic technology is particularly useful in studying oncological diseases due to the correlation between cancer cell migration and the gradient of various chemokine concentrations. Notable recent developments in microfluidics include 3D microfluidic chips and microfluidic devices for managing chemotactic migration of HNSCC cells. Furthermore, it is easier to use and enables research of HNSCC that closely mimics human physiology compared to animal testing [45].

Therefore, tumor-on-a-chip technology represents a valuable tool for personalized evaluation of the efficacy of various antitumor agents, either individually or in combination. It allows for dynamic monitoring of how tissue samples from HNSCC patients respond to different treatments. The progress in microfluidic platforms holds the potential to improve patient outcomes by enabling the selection of the most effective personalized treatment strategies. Some studies comparing 2D and 3D microfluidic device models are summarized in Table 3C.

**Table 3.** Existing models of head and neck cancers (HNCs) have been reported in literature.

| Models | 2D vs. 3D Geometry | Primary vs. Cell Lines | Drugs Simulant | Aim | Authors and Ref. |
|---|---|---|---|---|---|
| (A) Spheroids | 2D: Monolayer control<br>3D: Forced floating and hanging drop methods | Primary: Tumor biopsy from HNSCC<br>Cell lines: CAL-27, FaDu | Cisplatin, 5-FU, 2-Gy radiation | To compare 2D and 3D methods as platforms for testing chemotherapy and radiotherapy | Hagemann et al. [46] |
| | 2D: Not studied<br>3D: Forced floating method | Primary: Patient-derived cancer-associated fibroblasts<br>Cell lines: LK0902, LK0917 | All-trans retinoic acid (ATRA) | To evaluate a 3D model as a therapy testing platform | Gorican et al. [47] |
| | 2D: Not studied<br>3D: Forced floating method | Primary: Patient-derived cancer-associated fibroblasts<br>Cell lines: LK0902, LK0917 | Cisplatin, cetuximab | To evaluate a 3D model as a platform for testing chemotherapy and immunotherapy | Magan et al. [48] |
| (B) Organotypic | 2D: Monolayer control<br>3D: The forced floating method was employed initially, followed by the transfer of the cells into Matrigel® | Primary: Tumor biopsy from H&N squamous cell carcinoma<br>Cell lines: MDA-HN2016-2, MDA-HN2016-18, MDA-2016-21 | Cisplatin, docetaxel | To compare 2D and 3D methods as platforms for evaluating chemotherapy and sensitivity | Tanaka et al. [49] |
| | 2D: Monolayer control<br>3D: Decellularized extracellular matrix from tongue tissue, sourced from mice and pigs alongside a Matrigel® matrix | Primary: Tongue squamous cell carcinoma and cancer-associated fibroblasts derived from patients<br>Cell lines: CAL-27 | Cisplatin | To compare 2D and 3D methods as platforms for chemotherapy screening and regenerative applications | Zhao et al. [50] |
| | 2D: Dynamic flow<br>3D: Collagen hydrogel adhesion chamber, dynamic flow, syringe pump | Primary: Human tubular lymphatic vessels and fibroblasts associated with cancer<br>Cell lines: HLEC2500, HorF2640 | Not studied | A dynamic culture technique employed as a platform for studying angiogenesis | Burghartz et al. [51] |

**Table 3.** *Cont.*

| Models | 2D vs. 3D Geometry | Primary vs. Cell Lines | Drugs Simulant | Aim | Authors and Ref. |
|---|---|---|---|---|---|
| (C) Microfluidic Devices | 2D: Unexposed control, dynamic flow 3D: Tissue chamber, dynamic flow, syringe pump | Primary: Human thyroid tissue samples Cell lines: Not studied | Etoposide (topoisomerase II inhibitor), SP600125 (JNK inhibitor) | A dynamic culture method, used as drug screening platform | Riley et al. [52] |
| | 2D: Unexposed control, dynamic flow 3D: Biopsy chamber, dynamic flow, syringe pump | Primary: Staging of human biopsies of laryngeal, oropharyngeal, and oral cavity tumors at T2 through T4 Cell lines: Not studied | Not studied | A dynamic culture method, used as maintenance platform | Bower et al. [53] |
| | 2D: Dynamic flow 3D: Collagen hydrogel adhesion chamber, dynamic flow, syringe pump | Primary: Human tubular lymphatic vessels and fibroblasts associated with cancer Cell lines: HLEC2500, HorF2640 | Not studied | A dynamic culture method, used as an angiogenesis platform | Lugo-Cintrón et al. [54] |

## 3. Experimentation with 3D Models of HNSCC

### 3.1. Thyroid Gland

In a study conducted by Peng Su, Chao Yue et al. [12], uniaxial compression tests were conducted on fresh porcine thyroid tissue at quasi-static strain rates of 0.005 $s^{-1}$ and 0.05 $s^{-1}$, with loading applied both perpendicular and parallel to the thyroid surface. These experiments were conducted using a biomechanical testing platform equipped with a Nano25 high-precision sensor to evaluate how strain rate and loading direction influence the mechanical properties of porcine thyroid tissue. The findings revealed that porcine thyroid tissue showed minimal strain rate sensitivity within the low strain rate range of 0.005 $s^{-1}$ to 0.05 $s^{-1}$. Furthermore, the loading direction had little effect on the tissue's mechanical properties, indicating that the tissue behaves as a homogeneous material. The mechanical characteristics of porcine thyroid tissue were also examined under quasi-static conditions. It was found that Young's modulus showed no significant variation across different strain rates and loading directions. The average Young's modulus was found to be approximately $2.233 \times 10^{-5}$ MPa for the small deformations and $3.108 \times 10^{-3}$ MPa for the large deformations. To analyze the mechanical properties of porcine thyroid tissue under quasi-static conditions, it was modeled as an incompressible, isotropic superelastic material. A hyperelastic constitutive model was developed using the Yeoh strain energy density function to describe the tissue behavior at a low strain rate. The three parameters of the Yeoh function were determined through fitting and were found to be: $C_{10} = 1.9 \times 10^{-3}$ MPa, $C_{20} = -2.3 \times 10^{-3}$ MPa, $C_{30} = 0.04$ MPa.

The stress–strain curves (Figure 5) derived from the simulation were generally consistent with the experimental data. However, some discrepancies were observed, likely due to factors that could not be fully replicated in the actual tests, such as localized deformations and uneven stress distributions. The quasi-static mechanical properties of the thyroid, obtained from uniaxial unconfined compression tests and represented by the developed hyperelastic constitutive model, are highly suitable for digital modeling of thyroid tissues. These findings are presented in Table 4A.

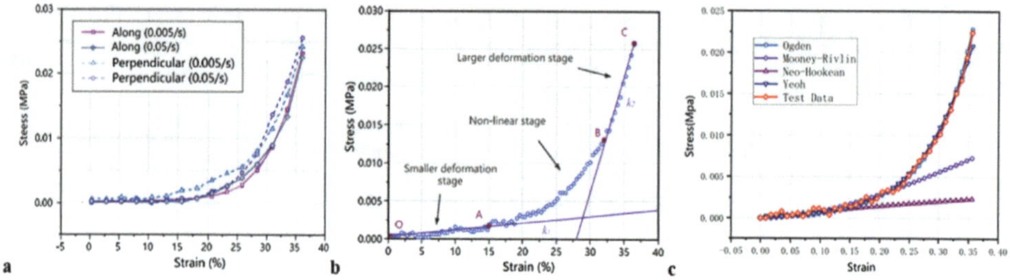


**Figure 5.** (**a**) The stress–strain curve for the quasi-static compression test; (**b**) Analysis of the mechanical properties of porcine thyroid gland tissue; (**c**) Fitting of the thyroid stress–strain curve to the constitutional model. (Reprinted with permission from Ref. [12]).

### 3.2. Head and Neck Cancer (HN-5) Cell Line

In a paper by M.H. Korayem et al. [55], experimental methodologies utilizing atomic force microscopy (AFM) were employed to investigate the physical and mechanical properties of the head and neck carcinoma (HN-5) cell line. Young's modulus was calculated by conducting repeated indentations at a minimum of 10 different points and utilizing two contact modes. The results showed that regions with lower elevation had a higher elasticity modulus, and vice versa. The average elasticity modulus for the cells was found to be 12 kPa. Furthermore, the adhesion force, which plays a key role in friction and manipulation, was experimentally measured. Similar to the elasticity modulus, maximum adhesion was recorded at the thinner edges of the cells, while the minimum adhesion was observed at the center of the cells. As adhesion increased, more force was required to detach the cells from the surface, leading to a corresponding increase in the manipulation force. In air medium and contact mode of the cantilever, the average adhesion value was recorded as 2.47 nN (Figure 6).

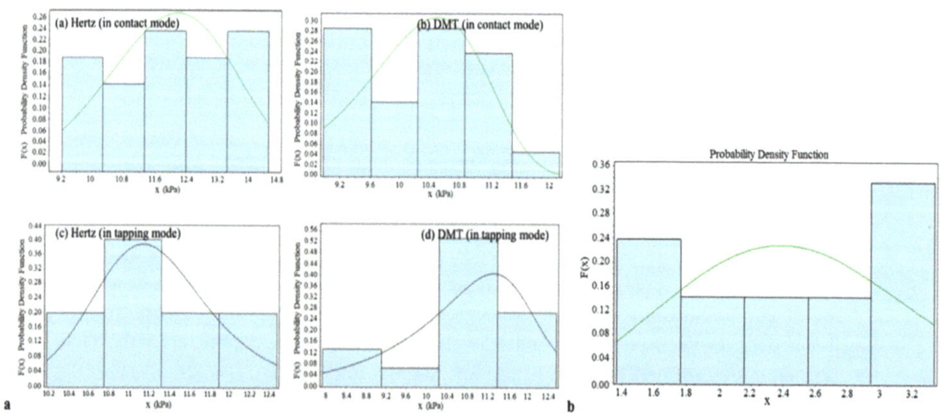


**Figure 6. Panel a**: (**a**) Normal distribution and histogram of Young's modulus calculation in contact mode with the Hertz model.; (**b**) DMT contact model results in contact mode; (**c**) Hertz contact model results in tapping mode; and (**d**) DMT contact model results in tapping mode; **Panel b**: The histogram displays the extracted values for the adhesion force measured in contact mode. (Reprinted with permission from Ref. [55]).

Another characteristic measured was the folding factor of the cell, which was assessed using two different methods, resulting in values of 1.19 and 1.40, respectively. It was concluded that both the spring constant and the damping coefficient are directly affected by the indentation depth. Following this, the creep function for a cell was derived, simulated using a basic viscoelastic model, such as the Kelvin–Voigt model (Figure 7):

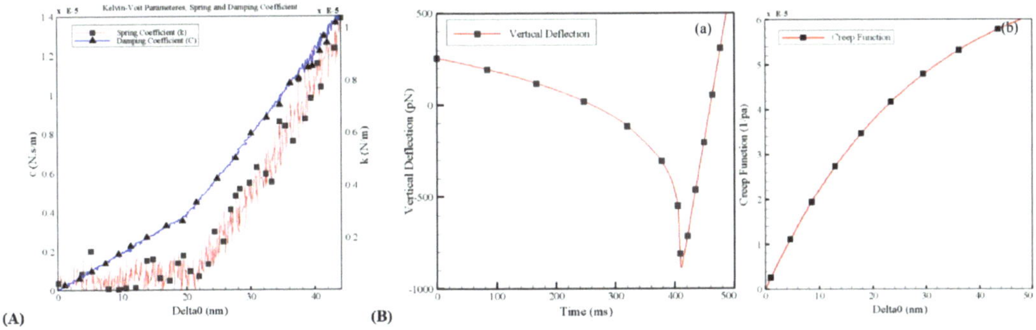


**Figure 7. Panel A**: Kelvin–Voigt components (spring constant and damping coefficient) of the HN-5 cell; **Panel B**: (**a**) Vertical deflection over time; (**b**) Creep function as a function of the oscillation amplitude of indentation. (Reprinted with permission from Ref. [55]).

In viscoelastic materials, the creep–compliance curve shows that the compliance (strain) of the material increases with time under constant stress. The region of interest in the creep test corresponds to the portion of delayed elastic strain. This implies that if the stress is removed, the sample will gradually return to its original state over time t. The results are presented in Table 4B.

### 3.3. Cervical Lymph Nodes

Cervical lymph nodes are commonly involved in metastatic head and neck cancers. Metastatic lymph nodes are usually firm, while benign nodes are softer. In clinical practice, palpation is still a standard technique used by ear, nose, and throat (ENT) specialists and oncologists to assess cervical lymphadenopathy, despite the inherent subjectivity of this method. The study conducted by Queeny Wing-Han Yuen et al. [56] aimed to provide a quantitative assessment of lymph node stiffness by measuring the tissue stiffness of pig lymph nodes using two methods: elastography for strain measurement of the entire lymph node and indentation for modulus determination of sliced lymph node specimens. The entire lymph nodes were embedded in agar–gelatin blocks for elastography, while only sliced specimens were used for indentation testing. No significant correlation was found between Young's modulus and the inverse strain ratio in both the peripheral and middle regions. This discrepancy may be due to the fact that the inverse strain ratio indicates the stiffness contrast between the lymph node and the phantom material, while Young's modulus reflects the absolute stiffness of the lymphatic tissue. When the modulus ratio was applied, a moderate correlation was observed between the two methods, likely influenced by factors such as elastography image quality, interfacial bonding, boundary conditions, tissue geometry, and size. The investigation revealed that the pig lymph nodes had distinct smooth boundaries, easily separated from surrounding connective tissues. However, some connective tissues remained attached to the lymph nodes when embedded in agar–gelatin blocks, potentially increasing the surface area for bonding with the phantom material. Elastography revealed that the stiffness of the middle region of the lymph nodes was like that of the background material, while the peripheral region was harder than the middle region. Conversely, the indentation test revealed that the central region was stiffer than the outer region. This discrepancy may be due to the direction of compression in elastography (parallel to the slice surface) versus indentation (perpendicular to the slice) (Figure 8).

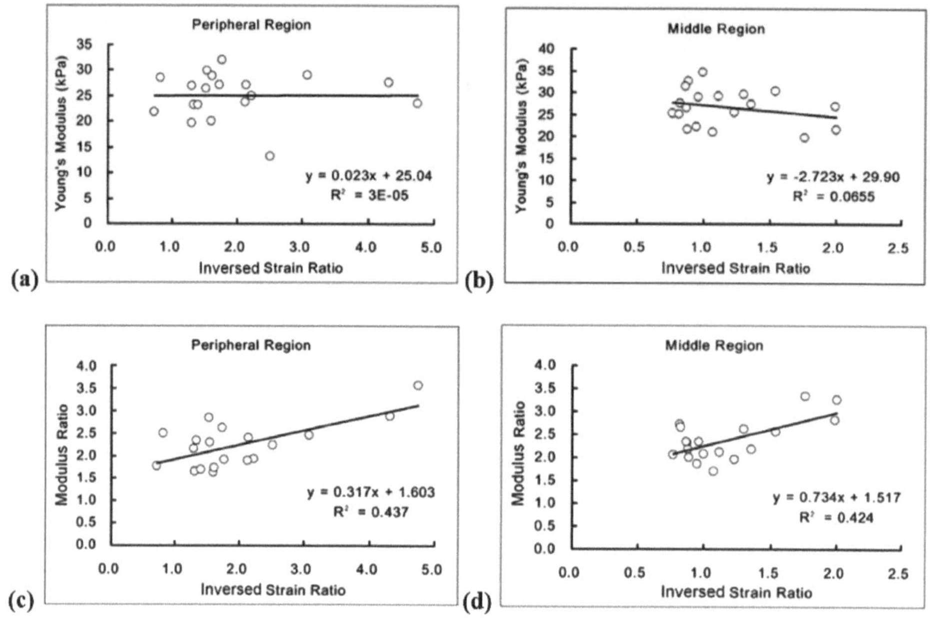


**Figure 8.** Correlation between Young's modulus/elastic modulus ratio and inverse strain ratio for peripheral and intermediate lymph nodes. (**a**,**b**) pertain to the results of Young's modulus measurements, while (**c**,**d**) relate to the modulus ratio findings. (Reprinted with permission from Ref. [56]).

Additionally, although strain measurements were taken at various sites of the lymph node to assess strain distribution, these did not perfectly align with the plane used for modulus measurements. The indentation system demonstrated satisfactory repeatability, with a prestudy evaluation on 12 silicone samples of varying stiffness showing an intraclass correlation coefficient (ICC) of 0.99, indicating a repeatability of 99%, and a repeatability coefficient (according to Bland et al. [57]) of 10.7 kPa. The observed difference in Young's modulus between the surrounding background material (11.78 ± 2.80 kPa) and the lymph node tissue (26.06 ± 6.03 kPa) can be attributed to the inherent stiffness differences, as indicated by this coefficient. Due to equipment constraints, the sliced specimens were relatively thick, exceeding 7 mm. Sample thickness is an important consideration, especially for pigs, as their lymph nodes may contain multiple nodelets, leading to significant internal tissue heterogeneity. Thinner slices are preferred, as they generally display more consistent properties throughout the tissue depth. In this study, a cutting technique was developed to create slice specimens with uniform thickness across a larger cross-sectional area (8–10 cm in width and length). Thicker sliced specimens were favored for the indentation test due to their superior quality compared to thinner slices. The study was conducted solely on normal lymph nodes obtained from market pigs assumed to be healthy. The results are presented in Table 4C. In conclusion, this study aimed to assess the stiffness of porcine lymph nodes by measuring strain through elastography and Young's modulus using a push-in test. Both methods highlighted significant differences in parameters between the peripheral and middle regions of the lymph node, with the results from the two tests showing a moderate correlation [56].

**Table 4.** Summary of mechanical properties extracted from the models in literature. (**A**) Young's modulus in the small ($E_1$) and large ($E_2$) deformation phase of the porcine thyroid (**a**); Yeoh hyperelasticity constitutive model evaluated by material parameters ($C_{10}$, $C_{20}$, $C_{30}$) and correlation coefficient ($R^2$) (**b**); Statistics on stress in stress–relaxation tests (**c**). (**B**) Young's modulus in contact and tapping modes for Hertz and DMT contact models (**a**); adhesion strength of HN-5 cells (**b**); folding factor of HN-5 cells based on surface method (**c**). (**C**) Results of Elastography and Indentation tests (mean ± SD).

| Type of Model | Mechanical Features | Type of Value | Value | Ref. |
| --- | --- | --- | --- | --- |
| (**A**) Thyroid Gland | (**a**) Young's modulus | Mean | $E_1$ (MPa) = $2.333 \times 10^{-5}$<br>$E_2$ (MPa) = $3.108 \times 10^{-3}$ | [12] |
| | (**b**) Hyperelasticity constitutive model | Yeoh | $C_{10}$/MPa = $1.9 \times 10^{-3}$<br>$C_{20}$/MPa = $-2.3 \times 10^{-3}$<br>$C_{30}$/MPa = 0.04<br>$R^2$ = 0.999 | |
| | (**c**) Stress–relaxation tests | Mean | Initial stress (MPa) = $2.433 \times 10^{-2}$<br>Last stress (MPa) = $3.693 \times 10^{-3}$ | |
| (**B**) Head and Neck Cancer (HN-5) Cell Line | (**a**) Young's modulus (kPa) | Mean | Contact/Hertz = 11.95<br>Contact/DMT = 10.29<br>Tapping/Hertz = 11.28 | [55] |
| | (**b**) The adhesion force | Mean | 2.47 nN | |
| | (**c**) Folding-surface method | - | Project area ($nm^2$) = 1873.02<br>Surface area ($nm^2$) = 2628.13<br>Folding factor (first method) = 1.19<br>Folding factor (second method) = 1.403 | |
| (**C**) Cervical Lymph Nodes | Elastography strain ratio | - | Peripheral region = 0.61 ± 0.32 *<br>Middle region = 0.93 ± 0.33 | [56] |
| | Indentation Young's modulus (kPa) | - | Peripheral region = 25.39 ± 6.14 *<br>Middle region = 26.73 ± 5.64 | |
| | Indentation modulus ratio | - | Peripheral region = 2.21 ± 0.60<br>Middle region = 2.33 ± 0.51 | |

* Indicates a significant difference ($p < 0.05$).

### 3.4. Laryngotracheal Cartilage

In a review written by Christine M. Pauken et al. [58], the literature on the mechanical, cellular, and proteomic properties of laryngotracheal cartilages was comprehensively examined to establish a foundational understanding. A summary of their findings is provided in Table 5.

The concepts outlined hold significant implications for laryngotracheal cartilage tissue engineering. Currently, there is limited understanding of the mechanical properties of these cartilages. Tissue stiffness, both under tensile and compressive conditions, is a key factor, especially considering that the stiffness of thyroid and arytenoid cartilages can affect vocal performance, particularly in aging tissues where ossification may alter their stiffness. Furthermore, the cricoid and tracheal cartilages need to maintain sufficient stiffness to keep the airway open. Unfortunately, the compressive and tensile properties of human cricoid, tracheal, arytenoid, and epiglottic cartilages remain largely unexplored. Other important material properties, such as bending modulus and joint lubrication, are also critical for cartilage function. The bending modulus at various points on the epiglottis is essential for its proper function, while effective lubrication is crucial for the movement of the cricoarytenoid and cricothyroid joints. Testing these cartilages should be linked to factors like cell density, glycosaminoglycan (GAG) concentration, the distribution of key proteins, collagen and elastin networks, and areas of ossification. A thorough understanding of these factors will greatly enhance the ability of professionals in regenerative medicine to reconstruct the laryngotracheal system [58].

**Table 5.** Summary of knowledge on biomechanical properties of Laryngotracheal Cartilage [58].

| Structure | Cartilage Type | Biomechanical Properties | Ref. |
|---|---|---|---|
| Thyroid cartilage | Hyaline | Undergoes forces from both intrinsic and extrinsic muscles<br>Increased stiffness due to the process of ossification<br>Interacts with the cricoid through a synovial joint that exhibits three different morphological variants | [59] |
| Cricoid cartilage | Hyaline | Has two pairs of synovial joints for connecting with the thyroid and arytenoid cartilages<br>A radial expansile force averaging 97.25N is necessary to break human cricoid cartilage<br>A study in horses indicates that the compressive properties of cricoid cartilage vary regionally | [60] |
| Epiglottic cartilage | Elastic | Parameters for rabbits are characterized by a Poisson's ratio of $0.250 \pm 0.115$, permeability of $8.01 \pm 5.16 \times 10^{-16}$ $m^4/N{\cdot}s$, and an aggregate modulus of $0.290 \pm 0.174$ MPa<br>The aggregate modulus of the epiglottis differs considerably from that of other elastic cartilages | [61] |
| Arytenoid cartilage | Hyaline and elastic | The bulk aggregate modulus for equine tissue is $0.42 \pm 0.11$ MPa, with a permeability of $1.303 \pm 0.191$ $mm^4/N{\cdot}s$ | [62] |
| Tracheal cartilage | Hyaline | The average tensile modulus at the abluminal surface is $13.6 \pm 1.5$ MPa<br>The tensile modulus tends to decrease as depth increases<br>The stiffness of tracheal cartilage increases as age advances<br>Differences in the tensile moduli and the viscosity coefficient of tracheal cartilage influence the subglottal acoustic spectra | [63] |

## 4. Comparison of In Vitro and In Vivo Models in HNSCC Research

The development of reliable models that closely replicate the tumor microenvironment (TME) is crucial for advancing cancer research and enhancing personalized medicine. While in vitro and in vivo models each have their own strengths and weaknesses, their integration is essential for achieving translational success. Recent advancements have improved the capacity of in vitro systems to mimic key features of in vivo conditions, adhering to the principles of the 3Rs (replacement, reduction, and refinement) to minimize the use of animal models.

In vitro models, such as 3D cultures, organoids, and bioprinting techniques, provide a controlled environment to study tumor biology, offering insights into drug responses, cell–cell interactions, and stromal remodeling. In Table 6 the main features of the most common 3D models used for HNSCC are compared.

For instance, Wafa Wahbi et al. [60] demonstrated the utility of Myogel-coated wells and 3D microfluidic chips in replicating the extracellular matrix (ECM) and tumor–immune interactions. These models facilitate the testing of patient-derived cells, enabling more precise development of personalized therapies. However, the lack of systemic factors, including angiogenesis and immune responses, represents a key limitation of in vitro approaches. Conversely, in vivo models, such as zebrafish xenografts, provide a more comprehensive representation of the tumor microenvironment, incorporating systemic factors like immune cell dynamics and vascularization. Zebrafish assays have shown a high concordance with clinical outcomes, particularly in testing chemotherapeutic, radiotherapeutic, and targeted therapies. By integrating these complementary models, researchers can enhance the physiological relevance of preclinical studies, paving the way for more effective, patient-specific therapeutic strategies.

**Table 6.** In vitro models of HNSCC: summary of main features adapted from Arutyunyan et al. [1].

| | Spheroids and Heterospheroids | Tissue-Engineered Models | Bioprinted Models | Organoids | Explants and Histocultures |
|---|---|---|---|---|---|
| Source | Patient-derived tissues, primary cell cultures, immortalized cell lines | Patient-derived tissues, primary cell cultures, immortalized cell lines | Patient-derived tissues, primary cell cultures, immortalized cell lines | Patient-derived tissues | Patient-derived tissues |
| Heterogeneity of tumor cellular composition | Depends on the source | Depends on the source | Depends on the source | Preserved | Preserved |
| ECM | - | Natural/synthetic polymers, decellularized tissue | Bioink based on hydrogels | Basement membrane matrix, collagen | Native |
| Tissue architecture, pathophysiological gradients | Partially reconstituted | - | Reconstituted | - | Preserved |
| In vitro culture duration | - | Limited | Limited | - | - |
| Difficulty of obtaining | Medium | Medium | High | High | Medium |
| Major advantages | The most commonly available 3D model | The benefit of analyzing ECM–cell interactions lies in the ability to develop a model with precise linear dimensions | Generating synthetic tumor tissue with defined spatial properties | The capability to support tumor cells at different differentiation stages while mimicking the tumor microenvironment | Tumor tissue with minimal manipulation |
| Specific disadvantages | Tends to merge into conglomerates, with challenges in size control | Many cells are needed for modeling | Modeling requires a substantial number of cells and advanced equipment | The efficiency of production is approximately 60–70% | Extended in vitro cultivation necessitates the use of supporting matrices or microfluidic devices |
| Mechanical properties | Variable, often lacking robust mechanical stability | Can be engineered to match specific mechanical properties (e.g., stiffness, elasticity) | Can be adjusted based on the bioink and printing conditions | Are often similar to native tissue | Preserved in the native tissue |

On the other hand, in vivo models, such as murine xenografts and zebrafish larvae, analyzed in an article written by Roosa Hujanen et al. [64], maintain the heterogeneity of primary tumors and enable the study of systemic interactions, including metastasis and vascular mimicry (VM). Zebrafish models have shown a high correlation with clinical outcomes, making them a cost-effective and ethical alternative to traditional mammalian models. For instance, studies in oral squamous cell carcinoma (OSCC) demonstrated a 77% alignment between zebrafish xenograft results and patient responses, underscoring the reliability of these models.

Despite these differences, both in vitro and in vivo systems share the goal of faithfully reproducing tumor behaviors to facilitate drug discovery and improve therapeutic strategies. The increasing correspondence between in vitro and in vivo findings highlights the potential for advanced in vitro models to complement or even replace certain in vivo approaches. By integrating in vitro and simplified in vivo models, researchers can better simulate the complexities of the TME while adhering to ethical research practices.

In conclusion, the synergy between in vitro and in vivo systems not only enhances our understanding of tumor biology but also provides a pathway toward reducing animal use in research. The continued refinement of these models will bridge the gap between preclinical findings and clinical applications, accelerating the development of effective and ethical cancer therapies [65].

## 5. Discussion and Future Prospects

Head and neck cancers comprise a diverse range of malignancies that arise from several anatomical areas, including the oral cavity, pharynx, larynx, nasal cavity, and salivary glands. Precisely identifying and characterizing cancerous tissues is crucial for accurate diagnosis, treatment strategy development, and enhancing patient outcomes. Three-dimensional (3D) in vitro models have emerged as promising tool to enhance our understanding and prediction of HNSCC tissue behavior, offering more physiologically relevant conditions that closely mimic the mechanical and structural properties of native tumor tissues compared to traditional two-dimensional (2D) cultures [66].

This review highlighted the critical role of mechanical properties in these 3D models and their characterization, emphasizing their importance in advancing HNSCC in vitro scientific research. Mechanical properties such as stiffness, elasticity, and dynamic behavior are crucial in replicating the native tumor microenvironment. For example, the stiffness of the extracellular matrix (ECM) influences cancer cell behavior, including proliferation, migration, and response to therapy. In HNSCCs, the tumor microenvironment is characterized by a heterogeneous ECM that affects tumor growth and metastatic potential. Three-dimensional models that accurately mimic these mechanical properties enable a more accurate study of tumor biology and the development of effective therapeutic strategies [67].

Various 3D culture techniques, including spheroids, organoids, hydrogels, and bioprinted tissues, have been developed to replicate the complex architecture and mechanical properties of HNC tissues. Each 3D model technique offers unique advantages and limitations in mimicking the head and neck cancer environment. For example, spheroids are easy to use and suitable for high-throughput screening but lack the complexity of native tumors. Organoids, while providing patient-specific models with greater complexity, are more expensive and require technical expertise. Three-dimensionally bioprinted models offer precise control over the spatial arrangement of cells and ECM components, making them powerful tools for studying cell–cell and cell–matrix interactions, drug responses, and tissue mechanics. However, bioprinting is technically complex and expensive, limiting its accessibility for large-scale studies. Hydrogels and ECM-mimicking scaffolds provide a supportive and customizable environment for cell growth, closely resembling the biochemical and mechanical properties of the native ECM. While highly biocompatible, their design and fabrication remain technically challenging, and the cost of materials is often high, restricting their use to specialized applications [68].

Despite the significant progress made, several challenges must be addressed to develop realistic 3D in vitro models for HNSCC research. The lack of standardized protocols affects reproducibility and comparability across studies. Current models often fail to fully capture the complexity of the tumor microenvironment, including immune system interactions, vascularization, and cross-talk between different cell types. Integrating multiple 3D models may provide a more dynamic and comprehensive system that better replicates the physiological tumor environment [69].

To further advance the field of 3D in vitro modeling for HNSCC, the integration of artificial intelligence (AI) tools, such as deep learning (DL) and machine learning (ML), represents a promising approach. These computational technologies have the potential to address some of the key limitations of 3D tumor models by improving model standardization, automating data analysis, and optimizing experimental design. Given the increasing importance of AI-driven tools in biomedical research, their role in refining 3D models should be explored in depth. Moreover, the lack of longitudinal studies and high-throughput applications in TME research has significantly hindered the clinical translation of therapies targeting mechanical properties [70]. Deep learning (DL) and machine learning (ML) can play a pivotal role in addressing these gaps by enabling real-time data analysis, predictive modeling, and automation of complex biological assessments [71].

For example, one of the key applications of ML in 3D in vitro models is in the automated analysis of organoid morphology and fluorescence-based imaging. Traditional manual assessments are often time-consuming and prone to variability, whereas ML-based tools, such as ML-based Organoid Analysis software (MOrgAna: the software has been tested with Python versions 3.7, 3.8, and 3.9), have demonstrated their ability to analyze structural and functional parameters of organoids with higher precision and reproducibility. These advancements contribute to reducing human bias and increasing the reliability of in vitro tumor models [72].

Beyond ML, deep learning, a subset of ML that uses artificial neural networks to learn, further refines these capabilities by enabling the automatic extraction of relevant features from complex datasets without requiring manual input. For example, the development of self-learning microscopes powered by DL allows for real-time adaptive imaging and automated detection of morphological changes in 3D cultures. This approach can significantly improve the reproducibility of experiments, making it easier to compare results across different laboratories [73].

In addition to improving morphological assessments, DL models hold promise in predicting mechanical properties of 3D constructs. By analyzing large datasets, these systems can identify correlations between matrix composition, stiffness, and tumor behavior, leading to more precise control over model design. Recent studies conducted by JungHo Kong et al. [74] have demonstrated that deep learning can accurately predict the mechanical properties of multi-material metamaterials, significantly reducing the time required for evaluation and enabling large-scale parallel computing. This capability allows for the rational design of structures that exhibit a broad range of elastic properties while meeting additional mechanical constraints, such as stress uniformity to enhance fracture and fatigue resistance. Similarly, in the context of 3D tumor models, these computational approaches can be leveraged to optimize scaffold stiffness, biomaterial composition, and mechanical microenvironment parameters to better mimic in vivo conditions.

Moreover, DL-driven image analysis can facilitate the integration of patient-derived 3D cultures into personalized medicine by assessing drug responses in a high-throughput and automated manner. The ability of DL models to process vast amounts of imaging and mechanical data enhances reproducibility and predictive accuracy, ultimately refining the development of in vitro tumor models. By incorporating mechanical constraints into DL frameworks, researchers can further bridge the gap between experimental and computational modeling, paving the way for more physiologically relevant 3D systems in cancer research and therapeutic development [75].

Despite these advantages, the implementation of DL and ML in 3D in vitro modeling still faces challenges. One of the primary limitations is the need for extensive annotated datasets for proper algorithm training. Additionally, computational demands and hardware requirements can pose barriers for many research laboratories. However, the establishment of standardized imaging databases for 3D cultures could accelerate progress in this field, enhancing model reproducibility and predictive accuracy. By integrating DL and ML approaches, researchers can overcome some of the existing limitations of 3D in vitro models, particularly in standardization, reproducibility, and high-throughput analysis. As these technologies continue to evolve, their application in tumor modeling is expected to refine in vitro systems, bridging the gap between preclinical research and clinical applications.

## 6. Conclusions

The development of 3D tumor models has significantly advanced research in the TME by providing more physiologically relevant platforms than traditional 2D cultures. However, their full potential in high-throughput drug screening and clinical translation is hindered by a lack of standardization in model generation, characterization, and validation. Different 3D culture systems, such as tumor organoids, spheroids, and bioprinted models, exhibit substantial variability in ECM composition, mechanical properties, and tumor–stroma interactions, leading to inconsistencies in experimental outcomes.

A major challenge in using these models is reproducibility, as variations in cell sourcing, ECM stiffness, and culture conditions make it difficult to compare results across studies. Additionally, the absence of standardized methods for measuring mechanical properties and assessing drug responses complicates the translation of TME-targeting therapies from preclinical models to clinical applications. Many 3D models also fail to fully integrate immune and stromal components, limiting their ability to replicate the complex tumor–stroma interactions that influence therapy resistance.

While 3D in vitro models have demonstrated their potential in head and neck squamous cell carcinoma (HNSCC) research, further advancements are needed to enhance their physiological relevance and predictive accuracy. One critical improvement involves implementing longitudinal studies to track tumor progression and treatment response over time, providing insights into resistance mechanisms and therapeutic efficacy. Additionally, integrating genomic, proteomic, and metabolomic data with 3D models could offer a more comprehensive understanding of tumor biology, facilitating the identification of new therapeutic targets. This multi-omics approach aligns with personalized medicine principles, allowing for the development of tailored treatment strategies.

By continuing to refine and integrate 3D model techniques, we can achieve more accurate and comprehensive insights into HNSCC biology. Advancements in standardization, multi-system integration, and high-throughput analysis will further strengthen these models, ultimately leading to more effective and personalized therapeutic strategies. As these technologies evolve, they hold significant potential for improving both preclinical research and clinical outcomes in HNSCC.

**Author Contributions:** Conceptualization, S.P. and A.E.; methodology, F.S.; software, M.C. and F.A.; validation, B.C., M.B. and I.G.; investigation, R.D.; resources, S.P. and A.E.; data curation, F.S.; writing—original draft preparation, A.E. and S.P.; writing—review and editing, R.D.; visualization, F.A.; supervision, B.C. and M.B.; project administration, B.C. and F.A.; funding acquisition, M.B. All authors have read and agreed to the published version of the manuscript.

**Funding:** The work reported in this publication was funded by the Italian Ministry of Health, RC-2023-08053922 "Nano-Electro-Chemo-Immuno Therapy (NECIT) to enhance head and neck cancer treatment". The work reported in this publication was partially funded by Ricerca Corrente funding from Italian Ministry of Health to IRCCS Policlinico San Donato.

**Informed Consent Statement:** This article does not contain any studies with human or animal subjects. Ethical approval is not applicable for this article.

**Data Availability Statement:** This study is based on previously published data, which are cited in the references. No new data were generated.

**Conflicts of Interest:** The authors have no conflicts of interest to declare.

## Abbreviations

The following abbreviations are used in this manuscript:

| | |
|---|---|
| AFM | Atomic Force Microscopy |
| AI | Artificial Intelligence |
| ATRA | All-Trans Retinoic Acid |
| CAFs | Cancer-Associated Fibroblasts |
| CAL | Cancer-Associated Line |
| CPCR | G Protein-Coupled Receptor |
| DL | Deep Learning |
| DMT Model | Derjaguin–Muller–Toporov Model |
| E | Young's Modulus |
| ECM | Extracellular Matrix |
| EGFR | Epidermal Growth Factor Receptor |
| ENT | Ear, Nose, Throat |
| EPC2 | Esophageal Progenitor Cell 2 |
| GAG | Glycosaminoglycan |
| HA | Hyaluronic Acid |
| HEMa | Human Epidermal Melanocytes, adult |
| HLEC | Human Lymphatic Endothelial Cell |
| HNCs | Head and Neck Cancers |
| HNSCC | Head and Neck Squamous Cell Carcinoma |
| ICC | Intraclass Correlation Coefficient |
| JNK | c-Jun N-Terminal Kinase |
| MDA | Anderson Cancer Center |
| MDSCs | Myeloid-Derived Suppressor Cells |
| ML | Machine Learning |
| MOrgAna | ML-based Organoid Analysis Software |
| NECIT | Nano-Electro-Chemo-Immuno Therapy |
| OKF | Oral Keratinocyte Four |
| OSCC | Oral Squamous Cell Carcinoma |
| PCL | Poly-ε-caprolactone |
| PDE | Patient-Derived Tumor Explant |
| PEG | Polyethylene Glycol |
| PEGPH20 | Pegylated Recombinant Human Hyaluronidase |
| PLCL | Poly(L-lactide-co-ε-caprolactone) |
| PLG | Poly(lactide-co-glycolide) |
| PVA | Polyvinyl Alcohol |
| SCC | Squamous Cell Carcinoma |
| TAMs | Tumor-Associated Macrophages |
| TME | Tumor Microenvironment |
| Tregs | T Cells |
| VGP | Vertical Growth Phase |

## References

1. Arutyunyan, I.; Jumaniyazova, E.; Makarov, A.; Fatkhudinov, T. In Vitro Models of Head and Neck Cancer: From Primitive to Most Advanced. *J. Pers. Med.* **2023**, *13*, 1575. [CrossRef]

2. Tinhofer, I.; Braunholz, D.; Klinghammer, K. Preclinical models of head and neck squamous cell carcinoma for a basic understanding of cancer biology and its translation into efficient therapies. *Cancers Head Neck* **2020**, *5*, 9. [CrossRef] [PubMed]
3. Esposito, A.; Ferraresi, A.; Vallino, L.; Garavaglia, B.; Dhanasekaran, D.N.; Isidoro, C. Three-Dimensional In Vitro Cell Cultures as a Feasible and Promising Alternative to Two-Dimensional and Animal Models in Cancer Research. *Int. J. Biol. Sci.* **2024**, *20*, 5293–5311. [CrossRef]
4. Urzì, O.; Gasparro, R.; Costanzo, E.; De Luca, A.; Giavaresi, G.; Fontana, S.; Alessandro, R. Three-Dimensional Cell Cultures: The Bridge between In Vitro and In Vivo Models. *Int. J. Mol. Sci.* **2023**, *24*, 12046. [CrossRef] [PubMed]
5. Tosca, E.M.; Ronchi, D.; Facciolo, D.; Magni, P. Replacement, Reduction, and Refinement of Animal Experiments in Anticancer Drug Development: The Contribution of 3D In Vitro Cancer Models in the Drug Efficacy Assessment. *Biomedicines* **2023**, *11*, 1058. [CrossRef] [PubMed]
6. Morrissey, B.; Blyth, K.; Carter, P.; Chelala, C.; Jones, L.; Holen, I.; Speirs, V. The Sharing Experimental Animal Resources, Coordinating Holdings (SEARCH) Framework: Encouraging Reduction, Replacement, and Refinement in Animal Research. *PLoS Biol.* **2017**, *15*, e2000719. [CrossRef] [PubMed]
7. Tenschert, E.; Kern, J.; Affolter, A.; Rotter, N.; Lammert, A. Optimisation of Conditions for the Formation of Spheroids of Head and Neck Squamous Cell Carcinoma Cell Lines for Use as Animal Alternatives. *Altern. Lab. Anim.* **2022**, *50*, 414–422. [CrossRef]
8. Behera, S.A.; Nanda, B.; Achary, P.G. Recent advancements and challenges in 3D bioprinting for cancer applications. *Bioprinting* **2024**, *43*, e00357. [CrossRef]
9. Rodrigues, J.; Heinrich, M.A.; Teixeira, L.M.; Prakash, J. 3D In Vitro Model (R)evolution: Unveiling Tumor-Stroma Interactions. *Trends Cancer* **2021**, *7*, 249–264. [CrossRef]
10. Kalli, M.; Poskus, M.D.; Stylianopoulos, T.; Zervantonakis, I.K. Beyond matrix stiffness: Targeting force-induced cancer drug resistance. *Trends Cancer* **2023**, *9*, 937–954. [CrossRef] [PubMed]
11. Massey, A.; Stewart, J.; Smith, C.; Parvini, C.; McCormick, M.; Do, K.; Cartagena-Rivera, A.X. Mechanical properties of human tumour tissues and their implications for cancer development. *Nat. Rev. Phys.* **2024**, *6*, 269–282. [CrossRef]
12. Su, P.; Yue, C.; Cui, L.; Zhang, Q.; Liu, B.; Liu, T. Quasi-Static Mechanical Properties and Continuum Constitutive Model of the Thyroid Gland. *J. Funct. Biomater.* **2022**, *13*, 283. [CrossRef]
13. Wirtz, D.; Konstantopoulos, K.; Searson, P.C. The physics of cancer: The role of physical interactions and mechanical forces in metastasis. *Nat. Rev. Cancer* **2011**, *11*, 512–522. [CrossRef] [PubMed]
14. Fuhrmann, A.; Staunton, J.R.; Nandakumar, V.; Banyai, N.; Davies, P.C.; Ros, R. AFM stiffness nanotomography of normal, metaplastic and dysplastic human esophageal cells. *Phys. Biol.* **2011**, *8*, 015007. [CrossRef]
15. Bobrowska, J.; Awsiuk, K.; Pabijan, J.; Bobrowski, P.; Lekki, J.; Sowa, K.M.; Rysz, J.; Budkowski, A.; Lekka, M. Biophysical and Biochemical Characteristics as Complementary Indicators of Melanoma Progression. *Anal. Chem.* **2019**, *91*, 9885–9892. [CrossRef] [PubMed]
16. Remmerbach, T.W.; Wottawah, F.; Dietrich, J.; Lincoln, B.; Wittekind, C.; Guck, J. Oral cancer diagnosis by mechanical phenotyping. *Cancer Res.* **2009**, *69*, 1728–1732. [CrossRef]
17. Van Helvert, S.; Friedl, P. Strain Stiffening of Fibrillar Collagen during Individual and Collective Cell Migration Identified by AFM Nanoindentation. *ACS Appl. Mater. Interfaces* **2016**, *8*, 21946–21955. [CrossRef] [PubMed]
18. Prabhune, M.; Belge, G.; Dotzauer, A.; Bullerdiek, J.; Radmacher, M. Comparison of mechanical properties of normal and malignant thyroid cells. *Micron* **2012**, *43*, 1267–1272. [CrossRef]
19. Desgrosellier, J.S.; Cheresh, D.A. Integrins in cancer: Biological implications and therapeutic opportunities. *Nat. Rev. Cancer* **2010**, *10*, 9–22. [CrossRef]
20. Arner, E.N.; Rathmell, J.C. Metabolic programming and immune suppression in the tumor microenvironment. *Cancer Cell* **2023**, *41*, 421–433. [CrossRef] [PubMed]
21. Li, J.; Zeng, Z.; Jiang, X.; Zhang, N.; Gao, Y.; Luo, Y.; Sun, W.; Li, S.; Ren, J.; Gong, Y.; et al. Stromal microenvironment promoted infiltration in esophageal adenocarcinoma and squamous cell carcinoma: A multi-cohort gene-based analysis. *Sci. Rep.* **2020**, *10*, 18589. [CrossRef]
22. Bonartsev, A.P.; Lei, B.; Kholina, M.S.; Menshikh, K.A.; Svyatoslavov, D.S.; Samoylova, S.I.; Sinelnikov, M.Y.; Voinova, V.V.; Shaitan, K.V.; Kirpichnikov, M.P.; et al. Models of head and neck squamous cell carcinoma using bioengineering approaches. *Crit. Rev. Oncol. Hematol.* **2022**, *175*, 103724. [CrossRef] [PubMed]
23. Costa, E.C.; Moreira, A.F.; de Melo-Diogo, D.; Gaspar, V.M.; Carvalho, M.P.; Correia, I.J. 3D tumor spheroids: An overview on the tools and techniques used for their analysis. *Biotechnol. Adv.* **2016**, *34*, 1427–1441. [CrossRef]
24. Vakhshiteh, F.; Bagheri, Z.; Soleimani, M.; Ahvaraki, A.; Pournemat, P.; Alavi, S.E.; Madjd, Z. Heterotypic tumor spheroids: A platform for nanomedicine evaluation. *J. Nanobiotechnol.* **2023**, *21*, 249. [CrossRef] [PubMed]
25. Kadletz, L.; Heiduschka, G.; Domayer, J.; Schmid, R.; Enzenhofer, E.; Thurnher, D. Evaluation of spheroid head and neck squamous cell carcinoma cell models in comparison to monolayer cultures. *Oncol. Lett.* **2015**, *10*, 1281–1286. [CrossRef] [PubMed]

26. Melissaridou, S.; Wiechec, E.; Magan, M.; Jain, M.V.; Chung, M.K.; Farnebo, L.; Roberg, K. The effect of 2D and 3D cell cultures on treatment response, EMT profile and stem cell features in head and neck cancer. *Cancer Cell Int.* **2019**, *19*, 16. [CrossRef]
27. Francois, A.; Dirheimer, L.; Chateau, A.; Lassalle, H.P.; Yakavets, I.; Bezdetnaya, L. A Macrophages-Enriched Head and Neck Tumor Spheroid Model to Study Foslip(®) Behavior in Tumor Microenvironment. *Int. J. Nanomed.* **2023**, *18*, 6545–6562. [CrossRef] [PubMed]
28. Saglam-Metiner, P.; Gulce-Iz, S.; Biray-Avci, C. Bioengineering-inspired three-dimensional culture systems: Organoids to create tumor microenvironment. *Gene* **2019**, *686*, 203–212. [CrossRef] [PubMed]
29. Driehuis, E.; Kretzschmar, K.; Clevers, H. Establishment of patient-derived cancer organoids for drug-screening applications. *Nat. Protoc.* **2020**, *15*, 3380–3409. [CrossRef]
30. Yao, Y.; Xu, X.; Yang, L.; Zhu, J.; Wan, J.; Shen, L.; Xia, F.; Fu, G.; Deng, Y.; Pan, M.; et al. Patient-Derived Organoids Predict Chemoradiation Responses of Locally Advanced Rectal Cancer. *Cell Stem Cell* **2020**, *26*, 17–26.e16. [CrossRef] [PubMed]
31. Moya-Garcia, C.R.; Okuyama, H.; Sadeghi, N.; Li, J.; Tabrizian, M.; Li-Jessen, N.Y.K. In vitro models for head and neck cancer: Current status and future perspective. *Front. Oncol.* **2022**, *12*, 960340. [CrossRef] [PubMed]
32. Rijal, G.; Bathula, C.; Li, W. Application of Synthetic Polymeric Scaffolds in Breast Cancer 3D Tissue Cultures and Animal Tumor Models. *Int. J. Biomater.* **2017**, *2017*, 8074890. [CrossRef] [PubMed]
33. Xu, K.; Ganapathy, K.; Andl, T.; Wang, Z.; Copland, J.A.; Chakrabarti, R.; Florczyk, S.J. 3D porous chitosan-alginate scaffold stiffness promotes differential responses in prostate cancer cell lines. *Biomaterials* **2019**, *217*, 119311. [CrossRef] [PubMed]
34. Colella, G.; Fazioli, F.; Gallo, M.; De Chiara, A.; Apice, G.; Ruosi, C.; Cimmino, A.; de Nigris, F. Sarcoma Spheroids and Organoids-Promising Tools in the Era of Personalized Medicine. *Int. J. Mol. Sci.* **2018**, *19*, 615. [CrossRef] [PubMed]
35. Kochanek, S.J.; Close, D.A.; Johnston, P.A. High Content Screening Characterization of Head and Neck Squamous Cell Carcinoma Multicellular Tumor Spheroid Cultures Generated in 384-Well Ultra-Low Attachment Plates to Screen for Better Cancer Drug Leads. *Assay Drug Dev. Technol.* **2019**, *17*, 17–36. [CrossRef] [PubMed]
36. Yao, Y.; Lin, W.; Zhang, Y. Fabrication of Tongue Extracellular Matrix and Reconstitution of Tongue Squamous Cell Carcinoma In Vitro. *J. Vis. Exp.* **2018**, *136*, 57235. [CrossRef]
37. Suliman, S.; Mustafa, K.; Krueger, A.; Steinmüller-Nethl, D.; Finne-Wistrand, A.; Osdal, T.; Hamza, A.O.; Sun, Y.; Parajuli, H.; Waag, T.; et al. Nanodiamond modified copolymer scaffolds affects tumour progression of early neoplastic oral keratinocytes. *Biomaterials* **2016**, *95*, 11–21. [CrossRef]
38. Almela, T.; Al-Sahaf, S.; Brook, I.M.; Khoshroo, K.; Rasoulianboroujeni, M.; Fahimipour, F.; Tahriri, M.; Dashtimoghadam, E.; Bolt, R.; Tayebi, L.; et al. 3D printed tissue engineered model for bone invasion of oral cancer. *Tissue Cell* **2018**, *52*, 71–77. [CrossRef] [PubMed]
39. Bulysheva, A.A.; Bowlin, G.L.; Petrova, S.P.; Yeudall, W.A. Enhanced chemoresistance of squamous carcinoma cells grown in 3D cryogenic electrospun scaffolds. *Biomed. Mater.* **2013**, *8*, 055009. [CrossRef] [PubMed]
40. Murphy, S.V.; Atala, A. 3D bioprinting of tissues and organs. *Nat. Biotechnol.* **2014**, *32*, 773–785. [CrossRef]
41. Kort-Mascort, J.; Bao, G.; Elkashty, O.; Flores-Torres, S.; Munguia-Lopez, J.G.; Jiang, T.; Ehrlicher, A.J.; Mongeau, L.; Tran, S.D.; Kinsella, J.M. Decellularized Extracellular Matrix Composite Hydrogel Bioinks for the Development of 3D Bioprinted Head and Neck in Vitro Tumor Models. *ACS Biomater. Sci. Eng.* **2021**, *7*, 5288–5300. [CrossRef]
42. Hirota, A.; AlMusawi, S.; Nateri, A.S.; Ordóñez-Morán, P.; Imajo, M. Biomaterials for intestinal organoid technology and personalized disease modeling. *Acta Biomater.* **2021**, *132*, 272–287. [CrossRef] [PubMed]
43. Wu, K.Z.; Adine, C.; Mitriashkin, A.; Aw, B.J.J.; Iyer, N.G.; Fong, E.L.S. Making In Vitro Tumor Models Whole Again. *Adv. Healthc. Mater.* **2023**, *12*, e2202279. [CrossRef] [PubMed]
44. Demers, I.; Donkers, J.; Kremer, B.; Speel, E.J. Ex Vivo Culture Models to Indicate Therapy Response in Head and Neck Squamous Cell Carcinoma. *Cells* **2020**, *9*, 2527. [CrossRef] [PubMed]
45. Xu, X.; Farach-Carson, M.C.; Jia, X. Three-dimensional in vitro tumor models for cancer research and drug evaluation. *Biotechnol. Adv.* **2014**, *32*, 1256–1268. [CrossRef]
46. Hagemann, J.; Jacobi, C.; Gstoettner, S.; Welz, C.; Schwenk-Zieger, S.; Stauber, R.; Strieth, S.; Kuenzel, J.; Baumeister, P.; Becker, S. Therapy Testing in a Spheroid-based 3D Cell Culture Model for Head and Neck Squamous Cell Carcinoma. *J. Vis. Exp.* **2018**, *134*, 57012. [CrossRef]
47. Goričan, L.; Gole, B.; Potočnik, U. Head and Neck Cancer Stem Cell-Enriched Spheroid Model for Anticancer Compound Screening. *Cells* **2020**, *9*, 1707. [CrossRef] [PubMed]
48. Magan, M.; Wiechec, E.; Roberg, K. CAFs affect the proliferation and treatment response of head and neck cancer spheroids during co-culturing in a unique in vitro model. *Cancer Cell Int.* **2020**, *20*, 599. [CrossRef]
49. Tanaka, N.; Osman, A.A.; Takahashi, Y.; Lindemann, A.; Patel, A.A.; Zhao, M.; Takahashi, H.; Myers, J.N. Head and neck cancer organoids established by modification of the CTOS method can be used to predict in vivo drug sensitivity. *Oral. Oncol.* **2018**, *87*, 49–57. [CrossRef]

50. Bower, R.; Green, V.L.; Kuvshinova, E.; Kuvshinov, D.; Karsai, L.; Crank, S.T.; Stafford, N.D.; Greenman, J. Maintenance of head and neck tumor on-chip: Gateway to personalized treatment? *Future Sci. OA* **2017**, *3*, Fso174. [CrossRef] [PubMed]
51. Burghartz, M.; Lennartz, S.; Schweinlin, M.; Hagen, R.; Kleinsasser, N.; Hackenberg, S.; Steußloff, G.; Scherzad, A.; Radeloff, K.; Ginzkey, C.; et al. Development of Human Salivary Gland-Like Tissue In Vitro. *Tissue Eng. Part A* **2018**, *24*, 301–309. [CrossRef] [PubMed]
52. Riley, A.; Green, V.; Cheah, R.; McKenzie, G.; Karsai, L.; England, J.; Greenman, J. A novel microfluidic device capable of maintaining functional thyroid carcinoma specimens ex vivo provides a new drug screening platform. *BMC Cancer* **2019**, *19*, 259. [CrossRef] [PubMed]
53. Lugo-Cintrón, K.M.; Ayuso, J.M.; Humayun, M.; Gong, M.M.; Kerr, S.C.; Ponik, S.M.; Harari, P.M.; Virumbrales-Muñoz, M.; Beebe, D.J. Primary head and neck tumour-derived fibroblasts promote lymphangiogenesis in a lymphatic organotypic co-culture model. *EBioMedicine* **2021**, *73*, 103634. [CrossRef] [PubMed]
54. Korayem, M.H.; Heidary, K.; Rastegar, Z. The head and neck cancer (HN-5) cell line properties extraction by AFM. *J. Biol. Eng.* **2020**, *14*, 10. [CrossRef] [PubMed]
55. Wing-Han Yuen, Q.; Zheng, Y.P.; Huang, Y.P.; He, J.F.; Chung-Wai Cheung, J.; Ying, M. In-vitro Strain and Modulus Measurements in Porcine Cervical Lymph Nodes. *Open Biomed. Eng. J.* **2011**, *5*, 39–46. [CrossRef] [PubMed]
56. Bland, J.M.; Altman, D.G. Statistical methods for assessing agreement between two methods of clinical measurement. *Lancet* **1986**, *1*, 307–310. [CrossRef]
57. Pauken, C.M.; Heyes, R.; Lott, D.G. Mechanical, Cellular, and Proteomic Properties of Laryngotracheal Cartilage. *Cartilage* **2019**, *10*, 321–328. [CrossRef]
58. Strek, P.; Skawina, A.; Petri, M.; Olszewski, E.; Nowogrodzka-Zagórska, M.; Waloch, J. The investigations of mechanical properties of ossificating thyroid cartilages of the human larynx. *Folia Morphol.* **1993**, *52*, 39–46.
59. Johnson, C.M.; Howell, J.T.; Mettenburg, D.J.; Rueggeberg, F.A.; Howell, R.J.; Postma, G.N.; Weinberger, P.M. Mechanical Modeling of the Human Cricoid Cartilage Using Computer-Aided Design: Applications in Airway Balloon Dilation Research. *Ann. Otol. Rhinol. Laryngol.* **2016**, *125*, 69–76. [CrossRef]
60. Yokoyama, S.; Kano, M.; Watanabe, M.; Ogawa, H.; Omori, K. Morphological and histologic examination of the epiglottis: Implications for improving epiglottic closure technique. *Ann. Otol. Rhinol. Laryngol.* **2006**, *115*, 23–29. [CrossRef] [PubMed]
61. Storck, C.; Juergens, P.; Fischer, C.; Wolfensberger, M.; Honegger, F.; Sorantin, E.; Friedrich, G.; Gugatschka, M. Biomechanics of the cricoarytenoid joint: Three-dimensional imaging and vector analysis. *J. Voice* **2011**, *25*, 406–410. [CrossRef]
62. Rains, J.K.; Bert, J.L.; Roberts, C.R.; Paré, P.D. Mechanical properties of human tracheal cartilage. *J. Appl. Physiol.* **1992**, *72*, 219–225. [CrossRef] [PubMed]
63. Hujanen, R.; Almahmoudi, R.; Salo, T.; Salem, A. Comparative Analysis of Vascular Mimicry in Head and Neck Squamous Cell Carcinoma: In Vitro and In Vivo Approaches. *Cancers* **2021**, *13*, 4747. [CrossRef] [PubMed]
64. Sucher, N. Searching for synergy in silico, in vitro and in vivo. *Synergy* **2014**, *1*, 30–42. [CrossRef]
65. Johnson, D.E.; Burtness, B.; Leemans, C.R.; Lui, V.W.Y.; Bauman, J.E.; Grandis, J.R. Head and neck squamous cell carcinoma. *Nat. Rev. Dis. Primers* **2020**, *6*, 92. [CrossRef] [PubMed]
66. Kim, J.E.; Reynolds, D.S.; Zaman, M.H.; Mak, M. Characterization of the mechanical properties of cancer cells in 3D matrices in response to collagen concentration and cytoskeletal inhibitors. *Integr. Biol.* **2018**, *10*, 232–241. [CrossRef]
67. Katt, M.E.; Placone, A.L.; Wong, A.D.; Xu, Z.S.; Searson, P.C. In Vitro Tumor Models: Advantages, Disadvantages, Variables, and Selecting the Right Platform. *Front. Bioeng. Biotechnol.* **2016**, *4*, 12. [CrossRef] [PubMed]
68. Wang, L.; Hu, D.; Xu, J.; Hu, J.; Wang, Y. Complex in vitro Model: A Transformative Model in Drug Development and Precision Medicine. *Clin. Transl. Sci.* **2023**, *17*, e13695. [CrossRef] [PubMed]
69. Sharifani, K.; Amini, M. Machine Learning and Deep Learning: A Review of Methods and Applications. *World Inf. Technol. Eng. J.* **2023**, *10*, 3897–3904.
70. Batis, N.; Brooks, J.M.; Payne, K.; Sharma, N.; Nankivell, P.; Mehanna, H. Lack of predictive tools for conventional and targeted cancer therapy: Barriers to biomarker development and clinical translation. *Adv. Drug Deliv. Rev.* **2021**, *176*, 113854. [CrossRef]
71. Gritti, N.; Lim, J.L.; Anlaş, K.; Pandya, M.; Aalderink, G.; Martínez-Ara, G.; Trivedi, V. MOrgAna: Accessible quantitative analysis of organoids with machine learning. *Development* **2021**, *148*, dev199611. [CrossRef] [PubMed]
72. Mienye, I.D.; Swart, T.G. A Comprehensive Review of Deep Learning: Architectures, Recent Advances, and Applications. *Information* **2024**, *15*, 755. [CrossRef]
73. Kong, J.; Lee, H.; Kim, D.; Han, S.K.; Ha, D.; Shin, K.; Kim, S. Network-based machine learning in colorectal and bladder organoid models predicts anti-cancer drug efficacy in patients. *Nat. Commun.* **2020**, *11*, 5485. [CrossRef]
74. Zhang, H.; Qie, Y. Applying Deep Learning to Medical Imaging: A Review. *Appl. Sci.* **2023**, *13*, 10521. [CrossRef]
75. Malhotra, R.; Singh, P. Recent advances in deep learning models: A systematic literature review. *Multimed. Tools Appl.* **2023**, *82*, 44977–45060. [CrossRef]

Journal of
*Functional Biomaterials*

MDPI

*Review*

# Piezoelectric Nanomaterials for Cancer Therapy: Current Research and Future Perspectives on Glioblastoma

**Zayne Knight [1], Amalia Ruiz [2,*] and Jacobo Elies [2,*]**

1 Centre for Pharmaceutical Engineering Science, School of Pharmacy, University of Bradford, Bradford BD7 1DP, UK
2 Institute of Cancer Therapeutics (ICT), Faculty of Life Sciences, University of Bradford, Bradford BD7 1DP, UK
* Correspondence: g.ruizestrada@bradford.ac.uk (A.R.); j.eliesgomez@bradford.ac.uk (J.E.); Tel.: +44-(0)-1274-232132 (J.E.)

**Abstract:** Cancer significantly impacts human quality of life and life expectancy, with an estimated 20 million new cases and 10 million cancer-related deaths worldwide every year. Standard treatments including chemotherapy, radiotherapy, and surgical removal, for aggressive cancers, such as glioblastoma, are often ineffective in late stages. Glioblastoma, for example, is known for its poor prognosis post-diagnosis, with a median survival time of approximately 15 months. Novel therapies using local electric fields have shown anti-tumour effects in glioblastoma by disrupting mitotic spindle assembly and inhibiting cell growth. However, constant application poses risks like patient burns. Wireless stimulation via piezoelectric nanomaterials offers a safer alternative, requiring ultrasound activation to induce therapeutic effects, such as altering voltage-gated ion channel conductance by depolarising membrane potentials. This review highlights the piezoelectric mechanism, drug delivery, ion channel activation, and current technologies in cancer therapy, emphasising the need for further research to address limitations like biocompatibility in whole systems. The goal is to underscore these areas to inspire new avenues of research and overcome barriers to developing piezoelectric nanoparticle-based cancer therapies.

**Keywords:** piezoelectric nanomaterials; cancer therapy; glioblastoma; voltage-gated ion channels; Piezo channels

## 1. Nanotechnology in Cancer Treatment

Cancer remains a significant global health challenge, with high mortality rates. In 2020, breast cancer had the highest incidence, with about 2.26 million cases worldwide [1]. By 2022, there were around 20 million new cases across 36 types in 115 countries [2], and this number is projected to increase by 77% by 2050 [3]. In the UK, 2021 data show around 393,000 new cancer diagnoses and 167,000 deaths annually. Although cancer death rates are declining, the rate of decline has slowed compared to the period from 2009 to 2019 [4].

Current cancer therapies often focus on symptom management rather than a definitive cure, especially for advanced or aggressive cancers. Traditional treatments like cytotoxic chemotherapy can negatively impact patients' quality of life due to their lack of specificity, causing side effects by targeting healthy cells along with cancerous ones [5]. This off-target interaction can lead to acute toxicity [6], necessitating higher doses and increasing patient risk. Combination therapies can mitigate these risks but require extensive development time [7–9]. Targeted therapies, particularly those using nanomaterials, offer promise by enhancing drug specificity, improving delivery, and overcoming physiological barriers, potentially reducing side effects and improving treatment efficiency [10].

Piezoelectricity is a property exhibited by certain materials that generate an electric potential upon applying an external physical force. Despite advancements in cancer therapy, the potential of piezoelectricity has not been thoroughly investigated. However, in recent years, piezoelectric nanotherapy has gained traction because it can minimise harm to healthy cells while actively targeting cancer cells. The novelty lies in the encapsulation of therapeutic materials, which generate radicals that induce cell death, as demonstrated in previous studies [11]. Nanomaterials can be classified as organic or inorganic [12]; however, when delivered into a biological system, it could be argued that all nanoparticles function as hybrids to encapsulate the active agent at the desired location (Figure 1).

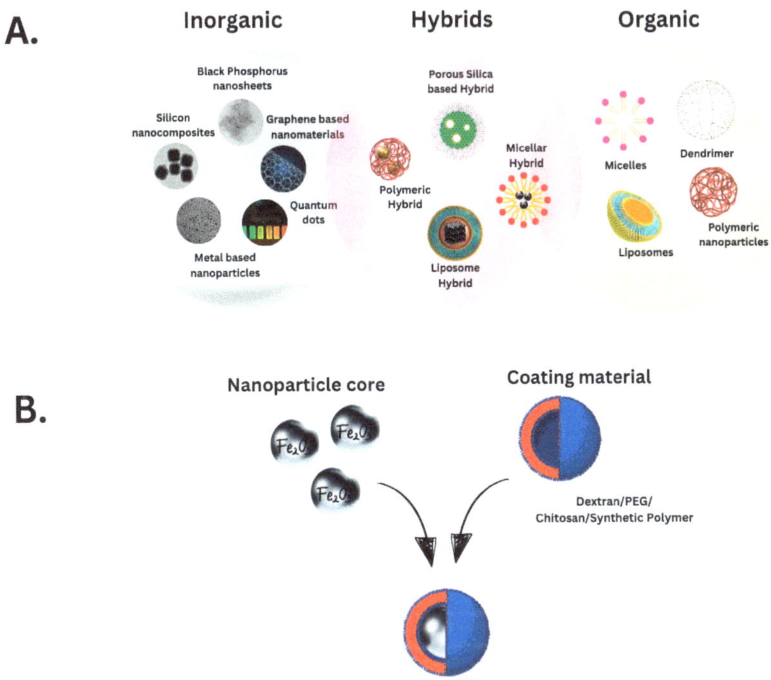


**Figure 1.** Nanomaterials classification. (**A**). Nanoparticles are broadly split into three classifications depending on their biological and engineering properties, and their use depends on the needs of the study or application. There are inorganic nanoparticles, which are made of metal or synthetic material. Organic nanoparticles are modelled on existing biological examples. Finally, hybrid nanoparticles are a mix of the two classifications and are mostly designed with a specific function in mind, unlike the other two classifications. (**B**). Piezoelectric nanoparticles are often hybrid nanomaterials (combination of inorganic and organic elements with a coating material) to ensure biocompatibility.

Nanoparticles are typically delivered within the tumour microenvironment (TME), but their delivery is affected by the body's barriers including cell membranes, epithelial layers, endothelial barriers, and the immune system. These barriers are categorised into four main types summarising nanoparticle delivery in cancer: blood, tumour, cells, and nuclear uptake [13]. Additionally, particle size is critically important in overcoming these barriers, noting that the typical size range for nanoparticles is around 5–200 nm. Smaller nanoparticles penetrate tumour tissue better, while larger nanoparticles have better retention [14]. This indicates the importance of carefully considering particle size when designing new piezoelectric nanoparticles for delivery.

Nanoparticles exert their effects through either passive or active targeting. Passive targeting involves the accumulation of nanoparticles in neoplastic tissue. Due to the high rate of neovascularisation and large pores in cancer cells, nanoparticles can exploit these characteristics, allowing them to leak from the blood vessels [15].

Active targeting is the direct interaction between ligands and receptors, facilitated by ligands bound to the surface of nanoparticles. These ligands selectively target molecules that are characteristically overexpressed on the surface of cancer cells [16]. Various agents, such as antibodies, peptides, amino acids, vitamins, and carbohydrates, can be incorporated into nanoparticles to achieve this targeting. This approach enables the active targeting of specific changes on the cancer cell surface. A recent development in this field is the use of metal-organic frameworks (MOFs), which offer greater control over this targeting mechanism [17]. MOFs are composed of organic linkers that bind to inorganic nodes, allowing them to interact with drugs through multiple mechanisms, including van der Waals forces, hydrogen bonding, and aggregation [18]. Unlike traditional carriers, MOFs can be engineered to encapsulate drugs with precision and high encapsulation efficiency, presenting significant opportunities for advancement in oncological applications [19].

This review provides an update on piezoelectric nanotherapeutics, focusing on whether the biophysical properties of piezoelectric nanomaterials can be used to design effective nanotherapy approaches for challenging tumours like glioblastoma. It highlights the classification of piezoelectric materials, both organic and inorganic, with their potential application in biomedicine, as summarized in Table 1, emphasizing the importance of assessing biocompatibility to avoid toxicity [20].

**Table 1.** Piezoelectric-specific materials and their applications in biomedicine. Many materials are piezoelectric and have electrostatic interactions that generate small electric fields for biological and engineering applications. The table provides an overview of the classification that may be utilised for purposes in the biomedical or biological field.

| Type of Nanomaterial | | Specific Material | | Potential Application in Biomedicine | Refs. |
|---|---|---|---|---|---|
| Synthetic Materials | Inorganic ceramics | Lead-based | Lead titanate | Electrochemical detection of nitrous oxide | [21–23] |
| | | | Lead lanthanum zirconate | Electro-optic applications. Ultrasound imaging, reduction in aperture, wireless device applications, stabilising additive. | [24,25] |
| | | | Lead zirconate titanate | Ceramic resonator for cancer biomarker detection and wireless monitoring applications. | [26–28] |
| | | | Lead magnesium niobate | Medical ultrasound imaging (biomedical measuring). | [29,30] |
| | | Lead-free | Barium titanate | Tissue engineering, bioelectrical sensing, cancer therapy, drug delivery, gene engineering. | [31–33] |
| | | | Lithium tantalate | Infrared detection and acoustic wave devices, glass and or bone engineering. | [34,35] |
| | | | Iron oxide | Drug delivery, iron supplementation, cancer therapy, gene carriers, macrophage polarisation. | [36–38] |
| | | | Zinc ferrite | Considered non-toxic. Cancer therapy (thermal ablation), antibacterial/antifungal, and inorganic/organic pollutant removal. | [39–41] |

**Table 1.** *Cont.*

| Type of Nanomaterial | | Specific Material | Potential Application in Biomedicine | Refs. |
|---|---|---|---|---|
| Synthetic Materials | Organic polymers | Poly (vinylidene difluoride) | Multifilament for vascular grafts, ligaments, and corneas. Also, drug and diffusion media. It can also be used as an encapsulation material. | [42–44] |
| | | Nylon | Hybridised materials such as skin dressings and composites for piezoelectric bone stimulation. | [45,46] |
| | | Polyacrylonitrile | Hybridisation with metallic materials as an antibacterial agent. It could be used in wound healing and prevention. Hydrophilic and highly elastic material. | [47,48] |
| | | Cellulose acetate | Tissue engineering as a primary scaffold or scaffold structures to osteoblast/fibroblast anchoring. | [49,50] |
| | Polymer composites | PVDF/PZT | It could be used for portable devices, mobile imaging, and electrical storage. | [51] |
| | | PVDF/ZnO | Organic electro-spun piezoelectric nanofibers. Self-powered sensors to monitor the cardiovascular walls of the heart. | [52] |
| | | PVDF/BT NPs | Increased electrical wireless stimulation in bone scaffolds for wound healing and oestogeneration. | [53] |
| | | PVDF/$MOS_2$ | Next-generation sensors for wireless biomedical applications. | [54] |
| Natural Materials | | Quartz crystals | Used in quartz crystal microbalance systems, which are used as wide-range biosensors. | [50,55] |
| | | Rochelle salt | To be developed as a 3D composite for prosthetics and smart sensing impact-prone professions (self-generative material). | [56,57] |
| | | Silk | Tissue engineering, cell coating, drug delivery, microfluidics, and formation of composite biomaterials. | [58,59] |
| | | Bone | An inherent piezoelectric material. Piezoelectrics contribute towards the promotion of regeneration and repair. | [60–62] |

The review also explores the principles of piezoelectricity and its potential therapeutic effects in cancer treatment, particularly for complex cancers such as glioblastoma. Additionally, it discusses future applications and perspectives, evaluates current technology, and addresses challenges in cancer therapeutics.

## 2. Piezoelectricity and Its Relevance in Physiology and Health

### 2.1. Piezoelectricity Principles and Mechanism

Piezoelectricity is a property of certain materials that enables them to convert mechanical stress into an electric field and vice versa. When mechanical stress is applied along the material's polarisation direction, it generates an electric field through a direct piezoelectric effect. Conversely, when an electric field is applied, the material undergoes mechanical deformation due to the inverse piezoelectric effect, releasing mechanical energy [63]. These materials are characterised by a non-centrosymmetric crystal structure, which makes them susceptible to mechanical stimuli that initiate a change in structure to displace electron balance. A net polarisation is created due to the imbalance of the electrical charge. Of the thirty-two crystal classes, 21 are non-centrosymmetric with 20 are piezoelectric as they become polarised on the application of mechanical stress. The remaining one-point group out of the 21 does not exhibit piezoelectricity due to the combination of symmetry elements. Ten out of the 20 piezoelectric point groups display a spontaneous polarization that exists even without an applied field or stress, making them polar or pyroelectric materials. Ferroelectric materials are polar dielectrics that can reverse and reorient their spontaneous polarization when exposed to an external electric field [64,65]. This happens due to an external influence that prioritises one polarisation state over the other. In these materials, domain walls dictate separate regions with polarisation orientations. This creates a motion in the material, turning it slightly under weak electric fields [66]. Additionally, any extra external force would increase the rate of this transition and result in a quick phase as the dipoles have been further displaced by the force generated. This creates asymmetrical symmetry within the structure, producing an electrical dipole from the opposingly charged ions. As such, these materials follow certain conditions to produce an electrical field. First, the material needs to have a dielectric property, a crystal structure with no centre of symmetry, and both positive and negative charged masses, which is a structure with an ionic crystal or molecular crystal composed of ionic clusters [67]. Figure 2 displays the mechanism of action of piezoelectric materials when mechanical force is applied and the consequences of the mechanical potential, previously reviewed in [68,69].

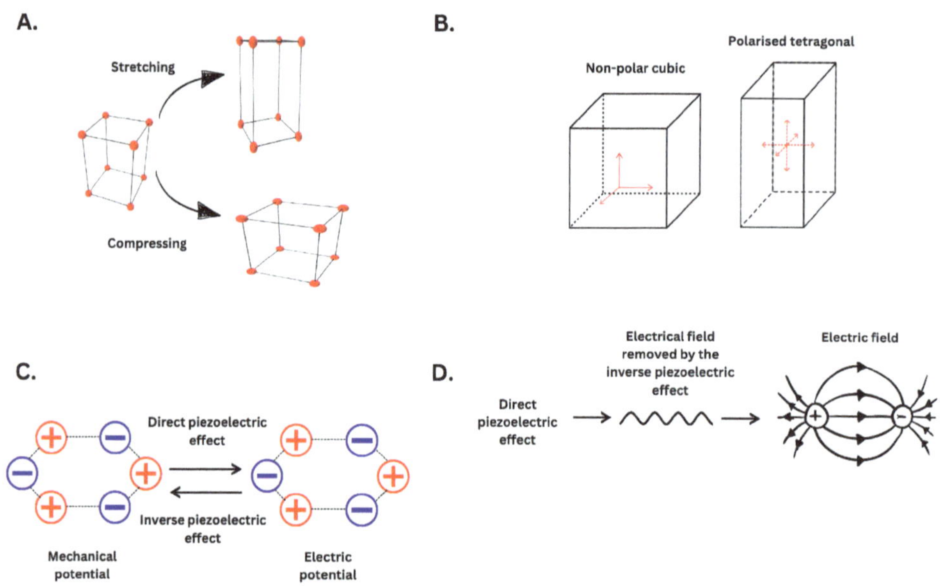


**Figure 2.** Overview of the basic piezoelectric mechanism and products of the mechanical strain. (**A**). displays a piezoelectric material under a certain mechanical stress with examples of the mechanical force that can act on the material. (**B**). displays the phase difference between activated and non-activated piezoelectric materials. The defined difference between whether a material is piezoelectric is if it is non-polar cubic or polarised tetragonal. This geometric direction displays the vibrational flow. If non-polar cubic, the centrosymmetric conformation is stable and stabilised, meaning there is no excess charge or instability between the dipoles. (**C**). shows the material in resting and the resulting dipole production with the two piezoelectric forces and how they act upon each other. Finally, (**D**). displays the production of the piezoelectric field, which is directly produced from the direct piezoelectric effect and the process of removal. Note that (**C**). applies only to a class that would be piezoelectric, not ferroelectric.

In general, once the mechanical force is applied. The atoms are displaced from their original position within the crystal lattice, resulting in a net electrical charge through the entire structure, which creates a counterbalance from the corresponding charges.

Barium titanate ($BaTiO_3$) is a well-studied ceramic non-lead-based nanoparticle and is a classic inorganic example in the research field [70]. It is defined as a perovskite-type ceramic, displaying the hallmarks of a piezoelectric material, which has been the focus of literature solely with a few combinations [33]. Some materials, like $BaTiO_3$, have different conformations and produce a higher piezoelectric effect due to the different crystal phases. If we use $BaTiO_3$ as an example of a piezoelectric material, it can display differing piezoelectric properties with different conformations depending on its geometric structure, such as cubic barium titanate (BTO), tetragonal unpolarised barium titanate (U-BTO), and tetragonal polarised barium titanate [71]. The morphology and size are the same; however, the electrical potentials are different due to the material's different characteristics. BTO produces 0 mV, U-BTO produces 425 mV, and P-BTO produces 886 mV. Regarding energy potential, piezoelectric nanoparticles will follow a basic rule, and their conformation will determine the electrical output of said material. These materials are in different states; BTO produces no energy because it is non-polar and, therefore, produces no electrical field as there is no dipole movement. The polarised form induces the dipole movement and shows a displacement of the overall symmetry. The polarised orthorhombic form has a higher potential energy than polarised due to a higher distortion in the symmetry, which additionally produces more of the potential inverse piezoelectric effect. Examples include lead zirconate titanate (PZT). The highest form is that of polarised rhombohedral, resulting in the lowest symmetry without breaking the functionality. Examples of these are lead titanate ceramics and ferroelectric films [72]. Barium titanate is a good example of all four of these phases. However, Figure 2B displays a simple diagram to provide what geometry results in piezoelectricity as it can conform to the higher energy states once polarised and tetragonal.

These materials can exhibit piezoelectric effects due to mechanical stress but also change their polarisation due to the thermal expansion when encountering temperature changes. As the temperature of the material changes, positive and negative polarisation charges are present on the surface of the crystal, which is termed the pyroelectric effect [73]. The thermodynamic equilibrium is broken and established due to the change in polarisation states, which causes the absorption and desorption of chemical species. This produces a piezo-catalytic effect from producing an electrolyte-heavy environment; this, however, would be hard to apply in a biological aspect due to the heating phase [74].

### 2.2. *Piezoelectricity in Biological Systems and Its Function*

Electrical surface charges have a role in cells and in regulating their functions. Throughout the body, there are piezoelectric organic structures that generate electrostatic interactions, which play a critical role in biological functions such as maintaining homeostasis, protein folding, cardiac muscle contraction, and ion channel charge dependencies [68]. In addition, the scientific community has been investigating the potential for piezoelectric materials in tissue regeneration in recent years, focusing on neural and bone regeneration. Piezoelectric-specific scaffolds that match the sizes of the target damaged tissue after implantation can provide electrical stimulation to promote regeneration [75].

Recent research has revealed that many bioactive materials exhibit piezoelectric properties due to their non-centrosymmetric alignment. Peptides, for instance, demonstrate significant spatial variation and movement, enabling the formation of complex structures through various bonding mechanisms. These structures can also be organised into nanostructures that display piezoelectric properties at the macroscopic level [76]. Some proteins, such as collagen, exhibit strong potential for electrostatic interactions and are known to possess piezoelectric interactions. Helical structures like collagen can twist or stretch, producing the piezoelectric effect. However, despite these underlying principles, the resultant effect leads to a weak piezoelectric response due to a low piezoelectric coefficient [77]. Another example is elastin, an extracellular matrix protein found in various connective tissues, which provides flexibility and elasticity. Under physical stress, elastin may exhibit electromechanical responses, including potential piezoelectric behaviour, which arises from its asymmetric molecular structure [75]. At the macroscopic level, this effect manifests through the organised alignment of these proteins within tissues, such as blood vessels or lungs, where their collective response to stress integrates into measurable biomechanical behaviours. As a result, these effects could influence the dilation and contraction of blood vessels and lung tissues, although the piezoelectric properties of elastin are not yet fully understood and require further investigation [78,79]. It has also been studied that this electrical charge generated by elastin may assist in regulating the migration and proliferation of vascular smooth muscle cells while also repairing blood vessels in vascular injury [79].

The cellular targets of piezoelectric influence would be indicated to any cellular or intracellular machinery that confers a change in electrostatic potential. Many of these are widely known, but comprehensive lists include neurons, muscle cells, and most other cells, which possess some form of electrostatic potential. One notable example is the cell membrane itself. Liu and colleagues discuss these principles in detail in their comprehensive review [80]. Phosphatidylserine is negatively charged, and the authors state that electrostatic interactions govern the localisation of peripheral proteins. Finally, electrostatics are defined in two territories: membranes of early secretory pathways in weakly charged regions and membranes of late secretory pathways. All this depends on the cytosolic leaflet charge potential. Following this and the previous example of collagen as a piezoelectric material, the signals generated by collagen can be transmitted through the extracellular matrix (ECM) to the voltage-gated channels in the cell membrane [81]. This suggests that extraneous piezoelectric materials can alter overall cell dynamics and cell-cell interactions with the intended target depending on potential voltage.

## 3. Applications of Piezoelectric Nanomaterials in Cancer Therapy

The main application of piezoelectric materials when dealing with cancer is to produce an end effect of ROS generation or a desired DNA-damaging agent. However, the nanoparticle needs to be delivered and targeted to trigger an increase in ROS generation, which will result in DNA damage and reduce the side effects of the therapy. This happens due to piezo-catalysis, which produces superoxide and hydroxyl radical formation, combined with glutathione depletion. This can be targeted specifically for cancer cells if conjugated and designed, resulting in high ROS formation within the cell and, as a consequence, cancer-specific apoptosis while avoiding healthy tissues surrounding the tumour [82]. This innovative therapeutic approach makes piezo-electric nanotherapy attractive for the treatment of solid tumours.

### 3.1. Piezo-Catalysis

The generation of ROS through piezoelectric material is a specific process and involves molecular reactions downstream in biological systems. Piezoelectric materials convert mechanical energy into an electrical field, with the opposite action to be true as well. Effective charge transfer contributes to redox catalytic activity, where piezoelectric materials release electrons to catalyse redox reactions and substrates. This is termed Piezo-catalysis, and the main source of action is from ROS radical formation [83]. These oxygen-containing substances increase oxidative potentials and free radicals containing unpaired electrons.

These include superoxide ions ($\bullet O_2^-$), hydroxyl radicals ($\bullet OH$), oxygen species containing singlet oxygens ($^1\Delta gO_2$) and hydroperoxide ($H_2O_2$) [84].

There are two theories of piezo-catalysis, as the full mechanism is not fully established. When the piezoelectric effect takes place, it allows catalysis of redox reactions. The enriched surface of the material activated by the dipole movement will shuttle electrons to reduce oxygen molecules to $O^{2-}$. In this state, the holes opened by stimulation allow oxidation of water molecules, which results in a net production of $\bullet OH$. This is known as the electric band theory [85].

The second theory is that of the screening charge effect. This theory argues that the piezo-catalytic reaction is determined by the surface screening charges, referred to as the screening charge effect [86]. When a piezoelectric material is subject to ultrasonic vibration, the potential induces opposite polarities and can be inferred as the dipole formation. Due to this effect, equal quantities of opposing charges are attached to the surfaces. This collection of charge eventually leads to absorption and dynamic release, enabling a piezo-catalytic reaction. Under mechanical strain, this undergoes periodic absorption and release until the free energy is completely transferred through the system. The negative screening charges driving these reactions are electrons generated by dissociating absorbed water molecules on the surface or donated by absorbed $\bullet OH$ species [87]. The positive screening, however, is the involvement of protons. This acts the same way as negative screening, and the theory works overall by the electrons and protons influencing each other when the mechanical stress is applied.

Regarding the piezo-catalysis mechanism in tumour treatment, piezoelectric nanoparticles can generate a small electrical field with anti-tumour therapeutic effects within the targeted system. This field-generating effect is known to reduce hypoxia, a common hallmark in many cancers [88]. Consequently, this reduction in hypoxia leads to a decrease in HIF$\alpha$ levels, which correlates with reduced metastasis and invasion.

This relationship is well-documented in the literature, as a successful reduction in hypoxia typically results in lower HIF$\alpha$ levels, thereby diminishing metastatic and invasive potential. When a piezoelectric material is introduced and subjected to mechanical force, an imbalanced charge state is produced on its surface. This excess charge results in two redox behaviours: one directly interacts with water molecules to produce oxygen, while the other suggests that the released charges can combine with water or oxygen to generate other ROS [87]. There is a further knock-on effect on the electrolyte as the electrolyte is attracted to the material surface due to the charge. This induces water splitting to produce oxygen. Additionally, the electrolytes with opposite polarity to the bound charges are involved in the redox reaction, producing more ROS. This whole process is a step reaction and will impact the tumour microenvironment (TME). An overview of this process is displayed in Figure 3.

Typically, cancer cells produce higher ROS levels than their normal counterparts due to an imbalance of antioxidants and oxidants. This low to moderate ROS level acts as a signal transducer for cellular proliferation, migration, invasion, and angiogenesis [89]. These differences arise from molecular changes in the electron transport chain within the mitochondria. Therefore, when selectively targeted with a piezo-catalytic inducer, the increased ROS levels surpass the survival threshold, leading to cell death as cancer cells have a reduced capacity for removing harmful metabolites. In the mitochondria, complexes I and III are the primary sites of oxygen reduction, where leaking produces superoxide. In normal cells, these are converted into hydrogen peroxide by superoxide dismutase 1 (SOD1) [90]. Hydrogen peroxide is then detoxified by glutathione peroxidase (GPX) and catalase (CAT) into water and oxygen [91]. When cancer cells are suddenly exposed to piezo-catalytic materials, they exceed their capacity for ROS removal, forcing them to undergo apoptosis or autophagy to survive the influx of oxygen radicals.

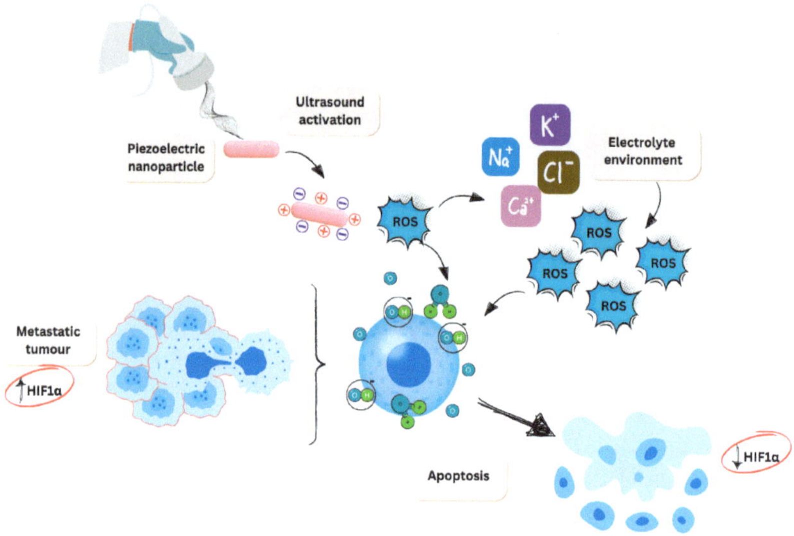


**Figure 3.** Overview of the piezo-catalysis mechanism in context to cancer cells. The figure displays that the mechanism ultimately results in apoptosis and a decrease in HIF-α. This is due to the hypoxia environment being charged to a more neutral level by the increased oxygen radicals. This process is a knock-on mechanistic approach. First, water splits to produce ROS, which affects the electrolyte environment to produce even more free radicals, which cause oxidative damage to the cells in question.

Materials that are piezo-catalytic in nature and exhibit the traditional piezoelectric effect have the effect of converting mechanical stress into electrical signals. These signals stimulate cells or interfere with the biological system's electrical field. The most notable influence is that of voltage-gated channels and biosensing, in which the piezoelectricity signal generates an effect to alter the state of signalling pathways [92]. This process does not catalyse reactions directly but promotes the production of effector molecules. This process is termed piezo-catalytic medicine as the process can indirectly be used for various applications in the medical field. Examples include connective tissue healing, remodelling of calcified tissue, and bone remodelling due to the piezoelectric nature of the bone. The exogenous charge from a piezoelectric biocompatible material can lead to osteoinduction; however, this is a relatively novel area, and the research is in its infancy [68].

Types of this therapy are already being employed in research for invasive but deep penetration treatments. An example of this is piezodynamic therapy (PzDT) investigated by Hoang and colleagues [93]. These materials are combined with ultrasound to separate the electrons and activate the piezoelectric effect, creating cytotoxic ROS redox reactions. The research involved MCF-7 breast cancer cells with a 2D PEGylated tungsten disulfide nanosheet and mouse xenografts. The investigation concluded that upon induction, the conclusion of the work generated a high volume of intracellular ROS contained in the mitochondria due to their chosen targeting molecule (FX11-LDHA inhibitor) while inducing apoptosis and suggesting that this investigation of the treatment method is successful and requires further investigation. A similar study by Gong and colleagues evaluated tetragonal barium titanate while using a combination of 5FU-based treatments for human colorectal carcinoma [32]. The study developed 3D organoids and mentioned performing "sonodynamic therapy", but the use of a piezoelectric material suggests that there is also a lack of agreement on this terminology. However, the investigation aimed to find a way to reduce the dose-dependent amount in colorectal cancer without relying on 5FU. The work concluded that the combination was equal to high-dose drugs despite a low dose of 5FU being used when the barium titanate nanoparticle was used. However, the paper does not highlight the classification of high or low doses. The investigation concludes that the cytotoxicity of 5FU can be reduced to provide a combined therapy equal to a high dose. This suggests that pioneering piezo-catalysis with a combined therapy is the way forward for more aggressive cancers, and we should not rely on a single treatment but multiple approaches.

### 3.2. *Ion Channel Activation*

Ion channels are essential for life, playing diverse biological roles such as cell-cell communication, excitability, proliferation, and apoptosis. They regulate cell membrane potentials by controlling the conductance of ions like $Ca^{2+}$, $Cl^-$, $K^+$, and $Na^+$ [94–97]. Table 2 displays a short overview of the voltage-dependent ion channels, their cellular role and mechanism of action to summarise potential changes that piezoelectric materials may result in after application [98–100].

**Table 2.** Short overview of relevant ion channels, detailing their cellular roles and mechanism of action by which piezoelectric nanomaterials can modulate ion channel activity.

| Ion Channel Class | Cellular Role | Mechanism of Action |
|---|---|---|
| Voltage-gated potassium channels | Regulate excitability and control the action potential waveform. Help with the secretion of hormones. | Activity regulated by calcium, voltage, and neurotransmitters |
| Voltage-gated chloride channels | Cell volume regulation, salt transport, and importantly, acidification of intracellular and extracellular components with cell cycle signalling. | Anion-selective and activated by intracellular calcium. |
| Acid-sensing ion channels | Permeable by $Na^+$ and serves to detect extracellular PH from neuronal response. | Gated by membrane depolarisation by transmembrane PH gradient |
| Volage-gated sodium channels | Allow movement of electrically charged particles. Dysfunctions of these, change the charge potentials of cells | Gated by depolarisation, and rapid inactivation, and are the first channels to respond to changes in voltage. |
| Voltage-gated calcium channels | Present in the membrane of highly excitable cells. Works as a secondary messenger with many functions across the cell. | Form hetero-oligomeric complexes with the α1 subunit providing extracellular binding sites. $Ca_v3$ type (T types) are low voltage-activated, unlike L types. |
| Piezo channels | Expressed in mechanically sensitive cells. Allow $Ca^{2+}$ influx and are observed in a variety of endothelial cells to sense physiological shear stress. | Allow the $Ca^{2+}$ influx in response to external force. The main function and action of this channel is that of mechanical transduction. |

Cells have an electric potential across their plasma membrane, known as the membrane potential (Vm), which ranges from −90 to −10 mV depending on the cell type and state [101,102]. This Vm is regulated by ion channel expression in cells, the ionic composition of the extracellular milieu, and the presence of bioelectric gradients, such as an electric field (EF), within a tissue. Changes in this potential are linked to depolarisation and hyperpolarisation. Cancer cells exhibit a more positive resting membrane potential, ranging from −30 to −20 mV, compared to other body cells [103]. This characteristic aligns them more closely with rapidly dividing cells, such as embryonic and stem cells, rather than with healthy, mature cells. Additionally, ion channels are often abnormally expressed in cancer tissues and cell lines. These hallmarks of cancer cells make tumour cells targetable using piezo-electric nanomaterials.

Ion channel dysregulation in cancer impairs key cellular processes, calcium signalling, cell volume regulation, membrane potential regulation, mechanosensitivity, and microenvironment regulation [104]. Oncochannelopathies is the term used to describe the group of cancer (or tumour processes) caused by the dysfunction of ion channel subunits (or their interacting proteins), including the oncogenic roles of ion channels [105]. Blocking these ion channels can inhibit cancer cell growth, highlighting the role of bioelectrical signalling as a key feature of cancer [106]. Substantial experimental evidence demonstrates ion channels' critical role in cellular proliferation, tumorigenesis, and metastasis. For instance, the Cav3.1 current is associated with the inhibition of proliferation and induction of apoptosis in MCF-7 human breast cancer cells [107]; and inhibition of Cav3 calcium channels decreases colorectal cancer cell proliferation [108]. In the context of glioblastoma, the downregulation of STIM1 and Orai1 results in a significant decrease in cell invasion [109]. These findings underscore the potential of targeting ion channels as a therapeutic strategy in cancer treatment.

To avoid redundancy, we will not delve into the intracellular signalling pathways associated with oncochannelopathies, as these have been extensively reviewed elsewhere [104,105,110–113]. Instead, this review will focus on three families of well-characterised ion channels: Voltage-gated Calcium Channels (VGCC), Piezo channels, and TRP channels. These ion channels are particularly relevant to this review due to their significance in glioblastoma and other types of cancer, and their modulation via piezoelectric nanomaterials. These channels possess inherent domains sensitive to changes in electrical potential or mechanical forces, which are key to their activation by piezoelectric nanomaterials. The subsequent paragraphs will summarize the biophysical properties of VGCC, Piezo channels, and TRP channels, which make them suitable targets for piezoelectric nanomaterials:

Voltage-gated Calcium Channels (VGCC or Cav channels) can be divided into two groups based on their voltage activation thresholds: high voltage-activated (HVA) and low voltage-activated (LVA) channels. Low voltage-activated $Ca^{2+}$ channels include Cav3.1-Cav3.3 channels, also known as T-type $Ca^{2+}$ channels. High voltage-activated $Ca^{2+}$ channels include Cav1.1-Cav1.4 (L-type channels) and Cav2.1-Cav2.3, which comprise the P/Q, N, and R-type channels [114].

The Cav family consists of 10 members, all sharing a similar pore-forming subunit (CaV$\alpha$1), composed of four domains. Each domain contains six transmembrane helices (S1–S6). Specifically, S1–S4 contribute to voltage sensing, while S5 and S6, along with each domain's P loop, form the channel's core. The S4 segment is particularly interesting as it contains regularly spaced arginine and lysine residues that sense changes in membrane voltage (Figure 4). This sensing leads to a conformational change that transitions the channel from a deactivated state to an activated, highly permeable $Ca^{2+}$ state [115].

Targeting the voltage-sensing domains in these channels can regulate ion channel activation. Agents such as piezoelectric nanomaterials could potentially be used to achieve this, allowing for direct control over ion influx and efflux systems. This approach could provide new therapeutic strategies for modulating cellular activities in various physiological and pathological conditions [116]. $Ca^{2+}$ influx across the plasma membrane occurs due to membrane depolarisation. This change in membrane potential is sensed by $Ca^{2+}$ voltage-gated channels, displaying an area of influence where piezoelectric materials can affect the fate of cells by interfering with the ion channel domains sensitive to the changes in membrane potential.

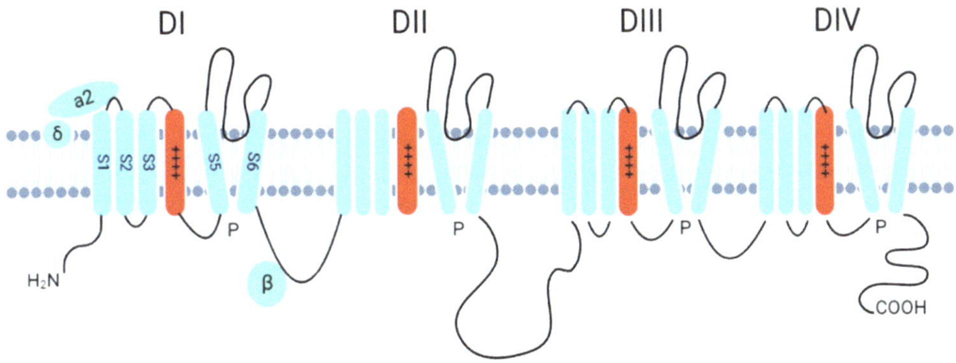


**Figure 4.** Structural domains of voltage-gated calcium channels (VGCCs). $Ca_V\alpha1$ schematic of four domains with six transmembrane units in each domain. The S4 is highlighted (red) as it contains positively charged amino acids that act as voltage sensors with the pores of the channels formed by the loop between S5 and S6. The $Ca_V\beta$ unit acts as a linker to interact with the domains and the domain linking between II–III.

There is substantial evidence supporting the role of VGCC in cancer. For instance, Cav1.2 and Cav1.3 channels have a direct effect on tumour cells, and blocking these currents reduces cell proliferation [117–119]. Additionally, blockade of L-type Ca current attenuates doxorubicin-induced cardiomyocyte apoptosis via suppression of the CaMKII-NF-κB pathway [120]. This suggests that nano-piezomaterials could potentially reduce the toxicity of chemotherapeutic drugs. These research findings demonstrate the significant role of piezosensitive ion channels in cancer. This review will focus on glioblastoma, where NMDA receptor dysregulation is common. NMDA receptors are involved not only in excitotoxic cell death but also in pathological cellular proliferation, contributing to the invasion and proliferation of glioblastoma cells and other types of cancer [121–124].

Targeting VGCCs that are downregulated in cancer could lead to new research opportunities. However, most current studies focus on upregulated channels. For example, voltage-gated sodium ion channels (VGSCs) are often overexpressed in many cancer types, promoting cell invasion and metastasis [125]. Another approach could be to overload these channels beyond their depolarisation limit. Calcium channels have received the most attention in this context. Alterations in ion channel expression can initiate, proliferate, and metastasise cancer cells [126]. Key pathways affected by these changes include mitogen-activated protein kinase (MAPK), ERK, JNK, Wnt/ß-catenin, PI3K/Akt, Notch, and the Rac and Rho pathways [127]. Studies have shown that changes in $Ca^{2+}$ and $K^+$ ion channels are directly involved in cell migration and EGFR signalling.

Calcium is particularly important because it plays a role in cancer initiation through epithelial-mesenchymal transitions (EMT). Targeting $Ca^{2+}$ channels could prevent cancer progression. For instance, PMCA4 has been shown to inhibit this pathway in gastric cancer. Further details on ion channel changes and their intracellular pathways in cancer are available in other reviews [128].

The discovery of new families of mechanically activated ion channels, such as PIEZOs, which play crucial physiological roles in mammals [129–133] has opened new avenues of inquiry into the roles of mechano-transduction in human health and disease and the development of novel therapeutic strategies aiming to modulate the activity of these ion channels.

Changes in Piezo1 have been identified in various cancers, with overexpression promoting invasion and metastasis in gastric cancers [134]. Piezo1 is also highly unregulated in thyroid and breast cancers, making it a promising target for a wide range of cancers. If Piezo1 ion channels could be targeted with piezoelectric biocompatible materials, it might have a therapeutic effect or provide insights into how these materials affect tumour progression.

Higher expression of Piezo1 is a hallmark of cancer cells. Knocking down caveolin1 or reducing cholesterol content inhibits Piezo1 expression [135]. Piezo 1 also promotes single-cell migration by modulating adhesion factors, notably the cytoskeleton protein F-actin, and forming invadopodia through calcium influx. This calcium influx affects downstream effectors such as ERK and Src. Additionally, elevated Piezo1 levels inhibit fibroblast formation, reducing adhesion with cadherins. In the context of piezoelectric nanoparticles, targeting Piezo1 mRNA could enhance the delivery effectiveness of an inhibitor if designed correctly. This approach could provide a combination therapy that uses an electrical field to depolarise any voltage-sensitive machinery.

The transient receptor potential (TRP) family of channels plays a critical role in various biological processes, including cell cycle regulation and cancer progression. Many TRP family members function as mechanosensory channels, making the TRP family a promising therapeutic target. Their involvement in multiple stages of cancer development and metastasis highlights their potential for therapeutic intervention [136,137].

TRPV6, for example, is well-documented for its high expression in various cancers, including those of the prostate, breast, colon, and oesophagus. The high expression is associated with metastasis and chemotherapy resistance [138]. Another example of the TRP family, TRPA1, is expressed in nociceptor neurons and acts as a chemosensory receptor for noxious compounds. Berrout and colleagues [139] investigated TRPA1 and concluded that it serves as a prognostic marker in cancer. Their research suggests that FGFR2 binds to TRPA1 to form a complex facilitated by ankyrin, which binds TRPA1 to the C-terminal proline-rich region of FGFR2. This interaction inhibits the channel, leading to a conformational change that promotes the proliferation and invasion of lung adenocarcinoma (LUAD).

However, further research is needed to determine if these findings can be translated into other cancer types. The study also implies that astrocytes target infiltrating LUAD cells by depleting TRPA1-expressing exosomal miRNA, thereby interrupting FGFR2 binding. Additional mechanistic insights are required to understand these interactions fully. The piezoelectric effect may influence both TRPV6 and TRPA1 channels, offering potential therapeutic applications alongside inhibitors or exciters. However, these options remain unexplored and can only be inferred from the current understanding of their mechanisms of action.

### 3.2.1. Evading Apoptosis

Calcium ion influx is required for cell cycle progression, and reducing the levels of extracellular $Ca^{2+}$ terminates progression via the G1 phase. Halting cells at the G1/S phase boundary and mitogens induce calcium entry pathways to drive cellular progression through the cell cycle. Of the voltage-gated $Ca^{2+}$ channels (VGCC), Cav3 channels are stated to be expressed in many cancer cell lines, and the increased expression exhibits increased S phase activity, which is inferred to result in higher DNA synthesis [140]. One major hallmark of cancer is evasion of apoptosis, in which cancer cells must utilise mechanisms to reduce $Ca^{2+}$ influx either by altering the signalling pathways or downregulating the calcium-permeable channels (Figure 5). Apoptosis-resistant phenotypes are characterised by a reduction in store-operated calcium entry (SOCE), which prevents calcium ion overload from pro-apoptotic stimuli. The effect reduces the efficiency of mitochondrial and cytoplasm apoptotic pathways. A study performed by Liu and colleagues [141] investigated glioblastoma survival with the introduction of amlodipine and discovered, on its introduction, activated $Ca^{2+}$ entry. This further enhances SOCE and inhibits YAP/TAZ in glioblastoma by activating Lat1/2 kinases. The conclusion from this work indicated that activating SOCE to suppress YAP/TAZ signalling to interfere with extracellular calcium L-type channels may be a reliable focus on reducing glioblastoma clinically and other cancers. Other examples of bioelectric control modulated by Orai/SOCE have been described in breast [142] and cervical [143] cancer growth and metastasis [128,144].

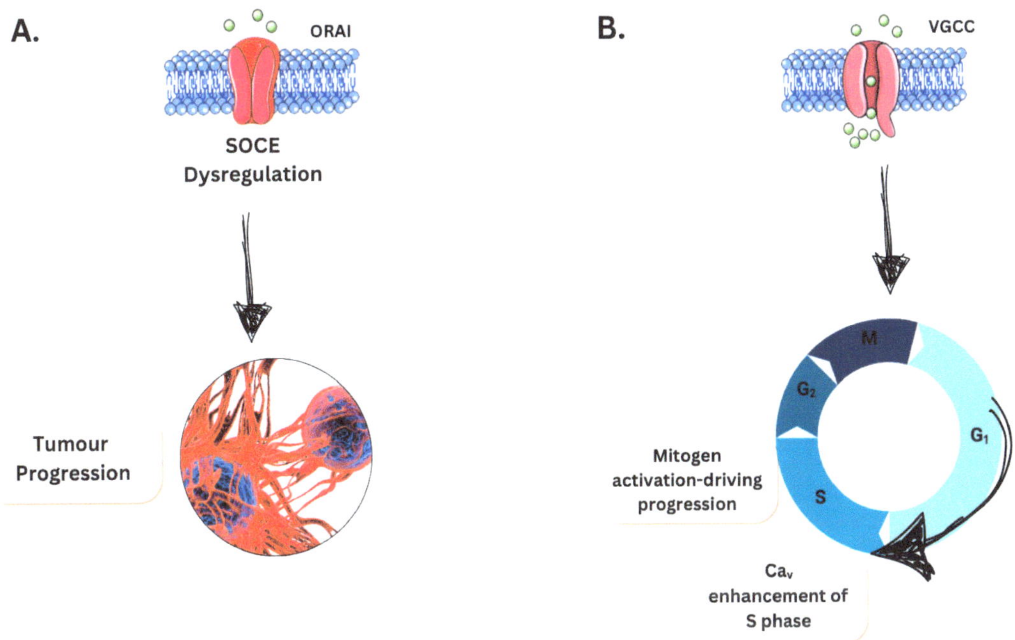


**Figure 5.** Scheme summarising main calcium-handling events on cancer cells. (**A**). Reduction of SOCE is associated with apoptotic-resistant phenotype and subsequent tumour progression. (**B**). Increased $Ca^{2+}$ influx via VGCC induces cell proliferation via promotion of S phase. These ion channels are ideal targets in piezoelectric nanotechnology.

### 3.2.2. Limitless Growth Potential

Focusing on a different hallmark to provide scope to voltage-gated ion channels is important to downstream mechanisms. The limitless replicative potential is a hallmark negatively influenced by $Ca^{2+}$ ions. Most somatic cells have a set limit to their replicative growth, known as the Hayflick limit, which varies by cell type [145]. This potential is determined by telomeres, which consist of several thousand repeats of 6 bp sequences that protect chromosome integrity. However, with each division, telomere shortens by 50–100 bp, depending on the cell type, eventually leaving the chromosome unprotected as the repeats are exhausted. This leads to replicative senescence in cells. Cancer cells, however, can extend this limit through the action of telomerase, which stabilises or synthesises telomeric DNA [146]. This extension of instability is facilitated by the influx of calcium through VGCC or TRP channels, promoting telomerase activation (Figure 6). This elevation of intracellular calcium has been investigated and confirmed in other types of senescence. Notably, Martin and Bernard [147] describe that the Cav1.3 L-type channel prevents a rise in rotenone-induced senescence in neuroblastoma SH-SH5Y cells. This intracellular increase also promotes the senescence-associated secretory phenotype (SASP), which has a knock-on effect on local inflammation. It promotes increased mitochondrial ROS via a drop in mitochondrial membrane potential. This enhances ROS production, adding to the potential for mutagenic damage in already altered DNA strands. During oncogenic senescence and telomere shortening, calcium is released from endoplasmic reticulum stores via the PLC/IP3/IP3R pathway [148]. This increased calcium is sustained for senescence, indicating that VGCC and activated machinery play a role in controlling this hallmark's progression in cancer types. This effect is particularly evident in cells that are not meant to divide and have short base repeats, such as neural cancers.

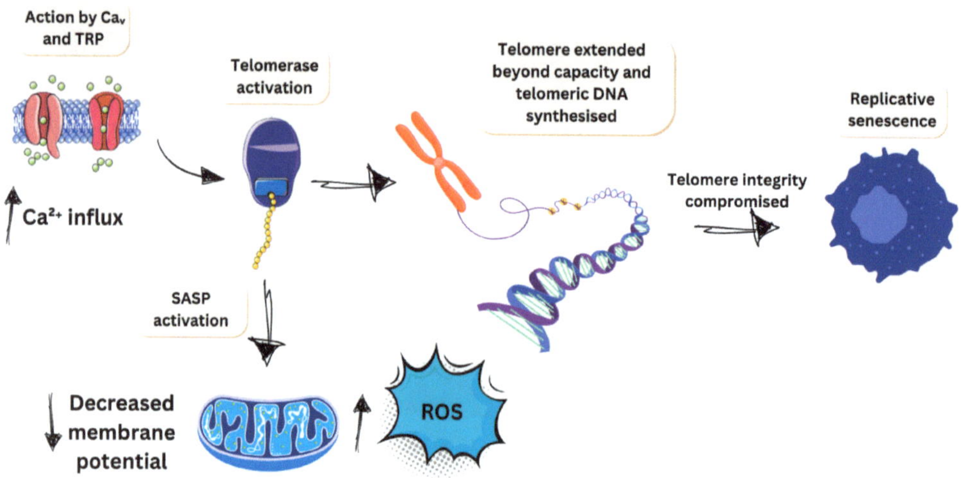


**Figure 6.** Scheme of somatic replicative senescence and oncogenic senescence in cancer cells. The figure illustrates key mechanisms that contribute to the limitless potential of cancer cells, highlighting the role of TRP and Cav channels in $Ca^{2+}$ release.

These areas are key for the potential expansion of research, as many studies give the mechanism of action of these ion channels in cancer development. Karska et al. [135] review this in detail, highlighting common cancers and the expression of ion channels closely associated with enhancing tumorigenesis. Mechanosensitive ion channels, such as Piezo and TRP families, are linked to mutations that facilitate tumour progression. Specifically, Piezo channels are activated by mechanical stretching of the cell membrane, while TRP channels are activated by changes in temperature, pressure or chemical environment [149,150].

### 3.3. Drug Delivery

The uniqueness of piezoelectric technologies in cancer is the application of wireless electrical stimulation, which has clear harmful effects and is not always readily accessible to a patient. Piezoelectric materials can be activated by ultrasound-based external pressure, which results in electrical stimulation by the direct piezoelectric effect [64]. This means the electrical stimulation can be directed to a specific tissue or cellular environment depending on the penetrating power that remotely generates an electrical charge. However, mechanical stimulation can include ultrasound, tide, water flow, wind, agitation, mechanical stirring, ball-milling, and vortex [151]. However, when critically appraising the mechanical stimulation sources, ultrasound is the most suited for biological systems unless activated beforehand and placed into the patient through a different delivery system.

The ultrasound wave is a mechanical wave with a frequency of >20 kHz, which needs a medium to travel. On initiation, it produces cavitation bubbles that provide mechanical pressure to these nanoparticles. Ultrasound can penetrate up to 5 cm in depth through tissue, and one unique ability of this technique, unlike the other stressors used for a direct piezoelectric effect, is that ultrasound can modulate the mechanical stress, manipulating the piezoelectric effect [152]. However, a more recent paper argues that this can be a depth of 4.5 cm by implanting membranes at different depths of porcine tissue, generating a high voltage of 8.22 V [153] This provides a medium for targeting cancers specifically by the area instead of cytotoxic chemotherapy or general radiotherapy methods, reducing adverse effects. The main clear advantage of piezoelectric nanoparticles regarding drug delivery is that the surface charge of the material regulates the cell membrane permeability. This has the additional ability to activate immune pathways, which are discussed further in Section 3.5 [154]. Interestingly, piezoelectric nanomaterials can be integrated with other delivery systems, such as polymers and hydrogels, to enhance their biocompatibility and efficiency [155,156]. However, further research is required to demonstrate their translation into clinical practice.

### 3.4. Electrodes for Tumour Treating Fields

Tumour treating fields (TTFields) are a novel cancer treatment modality that uses alternating electric fields of intermediate frequency (100–500 kHz) and low-intensity electric fields (1–3 V/cm) to disrupt cell division [157]. The frequency range could be selected based on the cancer type and sensitivity [158]. TTFields are typically applied by attaching electrodes to the target area to generate an electric field, with the frequency adjusted accordingly. This therapy is approved for glioblastoma patients at a frequency of 200 kHz [159]. The current used to create the field generates heat, and exceeding certain thresholds can be harmful. The reported maximum safe current density is 31 mA/cm$^2$ RMS, while the threshold for causing burns is 100 mA/cm$^2$ RMS. The skin can sustain thermal injuries at temperatures above 41 °C, with a critical injury threshold at 44 °C. Foster et al. provided a detailed analysis of heat distribution, skin type, thermal frequency, and exposure time to assess these risks [160].

Although the exact mechanism is not fully understood, TTFields are effective on mitotic cells because they target the mitotic spindle and microtubules [161,162]. Mitotic cells are highly polar, making them susceptible to externally applied electric fields, which disrupt spindle formation and activate the spindle assembly checkpoint (SAC). This leads to apoptosis, similar to the mechanism of action of microtubule-targeting agents, such as vinca alkaloids, taxanes, and epothilones. Also, TTfields can disrupt subcellular organelles, promote autophagy, and perturb cell membranes of cancer cells [163].

An alternative hypothesis suggests that the hourglass shape formed during anaphase causes the electric field to push charges and dipoles towards the cleavage furrow [164]. The non-uniform electrical field interferes with this process, extending the mitosis phase. Lee and collaborators describe this as dipole alignment by TTFields, which inhibits tubulin polymerisation, ultimately resulting in metaphase arrest due to improper spindle formation [165]. This further leads to abnormal chromosome segregation and cell death.

TTFields can also lead to replication stress, as demonstrated by Karanam and colleagues [166]. Their study shows that the effect of TTFields can be measured by observing polymerase progression. TTFields directly induce replication stress by decreasing the speed of DNA replication and increasing the duration of R-loop formation compared to treatments without TTFields. Figure 7 summarises these two theories, clarifying a key point of reference for the mechanism of action [159,164,167].

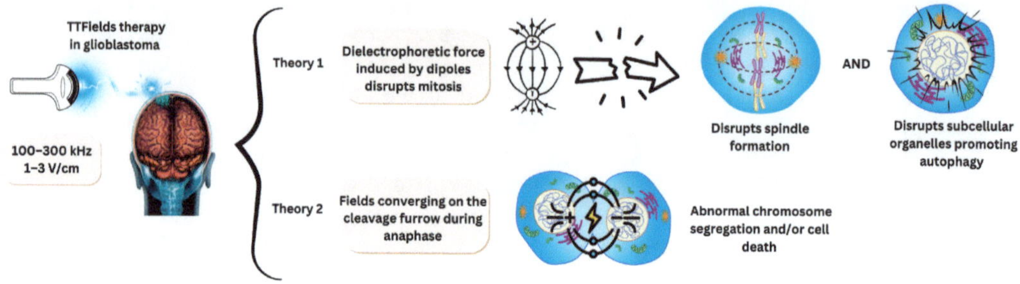


**Figure 7.** Overview of current theories explaining tumour treating fields in glioblastoma. These two individual theories focus on tubulin and mitotic spindle disruption resulting in cell death.

### 3.5. Nano-Piezoelectric Immunotherapy

Alongside the potential to cause cell death in cancer cells via radical formation, piezoelectric materials also have been shown to play a role in tumour immunotherapy. Piezoelectric materials are known to activate the immune system by modulating electrical signals, which directly alter the behaviour of immune cells via electrical mediation [73].

A study performed by Kong et al. [168] demonstrated that localised charge enhances the M1 polarisation of macrophages. The study continued to explain that ultrasounds induced a voltage potential, resulting in an influx of $Ca^{2+}$. This then activated the $Ca^{2+}$-CAMK2A-NF-κB cascade, which is involved in survival and death and relies on intraocular $Ca^{2+}$ to be activated [120]. This resulted in a proinflammatory response from M1 macrophages. This piezoelectric response both enhances M1 polarisation and inhibits M2 macrophages. M1 macrophages overexpress CD80, CD86, and CD16/33. These create pro-inflammatory cytokines, which drive immune recruitment and, in this context, a tumour immune response [169]. M2 macrophages express anti-inflammatory factors (IL-10), CCL17, and CCL22. These factors all recruit T-regs, which suppress the immune response by recruiting $CD4^+$, which subsequently suppresses $CD8^+$ cytotoxic T lymphocyte function but aids in tissue repair and homeostasis [170]. Overall, the piezoelectric response causes a hike in M1 macrophages, which promote immune responses but suppress M2 macrophages, which would promote a tumour microenvironment and further suppress angiogenesis. An overview of this mechanism of action can be observed in Figure 8.

Another example of nano-piezoelectric immunotherapy was developed by Miao et al. [171]. This study utilised $BaTiO_3$ conjugated glucan nanoparticles ($BaTiO_3$@Glu NPs) and focused on ROS production. Glucan was used as an immunological adjuvant to enhance the immune response. The study specifically examined the efficacy of $BaTiO_3$@Glu NPs in RAW264.7 macrophages and colon cancer cells, demonstrating findings consistent with those from previous studies [168]. Nanoparticle uptake following ultrasound stress led to increased levels of proinflammatory cytokines, including tumour necrosis factor-alpha (TNF-α) and interleukin 12 (IL-12). Additionally, there was an increase in CD86 and major histocompatibility complex class 2 (MHC II) biomarkers, indicating that glucan contributed to the observed MHC II and CD86 responses. This study provides insights into enhancing the nano-piezoelectric immunotherapeutic effect by activating macrophage responses through $Ca^{2+}$ influx and using glucan as an immunological adjuvant to boost the existing immunological effects of M1 macrophages. This piezoelectric mechanism of action is depicted in Figure 9, together with other three potential mechanisms by which piezoelectric nanomaterials can be designed as a therapeutic tool in glioblastoma.

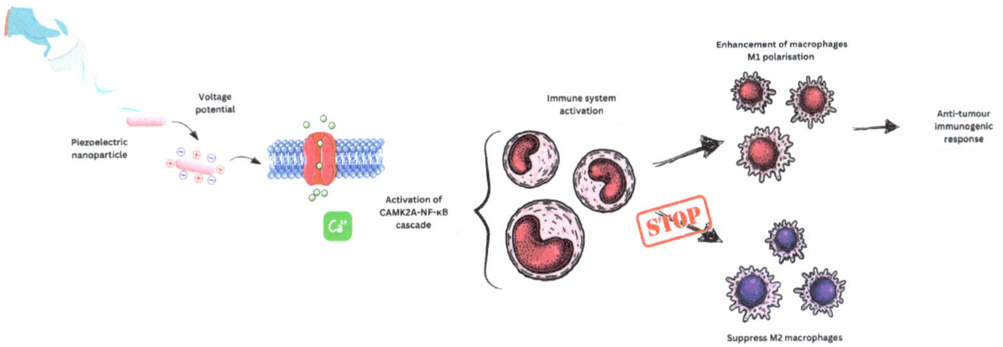


**Figure 8.** Macrophage activation upon introduction of the piezoelectric nanoparticle. This scheme illustrates the M1 macrophage polarisation pathway. The electrical stimulation via the electrical field produced as a knock-on effect by the ultrasound creates a pro-inflammatory effect in the host. This activates a cascade to inhibit M2 macrophages, mitigating the inflammatory response while enhancing the M2 response. An action needed greatly for cancer-specific immunity and recognition.

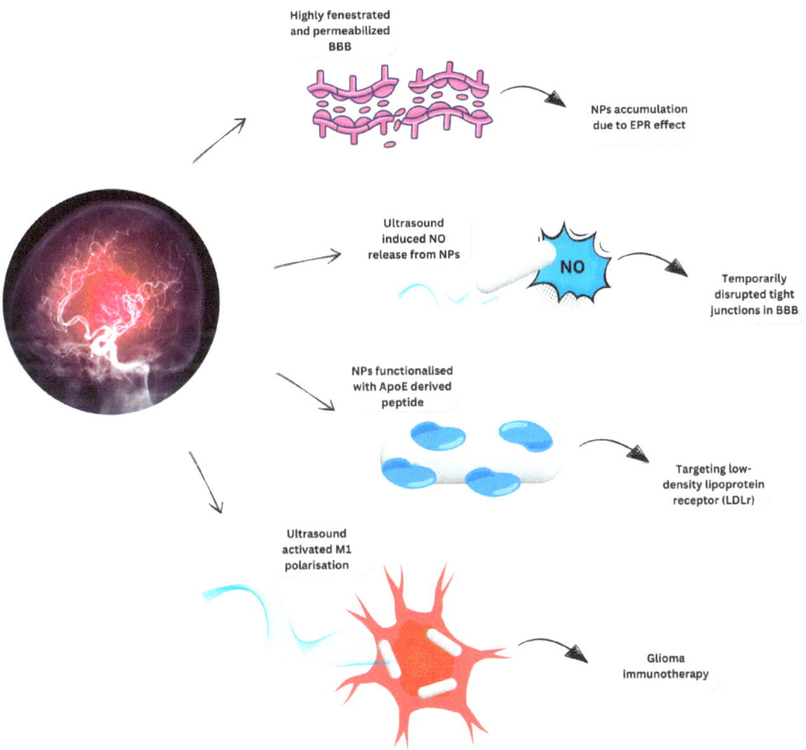


**Figure 9.** Mechanisms of Piezoelectric Nanoparticles in Targeted Glioblastoma Treatment. From top to bottom: (1) Accumulation of nanoparticles (NP) due to the enhanced permeability and retention (EPR) effect; (2) Disruption of BBB via NP-dependent nitric oxide (NO) release; (3) Targeting low-density lipoprotein receptors (LDLr); and (4) Ultrasound-activated M1 polarisation, in which $BaTiO_3$@Glu NPs increase MHC 2 response, leading to an enhanced CD4+ lymphocytes-dependent antigen-specific immune response.

Based on the studies discussed above, Table 3 summarises the main properties, size ranges, advantages, and limitations of key piezoelectric materials used in cancer therapy.

**Table 3.** Summary of key piezoelectric materials for cancer therapy, highlighting their main properties, size ranges, advantages, and limitations.

| Piezoelectric Nanomaterial | Size Range | Advantage | Limitation | Reference |
|---|---|---|---|---|
| Barium Titanate nanoparticles | 50–300 nm | -High Piezoelectric coefficient<br>-Can be surface functionalised | -Possible inflammatory response | [155,172–177] |
| Zinc Oxide nanoparticles | 30–150 nm | -Biocompatible and biodegradable<br>-Good piezoelectric responses | -Potential toxicity at high concentration | [155,178–180] |
| Polyvinylidene Fluoride (PVDF) nanofibers and nanoparticles | 20–100 nm | -Flexible and biocompatible | -Limited piezoelectric response compared to inorganic materials | [181,182] |
| Polyvinylidene fluoride-trifluoroethylene (PVDF-TrFE) micro particles | 2–6 µm | -Flexible, high piezoelectric output, | - Requires specific processing to enhance piezoelectric response | [183–185] |

### 3.6. Piezoelectric Nanomaterials for Glioblastoma Treatment

Glioblastoma (GBM) is one of the most prevalent malignant brain tumours in adults, accounting for 30–40% of all such cases [186]. Current management of GBM involves maximal safe surgical resection followed by radiation and chemotherapy. However, the prognosis remains poor, with a median survival rate of 14.6 months from diagnosis [187]. This poor outcome is primarily due to resistance to existing therapies, which leads to recurrence. Consistently, there is a pressing need for novel therapeutic strategies to manage glioblastoma recurrence.

It has been reported that systemically administrated piezoelectric nanoparticles were used to cross BBB and ultrasound-driven dopamine release to activate dopaminergic neuron like cells [188]. This novel report discusses the ability of piezoelectric nanoparticles to cross the BBB via nitric oxide release to temporarily disrupt the tight junctions in the BBB and favour brain penetration. A similar mechanism can be employed to design an ultrasound-responsive, on-demand drug delivery system for the treatment of GBM.

In an interesting study, polymeric piezoelectric nanoparticles were explored as a novel immunotherapy agent to reprogram the glioma-associated microglia from a tumour-supportive M2 phenotype to an antitumour M1 phenotype. Here, they used the wireless electrical signal produced by the camouflaged piezoelectric nanoparticles (piezoelectric nanoparticles coated with GBM cell membrane extracts) to locally generate electrical cues on GAM membranes, activating their M1 phenotype and ultimately triggering a promising anticancer activity against GBM (Miao et al. [171]. Although current glioblastoma treatments face challenges like drug resistance, poor blood-brain barrier (BBB) permeability, and lack of tumour specificity, some pioneering studies have developed cationic fluorescent anticancer agents that can penetrate the BBB and induce paraptosis and ferroptosis in GBM cells by targeting mitochondria and causing non-apoptotic cell death [189].

## 4. Advantages and Current Challenges

The advantages of piezoelectric nanomaterials in cancer therapy are numerous. They can be engineered to target cancer cells, reducing harm to healthy tissues specifically. As described above, they can convert mechanical energy, such as ultrasound vibrations, into electrical energy. This property can be harnessed to generate reactive oxygen species (ROS) that can kill cancer cells, offering a non-invasive treatment option. Piezoelectric nanomaterials can be combined with other treatments like chemotherapy to enhance effectiveness. They also present the potential advantages of helping to overcome resistance in cancer cells, improving treatment success, and improving tumour visualization, aiding in diagnosis and monitoring.

The primary challenge in using piezoelectric materials for cancer treatment is the toxicology of the materials currently in use. As shown in Table 1, biocompatibility is critical for the therapeutic application of piezoelectric materials. For instance, lead-based materials are unlikely to be used unless a comprehensive toxicological profile is established. Many studies have investigated the treatment of cancers using piezoelectric materials like barium titanate. Ahamed et al. [173] observed cytotoxicity in lung cancer cells (A549 cells) due to oxidative stress and free radical production. Similar studies have been conducted on other cancers and the development of piezoelectric materials. For example, Srinivasa Rao et al. [190] investigated the use of a drug delivery system with a piezoelectric mechanism as the basis for micropump delivery into a patient's body. Despite these advancements, most studies are conducted in closed systems or on individual cell lines. While these studies provide valuable insights into the behaviour of piezoelectric materials in controlled environments, they do not demonstrate how these materials interact with multiple systems. They also fail to provide comprehensive toxicological data on whole systems, including the antitumor effects and dose-response relationships. This indicates that further research is needed to scale up studies with 3D and animal models to obtain detailed toxicology reports.

### 4.1. *Challenges of Using Piezoelectric Nanomaterials in Glioblastoma*

Glioblastoma is the most common primary brain tumour, classified as a grade IV glioma, and accounts for 60–70% of malignant brain tumours. The life expectancy for patients is approximately 12–18 months [191]. The current standard of treatment includes surgical resection followed by radiotherapy and temozolomide. Glioblastoma persists despite treatment because it infiltrates deep into the brain, making additional resection impossible without fatal consequences [192]. This highlights the need for alternative treatments, such as using piezoelectric nanoparticles to target aberrant voltage-gated ion channels. However, challenges such as the blood-brain barrier (BBB) and the need for biocompatible nanoparticles must be addressed.

The BBB, composed of microvascular endothelial cells, acts as a barrier while communicating with astrocytes and pericytes. This anatomical feature creates tight junctions between endothelial cells, forming pores with diameters of 1.4 nm–1.8 nm [193]. Therefore, piezoelectric nanoparticles must be small enough to pass through these tight junctions and navigate the unique immune environment of the BBB and brain. Modulating the BBB is a significant task, with studies focusing on using tight junction modulating agents, drug efflux transport inhibitors, and ultrasound. Developing these methods further could allow the conjugation of piezoelectric nanoparticles, enabling comparisons with standard nanoparticles like gold to explore their therapeutic potential.

### 4.2. *Therapeutic Benefit of Using Tumour-Treating Fields*

Many tumour types, such as glioblastoma, are difficult to treat and have a very poor prognosis. Targeting these areas specifically is a significant challenge. Current treatment methods often produce side effects that are detrimental to the patient. An interesting follow-up clinical study demonstrated that tumour-treating fields (TTFields) have been applied to glioblastoma patients, however, the average survival remains under two years, with a maximum extension of one additional year (Stupp et al. [194]. Olatunji and colleagues investigated the outcome of Stupp and collaborators' investigation of using the tumour-treating field in current glioblastoma therapy [195]. Combining the standard treatment of glioblastoma and tumour treating fields, the effect was an extension of median survival by 4.9 months. They also noted that this increased the quality of life for the patient with no substantial rise in the rate of adverse effects. This was a randomised trial consisting of 695 patients, with those patients already having completed initial radiochemotherapy. While this combined therapy has its limitations, targeting the brain via a portable device does confirm clinical success. It proves that for future work, the use of TTFields improves therapeutic outcomes in glioblastoma patients. This principle is focused on glioblastoma; however, it may be a useful therapeutic tool for other persistent cancers if piezoelectric nanoparticles are developed for deep tissues.

Using piezoelectric nanomaterials offers a novel approach to addressing the challenge of treating cancer as a whole rather than targeting specific tumour types. Yu et al. [196] describe the benefits of piezocatalysis in detail, emphasising how these benefits optimise current targeting strategies. Nanoparticles smaller than 100 nm suggest favourable endocytic cell uptake. Additionally, 1D and 2D structures exhibit a greater piezoelectric response than 3D morphology. Combining these effects with conjugation and drug delivery is likely to produce a more significant therapeutic response.

This treatment method also offers a safer alternative to using cytotoxic agents. Marino and colleagues suggest this perceived safety in breast cancer cells, noting that despite being wire-based, the effects simulate mobile conditions similarly [172]. They found that cancer cells can be countered by applying electrical stimulation to develop multifunctional nanosystems. Their study concluded that electrical stimulation enhanced the cytotoxic effects of chemotherapy drugs, potentially allowing for lower dose concentrations and reducing harmful effects for patients.

## 5. Conclusions and Future Perspectives

This review highlights the promising potential of piezoelectric nanomaterials as a novel treatment method for various solid cancers. As an emerging area of research, the application of piezoelectric nanomaterials is still in its infancy and much remains to be explored. The benefits of this approach in the context of patient treatment are not yet fully understood. However, the potential advantages are significant, including the possibility of reducing or even eliminating the need for cytotoxic drugs. Additionally, piezoelectric nanomaterials could be combined with other treatment modalities, such as photothermal therapy, magnetic hyperthermia, chemotherapy and/or radiotherapy to enhance therapeutic outcomes.

Developing piezoelectric nanomaterials for cancer therapy could lead to wide-ranging applications, potentially increasing survival rates for tumour types currently considered untreatable with standard therapies. Also, combination therapies such as piezo-photodynamic therapy and piezo-magnetic hyperthermia hold significant potential in cancer treatment. New avenues of research could be opened to explore the application of piezoelectric materials as biosensors for the early detection of cancer by measuring the fundamental frequency variations of the piezoelectric resonator. The physicochemical properties of these materials also support their application in precision medicine approaches using label-free and cost-effective solutions. Their electronic properties can be further explored to design point-of-care devices monitoring biomarkers beyond blood or urine fluids for specific healthcare needs in real time.

The nanoscale piezoelectric effect offers a unique mechanism that could revolutionise the field of cancer therapeutics. However, several challenges remain, particularly in understanding the delivery, targeting, and mechanisms of action within cellular models.

Future research should address these challenges to define the practical limitations and optimise the use of piezoelectric nanomaterials in clinical settings. Investigations into the precise mechanisms of action, effective delivery systems, and targeted approaches will be crucial. Additionally, exploring the combination of piezoelectric nanomaterials with existing therapies could provide synergistic effects, further enhancing their therapeutic potential. Finally, a safe-by-design approach in developing these materials will ensure a faster translation into the clinic, a reduction of human and environmental risks and an improved socioeconomic impact. With this approach, the development of biocompatible and biodegradable materials can also contribute to the development of wearable point-of-care devices that can monitor patient biomarkers for early detection or the progression of cancer in real time, significantly impacting patient management by clinicians.

In conclusion, while the use of piezoelectric nanomaterials in cancer treatment is still in the early stages of development, the potential benefits are substantial. Continued research and development in this area could lead to significant advancements in cancer therapy, offering new hope for patients with difficult-to-treat tumours.

**Author Contributions:** Z.K.: writing—original draft and editing; A.R.: review & editing; and J.E.: conceptualization, supervisory guidance, review & editing. All authors have read and agreed to the published version of the manuscript.

**Funding:** This work received no external funding.

**Institutional Review Board Statement:** Not applicable.

**Informed Consent Statement:** Not applicable.

**Data Availability Statement:** No new data were created or analyzed in this study. Data sharing is not applicable to this article.

**Acknowledgments:** Z.K.'s research was supported by the Brad-ATTAIN PhD studentship, University of Bradford (UK). The authors gratefully acknowledge Arathyram Ramachandra Kurup Sasikala for her insights into the conceptualization of the review.

**Conflicts of Interest:** The authors declare no conflicts of interest.

## References

1. Păduraru, D.N.; Ion, D.; Niculescu, A.-G.; Mușat, F.; Andronic, O.; Grumezescu, A.M.; Bolocan, A. Recent Developments in Metallic Nanomaterials for Cancer Therapy, Diagnosing and Imaging Applications. *Pharmaceutics* **2022**, *14*, 435. [CrossRef] [PubMed]
2. Bray, F.; Laversanne, M.; Sung, H.; Ferlay, J.; Siegel, R.L.; Soerjomataram, I.; Jemal, A. Global cancer statistics 2022: GLOBOCAN estimates of incidence and mortality worldwide for 36 cancers in 185 countries. *CA A Cancer J. Clin.* **2024**, *74*, 229–263. [CrossRef] [PubMed]
3. WHO. Global Cancer Burden Growing, Amidst Mounting Need for Services. Available online: https://www.who.int/news/item/01-02-2024-global-cancer-burden-growing--amidst-mounting-need-for-services (accessed on 7 November 2024).
4. Macmillan. Cancer Statistics in the UK. Available online: https://www.macmillan.org.uk/about-us/what-we-do/research/cancer-statistics-fact-sheet (accessed on 7 November 2024).
5. Anand, U.; Dey, A.; Chandel, A.K.S.; Sanyal, R.; Mishra, A.; Pandey, D.K.; De Falco, V.; Upadhyay, A.; Kandimalla, R.; Chaudhary, A.; et al. Cancer chemotherapy and beyond: Current status, drug candidates, associated risks and progress in targeted therapeutics. *Genes Dis.* **2023**, *10*, 1367–1401. [CrossRef] [PubMed]
6. Huang, R.; Zhou, P.-K. DNA damage repair: Historical perspectives, mechanistic pathways and clinical translation for targeted cancer therapy. *Signal Transduct. Target. Ther.* **2021**, *6*, 254. [CrossRef]

7. Zeien, J.; Qiu, W.; Triay, M.; Dhaibar, H.A.; Cruz-Topete, D.; Cornett, E.M.; Urits, I.; Viswanath, O.; Kaye, A.D. Clinical implications of chemotherapeutic agent organ toxicity on perioperative care. *Biomed. Pharmacother.* **2022**, *146*, 112503. [CrossRef]
8. Wopat, H.; Harrod, T.; Brem, R.F.; Kaltman, R.; Anderson, K.; Robien, K. Body composition and chemotherapy toxicity among women treated for breast cancer: A systematic review. *J. Cancer Surviv.* **2024**, *18*, 1356–1369. [CrossRef]
9. van den Boogaard, W.M.C.; Komninos, D.S.J.; Vermeij, W.P. Chemotherapy Side-Effects: Not All DNA Damage Is Equal. *Cancers* **2022**, *14*, 627. [CrossRef]
10. Gavas, S.; Quazi, S.; Karpiński, T.M. Nanoparticles for Cancer Therapy: Current Progress and Challenges. *Nanoscale Res. Lett.* **2021**, *16*, 173. [CrossRef]
11. Chen, H.-A.; Lu, Y.-J.; Dash, B.S.; Chao, Y.-K.; Chen, J.-P. Hyaluronic Acid-Modified Cisplatin-Encapsulated Poly(Lactic-co-Glycolic Acid) Magnetic Nanoparticles for Dual-Targeted NIR-Responsive Chemo-Photothermal Combination Cancer Therapy. *Pharmaceutics* **2023**, *15*, 290. [CrossRef]
12. Sun, L.; Liu, H.; Ye, Y.; Lei, Y.; Islam, R.; Tan, S.; Tong, R.; Miao, Y.-B.; Cai, L. Smart nanoparticles for cancer therapy. *Signal Transduct. Target. Ther.* **2023**, *8*, 418. [CrossRef]
13. Xu, J.; Song, M.; Fang, Z.; Zheng, L.; Huang, X.; Liu, K. Applications and challenges of ultra-small particle size nanoparticles in tumor therapy. *J. Control. Release* **2023**, *353*, 699–712. [CrossRef]
14. Yu, W.; Liu, R.; Zhou, Y.; Gao, H. Size-Tunable Strategies for a Tumor Targeted Drug Delivery System. *ACS Central Sci.* **2020**, *6*, 100. [CrossRef] [PubMed]
15. Yao, Y.; Zhou, Y.; Liu, L.; Xu, Y.; Chen, Q.; Wang, Y.; Wu, S.; Deng, Y.; Zhang, J.; Shao, A. Nanoparticle-Based Drug Delivery in Cancer Therapy and Its Role in Overcoming Drug Resistance. *Front. Mol. Biosci.* **2020**, *7*, 193. [CrossRef] [PubMed]
16. Abrishami, A.; Bahrami, A.R.; Nekooei, S.; Saljooghi, A.S.; Matin, M.M. Hybridized quantum dot, silica, and gold nanoparticles for targeted chemo-radiotherapy in colorectal cancer theranostics. *Commun. Biol.* **2024**, *7*, 393. [CrossRef]
17. Aggarwal, V.; Solanki, S.; Malhotra, B.D. Applications of metal-organic framework-based bioelectrodes. *Chem. Sci.* **2022**, *13*, 8727–8743. [CrossRef]
18. Shano, L.B.; Karthikeyan, S.; Kennedy, L.J.; Chinnathambi, S.; Pandian, G.N. MOFs for next-generation cancer therapeutics through a biophysical approach-a review. *Front. Bioeng. Biotechnol.* **2024**, *12*, 1397804. [CrossRef]
19. Singhal, M.; Riches-Suman, K.; Pors, K.; Addicoat, M.A.; Ruiz, A.; Nayak, S.; Elies, J. Encapsulation and Delivery of Mitoxantrone Using Zirconium-Based Metal–Organic Frameworks (MOFs) and Their Cytotoxic Potential in Breast Cancer Cells. *Appl. Sci.* **2024**, *14*, 1902. [CrossRef]
20. Bairagi, S.; Islam, S.U.; Shahadat, M.; Mulvihill, D.M.; Ali, W. Mechanical energy harvesting and self-powered electronic applications of textile-based piezoelectric nanogenerators: A systematic review. *Nano Energy* **2023**, *111*, 108414. [CrossRef]
21. Zaka, A.; Liaqat, R.; Mehmood, S.; Haider, A.; Iqbal, M.; Mansoor, M.A. Single Source Precursor Synthesis of Lead Titanate (PbTiO3) for the Electrochemical Detection of Nitric Oxide (NO). *J. Electrochem. Soc.* **2024**, *171*, 057518.
22. Vijayakanth, T.; Shankar, S.; Finkelstein-Zuta, G.; Rencus-Lazar, S.; Gilead, S.; Gazit, E. Perspectives on recent advancements in energy harvesting, sensing and bio-medical applications of piezoelectric gels. *Chem. Soc. Rev.* **2023**, *52*, 6191–6220. [CrossRef]
23. Wu, L.; Gao, H.; Han, Q.; Guan, W.; Sun, S.; Zheng, T.; Liu, Y.; Wang, X.; Huang, R.; Li, G. Piezoelectric materials for neuroregeneration: A review. *Biomater. Sci.* **2023**, *11*, 7296–7310. [CrossRef] [PubMed]
24. Chen, X.; Chen, R.; Chen, Z.; Chen, J.; Shung, K.K.; Zhou, Q. Transparent Lead lanthanum zirconate titanate (PLZT) ceramic fibers for High-frequency Ultrasonic Transducer Applications. *Ceram. Int.* **2016**, *42*, 18554–18559. [CrossRef] [PubMed]
25. Rathee, G.; Bartwal, G.; Rathee, J.; Mishra, Y.K.; Kaushik, A.; Solanki, P.R. Emerging Multimodel Zirconia Nanosystems for High-Performance Biomedical Applications. *Adv. NanoBiomed Res.* **2021**, *1*, 2100039. [CrossRef]
26. Su, L.; Zou, L.; Fong, C.C.; Wong, W.L.; Wei, F.; Wong, K.Y.; Wu, R.S.; Yang, M. Detection of cancer biomarkers by piezoelectric biosensor using PZT ceramic resonator as the transducer. *Biosens. Bioelectron.* **2013**, *46*, 155–161. [CrossRef]
27. Guan, Y.; Bai, M.; Wang, Q.; Liu, L.; Yu, S.; Kong, B.; Lv, F.; Guo, M.; Liu, G.; Li, L.; et al. A self-powered wearable piezoelectric nanogenerator for physiological monitoring based on lead zirconate titanate/microfibrillated cellulose@polyvinyl alcohol (PZT/MFC@PVA) composition. *Chem. Eng. J.* **2023**, *460*, 141598. [CrossRef]
28. Wang, J.-B.; Wu, J.; Zhang, J.; Guan, L.-A.; Feng, H.-B.; Zhu, K.-Y.; Zhang, Y.; Sun, H.; Cheng, Y.-D.; Zhang, L. Bibliometric and Visualized Analysis of Piezoelectric Materials in Biomedical Application. *ACS Appl. Electron. Mater.* **2024**, *6*, 1562–1573. [CrossRef]
29. Zhou, Q.; Lam, K.H.; Zheng, H.; Qiu, W.; Shung, K.K. Piezoelectric single crystal ultrasonic transducers for biomedical applications. *Prog. Mater. Sci.* **2014**, *66*, 87–111. [CrossRef]
30. Park, J.S.; Huh, K.Y.; Kim, M.-S.; Jung, S.Y.; Park, J.H.; Kim, S.J.; Jang, H.W.; Hwang, K.S.; Kim, H.N.; Kim, T.G.; et al. A relaxor-ferroelectric PMN-PZT thin-film-based drop-on-demand printhead for bioprinting applications with high piezoelectricity and low heat dissipation. *Sens. Actuators B Chem.* **2024**, *417*, 136194. [CrossRef]

31. Sood, A.; Desseigne, M.; Dev, A.; Maurizi, L.; Kumar, A.; Millot, N.; Han, S.S. A Comprehensive Review on Barium Titanate Nanoparticles as a Persuasive Piezoelectric Material for Biomedical Applications: Prospects and Challenges. *Small* **2023**, *19*, 2206401. [CrossRef]
32. Gong, Z.; Mao, Y.; Liu, Y.; Hu, X.; Zhang, Y.; Zhu, L.; Guo, S.; Ding, Z.; Zhang, L. Sono-promoted piezocatalysis and low-dose drug penetration for personalized therapy via tumor organoids. *J. Colloid. Interface Sci.* **2024**, *675*, 192–206. [CrossRef]
33. Xiang, Z.; Xu, L.; Shan, Y.; Cui, X.; Shi, B.; Xi, Y.; Ren, P.; Zheng, X.; Zhao, C.; Luo, D.; et al. Tumor microenviroment-responsive self-assembly of barium titanate nanoparticles with enhanced piezoelectric catalysis capabilities for efficient tumor therapy. *Bioact. Mater.* **2024**, *33*, 251–261. [CrossRef] [PubMed]
34. Xiao, X.; Liang, S.; Si, J.; Xu, Q.; Zhang, H.; Ma, L.; Yang, C.; Zhang, X. Performance of LiTaO3 Crystals and Thin Films and Their Application. *Crystals* **2023**, *13*, 1233. [CrossRef]
35. DeCeanne, A.V.; Fry, A.L.; Wilkinson, C.J.; Dittmer, M.; Ritzberger, C.; Rampf, M.; Mauro, J.C. Experimental analysis and modeling of the Knoop hardness of lithium disilicate glass-ceramics containing lithium tantalate as a secondary phase. *J. Non-Cryst. Solids* **2022**, *585*, 121540. [CrossRef]
36. Dadfar, S.M.; Roemhild, K.; Drude, N.I.; von Stillfried, S.; Knüchel, R.; Kiessling, F.; Lammers, T. Iron oxide nanoparticles: Diagnostic, therapeutic and theranostic applications. *Adv. Drug Deliv. Rev.* **2019**, *138*, 302–325. [CrossRef]
37. Montiel Schneider, M.G.; Martín, M.J.; Otarola, J.; Vakarelska, E.; Simeonov, V.; Lassalle, V.; Nedyalkova, M. Biomedical Applications of Iron Oxide Nanoparticles: Current Insights Progress and Perspectives. *Pharmaceutics* **2022**, *14*, 204. [CrossRef]
38. Aisida, S.O.; Akpa, P.A.; Ahmad, I.; Zhao, T.-K.; Maaza, M.; Ezema, F.I. Bio-inspired encapsulation and functionalization of iron oxide nanoparticles for biomedical applications. *Eur. Polym. J.* **2020**, *122*, 109371. [CrossRef]
39. Garg, J.; Chiu, M.N.; Krishnan, S.; Kumar, R.; Rifah, M.; Ahlawat, P.; Jha, N.K.; Kesari, K.K.; Ruokolainen, J.; Gupta, P.K. Emerging Trends in Zinc Ferrite Nanoparticles for Biomedical and Environmental Applications. *Appl. Biochem. Biotechnol.* **2024**, *196*, 1008–1043. [CrossRef]
40. Haghniaz, R.; Rabbani, A.; Vajhadin, F.; Khan, T.; Kousar, R.; Khan, A.R.; Montazerian, H.; Iqbal, J.; Libanori, A.; Kim, H.-J.; et al. Anti-bacterial and wound healing-promoting effects of zinc ferrite nanoparticles. *J. Nanobiotechnol.* **2021**, *19*, 38. [CrossRef]
41. Aisida, S.O.; Ali, A.; Oyewande, O.E.; Ahmad, I.; Ul-Hamid, A.; Zhao, T.-K.; Maaza, M.; Ezema, F.I. Biogenic synthesis enhanced structural, morphological, magnetic and optical properties of zinc ferrite nanoparticles for moderate hyperthermia applications. *J. Nanopart. Res.* **2021**, *23*, 47. [CrossRef]
42. Concha, V.O.C.; Timóteo, L.; Duarte, L.A.N.; Bahú, J.O.; Munoz, F.L.; Silva, A.P.; Lodi, L.; Severino, P.; León-Pulido, J.; Souto, E.B. Properties, characterization and biomedical applications of polyvinylidene fluoride (PVDF): A review. *J. Mater. Sci.* **2024**, *59*, 14185–14204. [CrossRef]
43. Martins, P.; Lopes, A.C.; Lanceros-Mendez, S. Electroactive phases of poly(vinylidene fluoride): Determination, processing and applications. *Prog. Polym. Sci.* **2014**, *39*, 683–706. [CrossRef]
44. Ismail, A.M.; El-Newehy, M.H.; El-Naggar, M.E.; Meera Moydeen, A.; Menazea, A.A. Enhancement the electrical conductivity of the synthesized polyvinylidene fluoride/polyvinyl chloride composite doped with palladium nanoparticles via laser ablation. *J. Mater. Res. Technol.* **2020**, *9*, 11178–11188. [CrossRef]
45. Shakiba, M.; Rezvani Ghomi, E.; Khosravi, F.; Jouybar, S.; Bigham, A.; Zare, M.; Abdouss, M.; Moaref, R.; Ramakrishna, S. Nylon—A material introduction and overview for biomedical applications. *Polym. Adv. Technol.* **2021**, *32*, 3368–3383. [CrossRef]
46. Eom, K.; Na, S.; Kim, J.-K.; Ko, H.; Jin, J.; Kang, S.J. Engineering crystal phase of Nylon-11 films for ferroelectric device and piezoelectric sensor. *Nano Energy* **2021**, *88*, 106244. [CrossRef]
47. Danagody, B.; Bose, N.; Rajappan, K. Electrospun polyacrylonitrile-based nanofibrous membrane for various biomedical applications. *J. Polym. Res.* **2024**, *31*, 119. [CrossRef]
48. Tao, J.; Wang, Y.; Zheng, X.; Zhao, C.; Jin, X.; Wang, W.; Lin, T. A review: Polyacrylonitrile as high-performance piezoelectric materials. *Nano Energy* **2023**, *118*, 108987. [CrossRef]
49. Seddiqi, H.; Oliaei, E.; Honarkar, H.; Jin, J.; Geonzon, L.C.; Bacabac, R.G.; Klein-Nulend, J. Cellulose and its derivatives: Towards biomedical applications. *Cellulose* **2021**, *28*, 1893–1931. [CrossRef]
50. Szewczyk, P.K.; Berniak, K.; Knapczyk-Korczak, J.; Karbowniczek, J.E.; Marzec, M.M.; Bernasik, A.; Stachewicz, U. Mimicking natural electrical environment with cellulose acetate scaffolds enhances collagen formation of osteoblasts. *Nanoscale* **2023**, *15*, 6890–6900.
51. Rakesh, M.; Babu, B.R.N.; Prakash, A.P.G.; Prema, N.S.; Gowda, A.C.; Madhukar, B.S.; Kashimatt, M.G.V.; Pradeep, T.M.; Kumar, B.V.S.; Madhusudan, P. Fabrication of lead zirconate titanate-based polyvinylidene fluoride polymer nano-composites: Microcrystalline, morphological and electrical studies. *J. Mater. Sci. Mater. Electron.* **2023**, *34*, 372. [CrossRef]
52. Chang, G.; Pan, X.; Hao, Y.; Du, W.; Wang, S.; Zhou, Y.; Yang, J.; He, Y. PVDF/ZnO piezoelectric nanofibers designed for monitoring of internal micro-pressure. *RSC Adv.* **2024**, *14*, 11775–11783. [CrossRef]
53. Shuai, C.; Liu, G.; Yang, Y.; Yang, W.; He, C.; Wang, G.; Liu, Z.; Qi, F.; Peng, S. Functionalized $BaTiO_3$ enhances piezoelectric effect towards cell response of bone scaffold. *Colloids Surf. B Biointerfaces* **2020**, *185*, 110587. [CrossRef]

54. Islam, M.N.; Rupom, R.H.; Adhikari, P.R.; Demchuk, Z.; Popov, I.; Sokolov, A.P.; Wu, H.F.; Advincula, R.C.; Dahotre, N.; Jiang, Y.; et al. Boosting Piezoelectricity by 3D Printing PVDF-$MoS_2$ Composite as a Conformal and High-Sensitivity Piezoelectric Sensor. *Adv. Funct. Mater.* **2023**, *33*, 2302946. [CrossRef]
55. Jandas, P.J.; Prabakaran, K.; Luo, J.; Derry Holaday, M.G. Effective utilization of quartz crystal microbalance as a tool for biosensing applications. *Sens. Actuators A Phys.* **2021**, *331*, 113020. [CrossRef]
56. He, Q.; Zeng, Y.; Jiang, L.; Wang, Z.; Lu, G.; Kang, H.; Li, P.; Bethers, B.; Feng, S.; Sun, L.; et al. Growing recyclable and healable piezoelectric composites in 3D printed bioinspired structure for protective wearable sensor. *Nat. Commun.* **2023**, *14*, 6477. [CrossRef]
57. Khan, A.; Joshi, R.; Sharma, M.K.; Huang, C.-J.; Yu, J.-H.; Wang, Y.-L.; Lin, Z.-H. The potential of organic piezoelectric materials for next-generation implantable biomedical devices. *Nano Trends* **2024**, *6*, 100032. [CrossRef]
58. Sahoo, J.K.; Hasturk, O.; Falcucci, T.; Kaplan, D.L. Silk chemistry and biomedical material designs. *Nat. Rev. Chem.* **2023**, *7*, 302–318. [CrossRef]
59. Lee, J.C.; Suh, I.W.; Park, C.H.; Kim, C.S. Polyvinylidene fluoride/silk fibroin-based bio-piezoelectric nanofibrous scaffolds for biomedical application. *J. Tissue Eng. Regen. Med.* **2021**, *15*, 869–877. [CrossRef]
60. Khare, D.; Basu, B.; Dubey, A.K. Electrical stimulation and piezoelectric biomaterials for bone tissue engineering applications. *Biomaterials* **2020**, *258*, 120280.
61. Joo, S.; Gwon, Y.; Kim, S.; Park, S.; Kim, J.; Hong, S. Piezoelectrically and Topographically Engineered Scaffolds for Accelerating Bone Regeneration. *ACS Appl. Mater. Interfaces* **2024**, *16*, 1999–2011. [CrossRef]
62. Liu, H.; Shi, Y.; Zhu, Y.; Wu, P.; Deng, Z.; Dong, Q.; Wu, M.; Cai, L. Bioinspired Piezoelectric Periosteum to Augment Bone Regeneration via Synergistic Immunomodulation and Osteogenesis. *ACS Appl. Mater. Interfaces* **2023**, *15*, 12273–12293. [CrossRef]
63. Yang, S.; Wang, Y.; Liang, X. Piezoelectric Nanomaterials Activated by Ultrasound in Disease Treatment. *Pharmaceutics* **2023**, *15*, 1338. [CrossRef] [PubMed]
64. Dolai, J.; Biswas, A.; Jana, N.R. Piezoelectric Nanoparticles for Ultrasound-Based Wireless Therapies. *ACS Appl. Nano Mater.* **2022**, *5*, 14038–14050. [CrossRef]
65. Mikolajick, T.; Park, M.H.; Begon-Lours, L.; Slesazeck, S. From Ferroelectric Material Optimization to Neuromorphic Devices. *Adv. Mater.* **2023**, *35*, 2206042. [CrossRef]
66. Nataf, G.F.; Guennou, M.; Gregg, J.M.; Meier, D.; Hlinka, J.; Salje, E.K.H.; Kreisel, J. Domain-wall engineering and topological defects in ferroelectric and ferroelastic materials. *Nat. Rev. Phys.* **2020**, *2*, 634–648. [CrossRef]
67. Wang, J.; Chu, Y.; Zhao, Z.; Zhang, C.; Chen, Q.; Ran, H.; Cao, Y.; Wu, C. Piezoelectric enhanced sulfur doped graphdiyne nanozymes for synergistic ferroptosis–apoptosis anticancer therapy. *J. Nanobiotechnol.* **2023**, *21*, 311. [CrossRef]
68. Kamel, N.A. Bio-piezoelectricity: Fundamentals and applications in tissue engineering and regenerative medicine. *Biophys. Rev.* **2022**, *14*, 717–733. [CrossRef]
69. Potnis, P.R.; Tsou, N.-T.; Huber, J.E.; Potnis, P.R.; Tsou, N.-T.; Huber, J.E. A Review of Domain Modelling and Domain Imaging Techniques in Ferroelectric Crystals. *Materials* **2011**, *4*, 417–447. [CrossRef]
70. Murugan, C.; Lee, H.; Park, S. Tumor-targeted molybdenum disulfide@barium titanate core–shell nanomedicine for dual photothermal and chemotherapy of triple-negative breast cancer cells. *J. Mater. Chem. B* **2023**, *11*, 1044–1056. [CrossRef]
71. Catalano, E. Recent and future applications of ultrasound-activated piezoelectric nanoparticles for anticancer treatment: Mini-review. *J. Phys. Conf. Ser.* **2023**, *2579*, 012005. [CrossRef]
72. Chen, S.; Zhu, P.; Mao, L.; Wu, W.; Lin, H.; Xu, D.; Lu, X.; Shi, J. Piezocatalytic Medicine: An Emerging Frontier using Piezoelectric Materials for Biomedical Applications. *Adv. Mater.* **2023**, *35*, 2208256. [CrossRef]
73. Wang, Y.; Zang, P.; Yang, D.; Zhang, R.; Gai, S.; Yang, P. The fundamentals and applications of piezoelectric materials for tumor therapy: Recent advances and outlook. *Mater. Horiz.* **2023**, *10*, 1140–1184. [CrossRef] [PubMed]
74. Li, S.; Zhao, Z.; Zhao, J.; Zhang, Z.; Li, X.; Zhang, J. Recent Advances of Ferro-, Piezo-, and Pyroelectric Nanomaterials for Catalytic Applications. *ACS Appl. Nano Mater.* **2020**, *3*, 1063–1079. [CrossRef]
75. Wu, Y.; Zou, J.; Tang, K.; Xia, Y.; Wang, X.; Song, L.; Wang, J.; Wang, K.; Wang, Z. From electricity to vitality: The emerging use of piezoelectric materials in tissue regeneration. *Burns Trauma* **2024**, *12*, tkae013. [CrossRef]
76. Yang, J.; Chen, M.; Lee, H.; Xu, Z.; Zhou, Z.; Feng, S.-P.; Kim, J.T. Three-Dimensional Printing of Self-Assembled Dipeptides. *ACS Appl. Mater. Interfaces* **2021**, *13*, 20573–20580. [CrossRef]
77. Sencadas, V.; Garvey, C.; Mudie, S.; Kirkensgaard, J.J.K.; Gouadec, G.; Hauser, S. Electroactive properties of electrospun silk fibroin for energy harvesting applications. *Nano Energy* **2019**, *66*, 104106. [CrossRef]
78. Jiang, P.; Yan, F.; Nasr Esfahani, E.; Xie, S.; Zou, D.; Liu, X.; Zheng, H.; Li, J. Electromechanical Coupling of Murine Lung Tissues Probed by Piezoresponse Force Microscopy. *ACS Biomater. Sci. Eng.* **2017**, *3*, 1827–1835. [CrossRef]
79. Zhang, Y.; Li, J.; Boutis, G.S. The coupled bio-chemo-electro-mechanical behavior of glucose exposed arterial elastin. *J. Phys. D Appl. Phys.* **2017**, *50*, 133001.

80. Liu, W.-L.; Zou, M.-Z.; Qin, S.-Y.; Cheng, Y.-J.; Ma, Y.-H.; Sun, Y.-X.; Zhang, X.-Z. Recent Advances of Cell Membrane-Coated Nanomaterials for Biomedical Applications. *Adv. Funct. Mater.* **2020**, *30*, 2003559. [CrossRef]
81. Jacob, J.; More, N.; Kalia, K.; Kapusetti, G. Piezoelectric smart biomaterials for bone and cartilage tissue engineering. *Inflamm. Regen.* **2018**, *38*, 2. [CrossRef]
82. Kang, Y.; Kang, Y.; Lei, L.; Lei, L.; Zhu, C.; Zhu, C.; Zhang, H.; Zhang, H.; Mei, L.; Mei, L.; et al. Piezo-photocatalytic effect mediating reactive oxygen species burst for cancer catalytic therapy. *Mater. Horiz.* **2021**, *8*, 2273–2285. [CrossRef]
83. Ran, M.; Xu, H.; Bao, Y.; Zhang, Y.; Zhang, J.; Xing, M. Selective Production of CO from Organic Pollutants by Coupling Piezocatalysis and Advanced Oxidation Processes. *Angew. Chem. Int. Ed.* **2023**, *62*, 202303728. [CrossRef] [PubMed]
84. Wang, X.-Q.; Wang, W.; Peng, M.; Zhang, X.-Z. Free radicals for cancer theranostics. *Biomaterials* **2021**, *266*, 120474. [CrossRef]
85. Wang, K.; Han, C.; Li, J.; Qiu, J.; Sunarso, J.; Liu, S. The Mechanism of Piezocatalysis: Energy Band Theory or Screening Charge Effect? *Angew. Chem.* **2022**, *134*, 202110429. [CrossRef]
86. Jin, C.-C.; Liu, D.-M.; Zhang, L.-X. An Emerging Family of Piezocatalysts: 2D Piezoelectric Materials. *Small* **2023**, *19*, 2303586. [CrossRef]
87. Wang, Y.; Xu, Y.; Dong, S.; Wang, P.; Chen, W.; Lu, Z.; Ye, D.; Pan, B.; Wu, D.; Vecitis, C.D.; et al. Ultrasonic activation of inert poly(tetrafluoroethylene) enables piezocatalytic generation of reactive oxygen species. *Nat. Commun.* **2021**, *12*, 3508. [CrossRef]
88. Duranti, C.; Arcangeli, A. Ion Channel Targeting with Antibodies and Antibody Fragments for Cancer Diagnosis. *Antibodies* **2019**, *8*, 33. [CrossRef]
89. Nakamura, H.; Takada, K. Reactive oxygen species in cancer: Current findings and future directions. *Cancer Sci.* **2021**, *112*, 3945–3952. [CrossRef]
90. Montllor-Albalate, C.; Kim, H.; Thompson, A.E.; Jonke, A.P.; Torres, M.P.; Reddi, A.R. Sod1 integrates oxygen availability to redox regulate NADPH production and the thiol redoxome. *Proc. Natl. Acad. Sci. USA* **2022**, *119*, 2023328119. [CrossRef]
91. Jomova, K.; Raptova, R.; Alomar, S.Y.; Alwasel, S.H.; Nepovimova, E.; Kuca, K.; Valko, M. Reactive oxygen species, toxicity, oxidative stress, and antioxidants: Chronic diseases and aging. *Arch. Toxicol.* **2023**, *97*, 2499–2574. [CrossRef]
92. Zhao, D.; Feng, P.-J.; Liu, J.-H.; Dong, M.; Shen, X.-Q.; Chen, Y.-X.; Shen, Q.-D. Electromagnetized-Nanoparticle-Modulated Neural Plasticity and Recovery of Degenerative Dopaminergic Neurons in the Mid-Brain. *Adv. Mater.* **2020**, *32*, 2003800. [CrossRef]
93. Truong Hoang, Q.; Huynh, K.A.; Nguyen Cao, T.G.; Kang, J.H.; Dang, X.N.; Ravichandran, V.; Kang, H.C.; Lee, M.; Kim, J.-E.; Ko, Y.T.; et al. Piezocatalytic 2D WS2 Nanosheets for Ultrasound-Triggered and Mitochondria-Targeted Piezodynamic Cancer Therapy Synergized with Energy Metabolism-Targeted Chemotherapy. *Adv. Mater.* **2023**, *35*, 2300437. [CrossRef] [PubMed]
94. Catterall, W.A. Structure and function of voltage-gated ion channels. *Annu. Rev. Biochem.* **1995**, *64*, 493–531. [CrossRef] [PubMed]
95. Nilius, B.; Droogmans, G. Ion channels and their functional role in vascular endothelium. *Physiol. Rev.* **2001**, *81*, 1415–1459. [CrossRef]
96. Bates, E. Ion Channels in Development and Cancer. *Annu. Rev. Cell Dev. Biol.* **2015**, *31*, 231–247. [CrossRef]
97. Kefauver, J.M.; Ward, A.B.; Patapoutian, A. Discoveries in structure and physiology of mechanically activated ion channels. *Nature* **2020**, *587*, 567–576. [CrossRef]
98. Huang, J.; Pan, X.; Yan, N. Structural biology and molecular pharmacology of voltage-gated ion channels. *Nat. Rev. Mol. Cell Biol.* **2024**, *25*, 904–925.
99. Palmisano, V.F.; Anguita-Ortiz, N.; Faraji, S.; Nogueira, J.J. Voltage-Gated Ion Channels: Structure, Pharmacology and Photopharmacology. *ChemPhysChem* **2024**, *25*, e202400162. [CrossRef]
100. Fang, X.-Z.; Zhou, T.; Xu, J.-Q.; Wang, Y.-X.; Sun, M.-M.; He, Y.-J.; Pan, S.-W.; Xiong, W.; Peng, Z.-K.; Gao, X.-H.; et al. Structure, kinetic properties and biological function of mechanosensitive Piezo channels. *Cell Biosci.* **2021**, *11*, 1–20. [CrossRef]
101. Levin, M.; Martyniuk, C.J. The bioelectric code: An ancient computational medium for dynamic control of growth and form. *Biosystems* **2018**, *164*, 76–93. [CrossRef]
102. Wright, S.H. Generation of resting membrane potential. *Adv. Physiol. Educ.* **2004**, *28*, 139–142. [CrossRef]
103. Ahmad, M.A.; Natour, Z.A.; Mustafa, F.; Rizvi, T.A. Electrical Characterization of Normal and Cancer Cells. *IEEE Access* **2018**, *6*, 25979–25986. [CrossRef]
104. Prevarskaya, N.; Skryma, R.; Shuba, Y. Ion channels and the hallmarks of cancer. *Trends Mol. Med.* **2010**, *16*, 107–121. [CrossRef] [PubMed]
105. Prevarskaya, N.; Skryma, R.; Shuba, Y. Ion Channels in Cancer: Are Cancer Hallmarks Oncochannelopathies? *Physiol. Rev.* **2018**, *98*, 559–621. [CrossRef]
106. Payne, S.L.; Levin, M.; Oudin, M.J. Bioelectric Control of Metastasis in Solid Tumors. *Bioelectricity* **2019**, *1*, 114–130. [CrossRef]
107. Ohkubo, T.; Yamazaki, J. T-type voltage-activated calcium channel Cav3.1, but not Cav3.2, is involved in the inhibition of proliferation and apoptosis in MCF-7 human breast cancer cells. *Int. J. Oncol.* **2012**, *41*, 267–275. [CrossRef]
108. Lopez-Charcas, O.; Benouna, O.; Lemoine, R.; Rosendo-Pineda, M.J.; Anguheven-Ledezma, T.G.; Sandoval-Vazquez, L.; Gallegos-Gomez, M.L.; Robles-Martinez, L.; Herrera-Carrillo, Z.; Ramírez-Aragón, M.; et al. Blockade of CaV3 calcium channels and induction of G0/G1 cell cycle arrest in colon cancer cells by gossypol. *Br. J. Pharmacol.* **2024**, *181*, 4546–4570. [CrossRef]

109. Motiani, R.K.; Hyzinski-García, M.C.; Zhang, X.; Henkel, M.M.; Abdullaev, I.F.; Kuo, Y.-H.; Matrougui, K.; Mongin, A.A.; Trebak, M. STIM1 and Orai1 mediate CRAC channel activity and are essential for human glioblastoma invasion. *Pflüg. Arch.-Eur. J. Physiol.* **2013**, *465*, 1249–1260. [CrossRef]
110. Roger, S.; Besson, P.; Le Guennec, J.Y. Involvement of a novel fast inward sodium current in the invasion capacity of a breast cancer cell line. *Biochim. Biophys. Acta* **2003**, *1616*, 107–111. [CrossRef]
111. Huber, S.M. Oncochannels. *Cell Calcium* **2013**, *53*, 241–255. [CrossRef]
112. Williams, S.; Bateman, A.; O'Kelly, I. Altered Expression of Two-Pore Domain Potassium (K2P) Channels in Cancer. *PLoS ONE* **2013**, *8*, e74589. [CrossRef]
113. Litan, A.; Langhans, S.A. Cancer as a channelopathy: Ion channels and pumps in tumor development and progression. *Front. Cell Neurosci.* **2015**, *9*, 86. [CrossRef] [PubMed]
114. Gandini, M.A.; Zamponi, G.W. Voltage-gated calcium channel nanodomains: Molecular composition and function. *FEBS J.* **2022**, *289*, 614–633. [CrossRef] [PubMed]
115. Pallone, T.L.; Khurana, S.; Cao, C. Voltage-Gated Calcium Channels: Structure and Function (CACNA). In *Encyclopedia of Signaling Molecules*; Choi, S., Ed.; Springer International Publishing: Cham, Switzerland, 2018; pp. 5942–5949. [CrossRef]
116. Marino, A.; Arai, S.; Hou, Y.; Sinibaldi, E.; Pellegrino, M.; Chang, Y.-T.; Mazzolai, B.; Mattoli, V.; Suzuki, M.; Ciofani, G. Piezoelectric Nanoparticle-Assisted Wireless Neuronal Stimulation. *ACS Nano* **2015**, *9*, 7678–7689. [CrossRef] [PubMed]
117. Phan, N.N.; Wang, C.Y.; Chen, C.F.; Sun, Z.; Lai, M.D.; Lin, Y.C. Voltage-gated calcium channels: Novel targets for cancer therapy. *Oncol. Lett.* **2017**, *14*, 2059–2074. [CrossRef]
118. McKerr, N.; Mohd-Sarip, A.; Dorrian, H.; Breen, C.; James, J.A.; McQuaid, S.; Mills, I.G.; McCloskey, K.D. CACNA1D overexpression and voltage-gated calcium channels in prostate cancer during androgen deprivation. *Sci. Rep.* **2023**, *13*, 4683. [CrossRef]
119. Bhargava, A.; Saha, S. T-Type voltage gated calcium channels: A target in breast cancer? *Breast Cancer Res. Treat.* **2019**, *173*, 11–21. [CrossRef]
120. Ikeda, S.; Matsushima, S.; Okabe, K.; Ikeda, M.; Ishikita, A.; Tadokoro, T.; Enzan, N.; Yamamoto, T.; Sada, M.; Deguchi, H.; et al. Blockade of L-type $Ca^{2+}$ channel attenuates doxorubicin-induced cardiomyopathy via suppression of CaMKII-NF-κB pathway. *Sci. Rep.* **2019**, *9*, 9850. [CrossRef]
121. Dalavaikodihalli Nanjaiah, N.; Ramaswamy, P.; Goswami, K.; Fathima, K.H.; Borkotokey, M. Survival of glioblastoma cells in response to endogenous and exogenous oxidative challenges: Possible implication of NMDA receptor-mediated regulation of redox homeostasis. *Cell Biol. Int.* **2019**, *43*, 1443–1452. [CrossRef]
122. North, W.G.; Liu, F.; Dragnev, K.H.; Demidenko, E. Small-cell lung cancer growth inhibition: Synergism between NMDA receptor blockade and chemotherapy. *Clin. Pharmacol. Adv. Appl.* **2019**, *11*, 15–23. [CrossRef]
123. Ramaswamy, P.; Aditi Devi, N.; Hurmath Fathima, K.; Dalavaikodihalli Nanjaiah, N. Activation of NMDA receptor of glutamate influences MMP-2 activity and proliferation of glioma cells. *Neurol. Sci.* **2014**, *35*, 823–829. [CrossRef]
124. González-Cota, A.L.; Martínez-Flores, D.; Rosendo-Pineda, M.J.; Vaca, L. NMDA receptor-mediated Ca(2+) signaling: Impact on cell cycle regulation and the development of neurodegenerative diseases and cancer. *Cell Calcium* **2024**, *119*, 102856. [CrossRef]
125. Angus, M.; Ruben, P. Voltage gated sodium channels in cancer and their potential mechanisms of action. *Channels* **2019**, *13*, 400–409. [CrossRef]
126. Sheth, M.; Esfandiari, L. Bioelectric Dysregulation in Cancer Initiation, Promotion, and Progression. *Front. Oncol.* **2022**, *12*, 846917. [CrossRef]
127. Guéguinou, M.; Harnois, T.; Crottes, D.; Uguen, A.; Deliot, N.; Gambade, A.; Chantôme, A.; Haelters, J.P.; Jaffrès, P.A.; Jourdan, M.L.; et al. SK3/TRPC1/Orai1 complex regulates SOCE-dependent colon cancer cell migration: A novel opportunity to modulate anti-EGFR mAb action by the alkyl-lipid Ohmline. *Oncotarget* **2016**, *7*, 36168–36184. [CrossRef]
128. Tajada, S.; Villalobos, C. Calcium Permeable Channels in Cancer Hallmarks. *Front. Pharmacol.* **2020**, *11*, 968. [CrossRef]
129. Coste, B.; Mathur, J.; Schmidt, M.; Earley, T.J.; Ranade, S.; Petrus, M.J.; Dubin, A.E.; Patapoutian, A. Piezo1 and Piezo2 are essential components of distinct mechanically activated cation channels. *Science* **2010**, *330*, 55–60. [CrossRef]
130. Guo, Y.R.; MacKinnon, R. Structure-based membrane dome mechanism for Piezo mechanosensitivity. *Elife* **2017**, *6*, e33660. [CrossRef]
131. Saotome, K.; Murthy, S.E.; Kefauver, J.M.; Whitwam, T.; Patapoutian, A.; Ward, A.B. Structure of the mechanically activated ion channel Piezo1. *Nature* **2018**, *554*, 481–486. [CrossRef]
132. Zhao, Q.; Zhou, H.; Chi, S.; Wang, Y.; Wang, J.; Geng, J.; Wu, K.; Liu, W.; Zhang, T.; Dong, M.-Q.; et al. Structure and mechanogating mechanism of the Piezo1 channel. *Nature* **2018**, *554*, 487–492. [CrossRef]
133. Wang, L.; Zhou, H.; Zhang, M.; Liu, W.; Deng, T.; Zhao, Q.; Li, Y.; Lei, J.; Li, X.; Xiao, B. Structure and mechanogating of the mammalian tactile channel PIEZO2. *Nature* **2019**, *573*, 225–229. [CrossRef]
134. De Felice, D.; Alaimo, A. Mechanosensitive Piezo Channels in Cancer: Focus on altered Calcium Signaling in Cancer Cells and in Tumor Progression. *Cancers* **2020**, *12*, 1780. [CrossRef] [PubMed]

135. Karska, J.; Kowalski, S.; Saczko, J.; Moisescu, M.G.; Kulbacka, J. Mechanosensitive Ion Channels and Their Role in Cancer Cells. *Membranes* **2023**, *13*, 167. [CrossRef] [PubMed]
136. Xu, J.; Wang, Z.; Niu, Y.; Tang, Y.; Wang, Y.; Huang, J.; Leung, E.L. TRP channels in cancer: Therapeutic opportunities and research strategies. *Pharmacol. Res.* **2024**, *209*, 107412. [CrossRef]
137. Marini, M.; Titiz, M.; Souza Monteiro de Araújo, D.; Geppetti, P.; Nassini, R.; De Logu, F. TRP Channels in Cancer: Signaling Mechanisms and Translational Approaches. *Biomolecules* **2023**, *13*, 1557. [CrossRef]
138. Fan, H.; Shen, Y.X.; Yuan, Y.-F. Expression and prognostic roles of TRPV5 and TRPV6 in non-small cell lung cancer after curative resection. *Asian Pac. J. Cancer Prev.* **2014**, *15*, 2559–2563.
139. Berrout, J.; Kyriakopoulou, E.; Moparthi, L.; Hogea, A.S.; Berrout, L.; Ivan, C.; Lorger, M.; Boyle, J.; Peers, C.; Muench, S.; et al. TRPA1-FGFR2 binding event is a regulatory oncogenic driver modulated by miRNA-142-3p. *Nat. Commun.* **2017**, *8*, 947. [CrossRef]
140. Hu, S.; Li, L.; Huang, W.; Liu, J.; Lan, G.; Yu, S.; Peng, L.; Xie, X.; Yang, L.; Nian, Y.; et al. CAV3.1 knockdown suppresses cell proliferation, migration and invasion of prostate cancer cells by inhibiting AKT. *Cancer Manag. Res.* **2018**, *10*, 4603–4614. [CrossRef]
141. Liu, Z.; Wei, Y.; Zhang, L.; Yee, P.P.; Johnson, M.; Zhang, X.; Gulley, M.; Atkinson, J.M.; Trebak, M.; Wang, H.-G.; et al. Induction of store-operated calcium entry (SOCE) suppresses glioblastoma growth by inhibiting the Hippo pathway transcriptional coactivators YAP/TAZ. *Oncogene* **2019**, *38*, 120–139. [CrossRef]
142. Yang, S.; Zhang, J.J.; Huang, X.Y. Orai1 and STIM1 are critical for breast tumor cell migration and metastasis. *Cancer Cell* **2009**, *15*, 124–134. [CrossRef]
143. Chen, Y.F.; Chiu, W.T.; Chen, Y.T.; Lin, P.Y.; Huang, H.J.; Chou, C.Y.; Chang, H.C.; Tang, M.J.; Shen, M.R. Calcium store sensor stromal-interaction molecule 1-dependent signaling plays an important role in cervical cancer growth, migration, and angiogenesis. *Proc. Natl. Acad. Sci. USA* **2011**, *108*, 15225–15230. [CrossRef]
144. Takayasu, T.; Kurisu, K.; Esquenazi, Y.; Ballester, L.Y. Ion Channels and Their Role in the Pathophysiology of Gliomas. *Mol. Cancer Ther.* **2020**, *19*, 1959–1969. [CrossRef] [PubMed]
145. Chan, M.; Yuan, H.; Soifer, I.; Maile, T.M.; Wang, R.Y.; Ireland, A.; O'Brien, J.J.; Goudeau, J.; Chan, L.J.G.; Vijay, T.; et al. Novel insights from a multiomics dissection of the Hayflick limit. *eLife* **2022**, *11*, e70283. [CrossRef] [PubMed]
146. Fletcher-Sananikone, E.; Kanji, S.; Tomimatsu, N.; Di Cristofaro, L.F.M.; Kollipara, R.K.; Saha, D.; Floyd, J.R.; Sung, P.; Hromas, R.; Burns, T.C.; et al. Elimination of Radiation-Induced Senescence in the Brain Tumor Microenvironment Attenuates Glioblastoma Recurrence. *Cancer Res.* **2021**, *81*, 5935–5947. [CrossRef] [PubMed]
147. Martin, N.; Bernard, D. Calcium signaling and cellular senescence. *Cell Calcium* **2018**, *70*, 16–23. [CrossRef]
148. Martin, N.; Zhu, K.; Czarnecka-Herok, J.; Vernier, M.; Bernard, D. Regulation and role of calcium in cellular senescence. *Cell Calcium* **2023**, *110*, 102701. [CrossRef]
149. Rosenbaum, T.; Morales-Lázaro, S.L.; Islas, L.D. TRP channels: A journey towards a molecular understanding of pain. *Nat. Rev. Neurosci.* **2022**, *23*, 596–610. [CrossRef]
150. Koivisto, A.-P.; Belvisi, M.G.; Gaudet, R.; Szallasi, A. Advances in TRP channel drug discovery: From target validation to clinical studies. *Nat. Rev. Drug Discov.* **2022**, *21*, 41–59. [CrossRef]
151. Lin, X.; Song, J.; Chen, X.; Yang, H. Ultrasound-Activated Sensitizers and Applications. *Angew. Chem. Int. Ed.* **2020**, *59*, 14212–14233. [CrossRef]
152. Leinenga, G.; Langton, C.; Nisbet, R.; Götz, J. Ultrasound treatment of neurological diseases—Current and emerging applications. *Nat. Rev. Neurol.* **2016**, *12*, 161–174. [CrossRef]
153. Shi, X.; Chen, Y.; Zhao, Y.; Ye, M.; Zhang, S.; Gong, S. Ultrasound-activable piezoelectric membranes for accelerating wound healing. *Biomater. Sci.* **2022**, *10*, 692–701.
154. Ramedani, A.; Sabzevari, O.; Simchi, A. Hybrid ultrasound-activated nanoparticles based on graphene quantum dots for cancer treatment. *Int. J. Pharm.* **2022**, *629*, 122373. [CrossRef] [PubMed]
155. Barcena, A.J.R.; Dhal, K.; Patel, P.; Ravi, P.; Kundu, S.; Tappa, K. Current Biomedical Applications of 3D-Printed Hydrogels. *Gels* **2024**, *10*, 8. [CrossRef] [PubMed]
156. Huang, D.; Cheng, Y.; Chen, G.; Zhao, Y. 3D-Printed Janus Piezoelectric Patches for Sonodynamic Bacteria Elimination and Wound Healing. *Research* **2023**, *6*, 0022. [CrossRef] [PubMed]
157. Wenger, C.; Miranda, P.C.; Salvador, R.; Thielscher, A.; Bomzon, Z.; Giladi, M.; Mrugala, M.M.; Korshoej, A.R. A Review on Tumor-Treating Fields (TTFields): Clinical Implications Inferred from Computational Modeling. *IEEE Rev. Biomed. Eng.* **2018**, *11*, 195–207. [CrossRef]
158. Kirson, E.D.; Gurvich, Z.; Schneiderman, R.; Dekel, E.; Itzhaki, A.; Wasserman, Y.; Schatzberger, R.; Palti, Y. Disruption of Cancer Cell Replication by Alternating Electric Fields. *Cancer Res.* **2004**, *64*, 3288–3295. [CrossRef]
159. Ornelas, A.S.; Porter, A.B.; Sharma, A.; Knox, M.G.; Marks, L.A.; Wingerchuk, D.M.; O'Carroll, C.B. What is the Role of Tumor-treating Fields in Newly Diagnosed Glioblastoma? *Neurologist* **2019**, *24*, 71. [CrossRef]

160. Foster, K.R.; Ziskin, M.C.; Balzano, Q. Time-temperature Thresholds and Safety Factors for Thermal Hazards from Radiofrequency Energy above 6 GHz. *Health Phys.* **2021**, *121*, 234–247. [CrossRef]
161. Arvind, R.; Chandana, S.R.; Borad, M.J.; Pennington, D.; Mody, K.; Babiker, H. Tumor-Treating Fields: A fourth modality in cancer treatment, new practice updates. *Crit. Rev. Oncol./Hematol.* **2021**, *168*, 103535. [CrossRef]
162. Moser, J.C.; Salvador, E.; Deniz, K.; Swanson, K.; Tuszynski, J.; Carlson, K.W.; Karanam, N.K.; Patel, C.B.; Story, M.; Lou, E.; et al. The Mechanisms of Action of Tumor Treating Fields. *Cancer Res.* **2022**, *82*, 3650–3658. [CrossRef]
163. Shams, S.; Patel, C.B. Anti-cancer mechanisms of action of therapeutic alternating electric fields (tumor treating fields [TTFields]). *J. Mol. Cell Biol.* **2022**, *14*, mjac047. [CrossRef]
164. Rominiyi, O.; Vanderlinden, A.; Clenton, S.J.; Bridgewater, C.; Al-Tamimi, Y.; Collis, S.J. Tumour treating fields therapy for glioblastoma: Current advances and future directions. *Br. J. Cancer* **2021**, *124*, 697–709. [CrossRef] [PubMed]
165. Le, H.T.; Staelens, M.; Lazzari, D.; Chan, G.; Tuszyński, J.A. Real-Time Monitoring of the Effect of Tumour-Treating Fields on Cell Division Using Live-Cell Imaging. *Cells* **2022**, *11*, 2712. [CrossRef] [PubMed]
166. Karanam, N.K.; Ding, L.; Aroumougame, A.; Story, M.D. Tumor treating fields cause replication stress and interfere with DNA replication fork maintenance: Implications for cancer therapy. *Transl. Res.* **2020**, *217*, 33–46. [CrossRef] [PubMed]
167. Sung, H.; Jo, Y.; Oh, G.; Gi, Y.; Kim, H.; Park, S.; Seo, J.; Yoon, M. Technical note: Evaluation of methods for reducing edge current density under electrode arrays for tumor-treating fields therapy. *Med. Phys.* **2022**, *49*, 4837–4844. [CrossRef]
168. Kong, Y.; Liu, F.; Ma, B.; Duan, J.; Yuan, W.; Sang, Y.; Han, L.; Wang, S.; Liu, H. Wireless Localized Electrical Stimulation Generated by an Ultrasound-Driven Piezoelectric Discharge Regulates Proinflammatory Macrophage Polarization. *Adv. Sci.* **2021**, *8*, 2100962. [CrossRef]
169. Yunna, C.; Mengru, H.; Lei, W.; Weidong, C. Macrophage M1/M2 polarization. *Eur. J. Pharmacol.* **2020**, *877*, 173090. [CrossRef]
170. Ye, T.; Zhang, X.; Dong, Y.; Liu, J.; Zhang, W.; Wu, F.; Bo, H.; Shao, H.; Zhang, R.; Shen, H. Chemokine CCL17 Affects Local Immune Infiltration Characteristics and Early Prognosis Value of Lung Adenocarcinoma. *Front. Cell Dev. Biol.* **2022**, *10*, 816927. [CrossRef]
171. Miao, Y.-B.; Ren, H.-X.; Zhang, G.; Song, F.-X.; Liu, W.; Shi, Y. Achieving precise non-invasive ROS spatiotemporal manipulation for colon cancer immunotherapy. *Chem. Eng. J.* **2024**, *481*, 148520. [CrossRef]
172. Marino, A.; Battaglini, M.; De Pasquale, D.; Degl'Innocenti, A.; Ciofani, G. Ultrasound-Activated Piezoelectric Nanoparticles Inhibit Proliferation of Breast Cancer Cells. *Sci. Rep.* **2018**, *8*, 6257. [CrossRef]
173. Ahamed, M.; Akhtar, M.J.; Khan, M.A.M.; Alhadlaq, H.A.; Alshamsan, A. Barium Titanate ($BaTiO_3$) Nanoparticles Exert Cytotoxicity through Oxidative Stress in Human Lung Carcinoma (A549) Cells. *Nanomaterials* **2020**, *10*, 2309. [CrossRef]
174. Yoon, Y.N.; Lee, D.-S.; Park, H.J.; Kim, J.-S. Barium Titanate Nanoparticles Sensitise Treatment-Resistant Breast Cancer Cells to the Antitumor Action of Tumour-Treating Fields. *Sci. Rep.* **2020**, *10*, 2560. [CrossRef] [PubMed]
175. Wang, P.; Tang, Q.; Zhang, L.; Xu, M.; Sun, L.; Sun, S.; Zhang, J.; Wang, S.; Liang, X. Ultrasmall Barium Titanate Nanoparticles for Highly Efficient Hypoxic Tumor Therapy via Ultrasound Triggered Piezocatalysis and Water Splitting. *ACS Nano* **2021**, *15*, 11326–11340. [CrossRef] [PubMed]
176. Zhan, L.; Xiao, C.; Li, C.; Zhai, J.; Yang, F.; Piao, J.; Ning, C.; Zhou, Z.; Yu, P.; Qi, S. Internal Wireless Electrical Stimulation from Piezoelectric Barium Titanate Nanoparticles as a New Strategy for the Treatment of Triple-Negative Breast Cancer. *ACS Appl. Mater. Interfaces* **2022**, *14*, 45032–45041. [CrossRef] [PubMed]
177. Marino, A.; Almici, E.; Migliorin, S.; Tapeinos, C.; Battaglini, M.; Cappello, V.; Marchetti, M.; De Vito, G.; Cicchi, R.; Pavone, F.S.; et al. Piezoelectric barium titanate nanostimulators for the treatment of glioblastoma multiforme. *J. Colloid. Interface Sci.* **2019**, *538*, 449–461. [CrossRef]
178. Racca, L.; Limongi, T.; Vighetto, V.; Dumontel, B.; Ancona, A.; Canta, M.; Canavese, G.; Garino, N.; Cauda, V. Zinc Oxide Nanocrystals and High-Energy Shock Waves: A New Synergy for the Treatment of Cancer Cells. *Front. Bioeng. Biotechnol.* **2020**, *8*, 577.
179. Truong Hoang, Q.; Ravichandran, V.; Nguyen Cao, T.G.; Kang, J.H.; Ko, Y.T.; Lee, T.I.; Shim, M.S. Piezoelectric Au-decorated ZnO nanorods: Ultrasound-triggered generation of ROS for piezocatalytic cancer therapy. *Chem. Eng. J.* **2022**, *435*, 135039. [CrossRef]
180. Han, Q.; Fang, Z.; Lin, R.; Chen, J.; Wei, X.; Gong, C.; Yang, Z.; Zou, P.; Zhu, J.; Xing, L.; et al. Piezo-photodynamic therapy of Au@PEG-ZnO nanostructures enabled with a battery-free wireless cancer therapeutic dot. *Nano Energy* **2024**, *125*, 109530. [CrossRef]
181. Xie, C.; Ding, R.; Wang, X.; Hu, C.; Yan, J.; Zhang, W.; Wang, Y.; Qu, Y.; Zhang, S.; He, P.; et al. A disulfiram-loaded electrospun poly(vinylidene fluoride) nanofibrous scaffold for cancer treatment. *Nanotechnology* **2020**, *31*, 115101. [CrossRef]
182. Milenković, S.; Virijević, K.; Živić, F.; Radojević, I.; Grujović, N. Composite Nanoarchitectonics of Electrospun Piezoelectric PVDF/AgNPs for Biomedical Applications, Including Breast Cancer Treatment. *Materials* **2024**, *17*, 3872. [CrossRef]
183. Silva Pedraza, Z.; Wang, Y.; Carlos, C.; Tang, Z.; Li, J.; Cai, W.; Wang, X. Development of Ferroelectric P(VDF-TrFE) Microparticles for Ultrasound-Driven Cancer Cell Killing. *ACS Appl. Mater. Interfaces* **2023**, *15*, 54304–54311. [CrossRef]

184. Montorsi, M.; Pucci, C.; De Pasquale, D.; Marino, A.; Ceccarelli, M.C.; Mazzuferi, M.; Bartolucci, M.; Petretto, A.; Prato, M.; Debellis, D.; et al. Ultrasound-Activated Piezoelectric Nanoparticles Trigger Microglia Activity Against Glioblastoma Cells. *Adv. Healthc. Mater.* **2024**, *13*, 2304331. [CrossRef] [PubMed]
185. Pucci, C.; Marino, A.; Şen, Ö.; De Pasquale, D.; Bartolucci, M.; Iturrioz-Rodríguez, N.; Di Leo, N.; De Vito, G.; Debellis, D.; Petretto, A.; et al. Ultrasound-responsive nutlin-loaded nanoparticles for combined chemotherapy and piezoelectric treatment of glioblastoma cells. *Acta Biomater.* **2022**, *139*, 218–236. [CrossRef] [PubMed]
186. Shah, S. Novel Therapies in Glioblastoma Treatment: Review of Glioblastoma; Current Treatment Options; and Novel Oncolytic Viral Therapies. *Med. Sci.* **2023**, *12*, 1. [CrossRef]
187. Perry, J.R.; Laperriere, N.; O'Callaghan, C.J.; Brandes, A.A.; Menten, J.; Phillips, C.; Fay, M.; Nishikawa, R.; Cairncross, J.G.; Roa, W.; et al. Short-Course Radiation plus Temozolomide in Elderly Patients with Glioblastoma. *N. Engl. J. Med.* **2017**, *376*, 1027–1037. [CrossRef]
188. Kim, T.; Kim, H.J.; Choi, W.; Lee, Y.M.; Pyo, J.H.; Lee, J.; Kim, J.; Kim, J.; Kim, J.-H.; Kim, C.; et al. Deep brain stimulation by blood–brain-barrier-crossing piezoelectric nanoparticles generating current and nitric oxide under focused ultrasound. *Nat. Biomed. Eng.* **2023**, *7*, 149–163. [CrossRef]
189. Wang, J.; Cao, M.; Han, L.; Shangguan, P.; Liu, Y.; Zhong, Y.; Chen, C.; Wang, G.; Chen, X.; Lin, M.; et al. Blood–Brain Barrier-Penetrative Fluorescent Anticancer Agents Triggering Paraptosis and Ferroptosis for Glioblastoma Therapy. *J. Am. Chem. Soc.* **2024**, *146*, 28783–28794. [CrossRef]
190. Srinivasa Rao, K.; Hamza, M.; Ashok Kumar, P.; Girija Sravani, K. Design and optimization of MEMS based piezoelectric actuator for drug delivery systems. *Microsyst. Technol.* **2020**, *26*, 1671–1679. [CrossRef]
191. Louis, D.N.; Perry, A.; Reifenberger, G.; von Deimling, A.; Figarella-Branger, D.; Cavenee, W.K.; Ohgaki, H.; Wiestler, O.D.; Kleihues, P.; Ellison, D.W. The 2016 World Health Organization Classification of Tumors of the Central Nervous System: A summary. *Acta Neuropathol.* **2016**, *131*, 803–820. [CrossRef]
192. Seker-Polat, F.; Pinarbasi Degirmenci, N.A.-O.X.; Solaroglu, I.; Bagci-Onder, T.A.-O. Tumor Cell Infiltration into the Brain in Glioblastoma: From Mechanisms to Clinical Perspectives. *Cancer* **2022**, *14*, 443. [CrossRef]
193. Noorani, I.; de la Rosa, J. Breaking barriers for glioblastoma with a path to enhanced drug delivery. *Nat. Commun.* **2023**, *14*, 5909. [CrossRef]
194. Stupp, R.; Taillibert, S.; Kanner, A.; Read, W.; Steinberg, D.; Lhermitte, B.; Toms, S.; Idbaih, A.; Ahluwalia, M.S.; Fink, K.; et al. Effect of Tumor-Treating Fields Plus Maintenance Temozolomide vs Maintenance Temozolomide Alone on Survival in Patients With Glioblastoma: A Randomized Clinical Trial. *Jama* **2017**, *318*, 2306–2316. [PubMed]
195. Olatunji, G.; Aderinto, N.A.-O.; Adefusi, T.; Kokori, E.; Akinmoju, O.; Yusuf, I.; Olusakin, T.; Muzammil, M.A. Efficacy of tumour-treating fields therapy in recurrent glioblastoma: A narrative review of current evidence. *Medicine* **2023**, *102*, e36421. [PubMed]
196. Yu, Q.; Shi, W.; Li, S.; Liu, H.; Zhang, J. Emerging Advancements in Piezoelectric Nanomaterials for Dynamic Tumor Therapy. *Molecules* **2023**, *28*, 3170. [CrossRef]

MDPI AG
Grosspeteranlage 5
4052 Basel
Switzerland
Tel.: +41 61 683 77 34

*Journal of Functional Biomaterials* Editorial Office
E-mail: jfb@mdpi.com
www.mdpi.com/journal/jfb